To Live and To Die:
When, Why, and How

To Live and To Die: When, Why, and How

Edited by

Robert H. Williams

Springer-Verlag   New York   Heidelberg   Berlin
1973

Acknowledgments

Lyrics appearing on pages 163 and 164: WHO AM I? by Leonard Bernstein copyright 1950 by Leonard Bernstein. Used by permission of G. Schirmer, Inc.

Lyrics appearing on pages 164 and 165, words and music by Lee Magid and Max Rich, by permission of the copyright holder

Alexis Music, Inc.
5750 Melrose Avenue
Hollywood, Ca. 90038

Library of Congress Cataloging in Publication Data

Williams, Robert Hardin.
    To live and to die.

    1. Medicine—Addresses, essays, lectures.
I. Title.
R117.W54   610'.1   73-2868

ISBN 0-387-06220-3 Springer-Verlag New York · Heidelberg · Berlin
ISBN 3-540-06220-3 Springer-Verlag Berlin · Heidelberg · New York

Preface

In the 1960's marked changes occurred throughout the world in philosophies and policies related to man's role in life. These changes, prompted predominantly by extensive increases in knowledge and population density, have produced increased pleasures as well as problems. The rising number of people and improved methods of communication and transportation have caused more relationships among people, with their pleasures, competitions, jealousies, conflicts of interest, oppressions, and crimes. Large assortments of drugs have been developed and are easily obtained. There are drugs to speed us up, slow us down, make us sleep, change our perspectives on life, promote propagation of life or prevent it, prolong life or terminate it, and modify the course of life in many ways. Also, numerous mechanical devices have been developed that influence the propagation of life, the termination of life, and the manner in which we live. Many people have changed their overall goals in life, and in particular have experienced major changes in attitudes and policies applying to sexual activity, marriage, birth control, abortion, welfare, children, old people, criminals, economics, social status, careers, education, euthanasia, and suicide. There also has been marked enlightenment concerning the effect of the chemical and physical status of the brain upon normal and abnormal thinking and behavior.

Some of these developments have produced anxieties, and in certain segments of the population they have caused feelings of insecurity, fear, frustration, resentment, protest, and violence. There has been a marked increase in discussions, publications, and activities in these various areas. There are strong demands for changes in customs, religious policies, and laws.

Since I have been very much interested in these subjects for many years, at the request of medical students and physicians in 1966 I began offering an annual course dealing with them. Included in the course have been presentations by prominent religious leaders, attorneys, psychologists, psychiatrists, neurologists, geneticists, marriage counselors, and other specialists, as well as by criminals and sexual deviates.

The contributing authors of this book have previously demonstrated a keen interest and excellent ability in their respective subjects—indeed, several have written books in their areas. They were invited to present major considerations, to emphasize their own concepts, to include discus-

v

sions of future patterns for living, and to provide some recommended reading. In the prologue I express some of my thoughts concerning many of the topics in the book. In the epilogue I emphasize concepts of some of the authors and add some of my own.

The widely varied topics pertain, directly or indirectly, to one or more components of the book's title—To Live and To Die: When, Why, and How. It is wise for us to contemplate repeatedly *why* we live, including the advantages and disadvantages of our living, for ourselves and for others. *How* we live and *how* we expect our progeny to live are related to the extent to which man controls the quality and quantity of life that is both propagated and terminated.

Some concepts that I and other authors have presented are unproven, but some tentative conclusions are indicated. Of course, there are many differences of opinion on these subjects among the public. A number of the concepts discussed in this book run counter to religious policies, to laws, and to traditional ideas, and elicit strong emotional reactions, pro and con. Although major changes in many of the areas are indicated, the public's interest and support are needed to achieve optimal progress. This means that the public must take an enlightened view of the net advantages of the changes and their related moral compatibilities. Therefore, much wise and considerate leadership is required, along with adequate time.

I wish to express my appreciation to the contributors and many others for their excellent cooperation and contributions.

Robert H. Williams, M.D.

Table of Contents

List of Contributors

JOHN DARRAH, L.L.B., Seattle-King County Public Defender, Seattle, Washington.

KINGSLEY DAVIS, PH.D., Ford Professor of Sociology and Comparative Studies, and Director of International and Urban Research, University of California, Berkeley, California.

ARTHUR J. DYCK, PH.D., Mary B. Saltonstall Professor of Population Ethics, School of Public Health, Member of the Faculty of the Divinity School, and Member of the Center for Population Studies, Harvard University, Boston, Massachusetts.

J. RUSSELL ELKINTON, M.D., Editor Emeritus, Annals of Internal Medicine; Emeritus Professor of Medicine, University of Pennsylvania, Philadelphia, Pennsylvania.

DANA L. FARNSWORTH, M.D., Henry K. Oliver Professor of Hygiene (Emeritus), and Consultant on Psychiatry in the School of Public Health, Harvard University, Boston, Massachusetts.

EDMOND H. FISCHER, PH.D., Professor of Biochemistry, University of Washington, Seattle, Washington.

JOSEPH FLETCHER, S.T.D., D. LITT., DOCTOR OF SACRED THEOLOGY, Visiting Professor of Medical Ethics, University of Virginia, Charlottesville, Virginia; Emeritus, Robert Treat Paine Professor, Episcopal Theological School (affiliated with Harvard University), Cambridge, Massachusetts.

DANIEL X. FREEDMAN, M.D., Professor and Chairman of the Department of Psychiatry, University of Chicago, Chicago, Illinois.

JOHN L. HAMPSON, M.D., Professor of Psychiatry, University of Washington, Seattle, Washington.

ELISABETH KÜBLER–ROSS, M.D., Medical Director, South Cook County Mental Health and Family Services, Chicago Heights, Illinois.

DAVID R. MACE, PH.D., Professor of Family Sociology, Behavioral Sciences Center, Bowman Gray School of Medicine, Winston-Salem, North Carolina.

W. WALTER MENNINGER, M.D., Clinical Director and Director of Residency Training, Topeka State Hospital; Senior Staff Psychiatrist, the Menninger Foundation, Topeka, Kansas; Consultant, Federal Bureau of Prisons, Washington, D.C.

GILBERT S. OMENN, M.D., Assistant Professor of Medicine in Medical Genetics, and Fellow of the National Genetics Foundation, University of Washington, Seattle, Washington.

E. MANSELL PATTISON, M.D., Associate Professor of Psychiatry and Human Behavior, University of California, and Deputy Director of Training, Orange County Department of Mental Health, Irvine, California.

LUVERN V. RIEKE, L.L.B., L.L.M., Professor of Law, University of Washington, and Executive Secretary of the Washington State Judicial Council, Seattle, Washington.

MICHAEL B. ROTHENBERG, M.D., Professor of Psychiatry and Pediatrics, University of Washington, and Head of the Division of Behavioral Sciences, Children's Orthopedic Hospital and Medical Center, Seattle, Washington.

ROBERT F. RUSHMER, M.D., Professor and Chairman of the Department of Bioengineering, and Director of the Center for Bioengineering, University of Washington, Seattle, Washington.

MELVIN M. TUMIN, PH.D., Professor of Sociology and Anthropology, Princeton University, Princeton, New Jersey.

J. LYNWOOD WALKER, PH.D., Assistant Dean for Continuing Education, Graduate Theological Union, University of California, Associate Professor of Religion and Psychology, American Baptist Seminary of the West, Berkeley, California.

ROBERT H. WILLIAMS, M.D., Professor of Medicine, and Head of the Division of Endocrinology and Metabolism, University of Washington, Seattle, Washington.

STEWART WOLF, M.D., Director of the Marine Biomedical Institute of the University of Texas Medical Branch at Galveston; Emeritus Head of the Department of Medicine and Regents Professor of Medicine and Psychiatry, University of Oklahoma, Oklahoma City, Oklahoma.

To Live and To Die: When, Why, and How

CHAPTER 1

PROLOGUE

ROBERT H. WILLIAMS

The net advantages and disadvantages in living or in dying for an individual, his family and friends, and society depend upon many factors, the most prominent of which are when, why, and how one lives or dies. In this chapter I present briefly some major considerations related to these factors. These concepts are some of my own and others regarding many of the major topics of this book. More detailed discussion of these and other important aspects of life are discussed in the subsequent chapters.

WHY LIVE AND WHY DIE?

Dying is inevitable because the genetic and biochemical patterns are set to assure it. There are times when the merits of dying outweigh those of living. Sometimes we have gone to unwise extremes in unduly delaying death. There are times to promote living and times to promote dying. Why live? The prime purpose for living is to engage in mentation, the act of thinking (Chapter 2), and to provide for mentation in one's progeny. A person who will never have mentation usually serves no desirable purpose in life, but he will experience no suffering. Pleasant mentation stimulates desire for living. Mentation associated with marked and persistent suffering prompts desire for death. Many people have gradations of suffering between these two extremes and experience respective differences in their desires for continued life or for death. Our living and our dying, as well as how much pleasure and suffering we experience, depend chiefly upon genetic patterns and environmental influences. Some persons are born with more than a 75 percent chance of being afflicted with certain mental or physical disorders that are known to cause considerable suffering. A vast array of environmental influences can produce agonies via such things as infections, poison, nutritional deficiencies, physical injuries, and emotional upsets.

Each person bases his plan of living on guidelines that he and others have formulated. He may err because of abnormalities in his mentation, and he may be misled by others. Our patterns of mentation depend upon the chemical and physical status of the brain (Chapter 2). Abnormalities

1

in these account for abnormal behavior. In turn, these abnormalities depend upon primary reactions in the brain, influences from other parts of the body, and environmental factors.

Many individuals believe that they are guided by their soul in dealing with spiritual, moral, and ethical problems. As discussed in Chapter 3, I regard the soul as a special aspect of mentation. With no mentation there presumably is no soul and no intercommunication with God.

SOME GUIDELINES FOR LIVING AND DYING

Guidelines for living are imposed by laws, religions, and public traditions, and important influences are exerted also by parents, teachers, spouses, clubs, societies, racial groups, and others. Religious policies and laws presumably have been formulated along lines considered to be for the good of society and for individuals, and many are beneficial but some cause unnecessary suffering. Deletions, additions, and modifications must be made in these policies in order to meet present and future needs. Unfortunately, progress has been extraordinarily slow (Fig. 1).

There are hundreds of religious groups with numerous policies and creeds, and each denomination maintains strongly that its creeds are the correct ones. This has led to bitter battles. Each religion has its good and

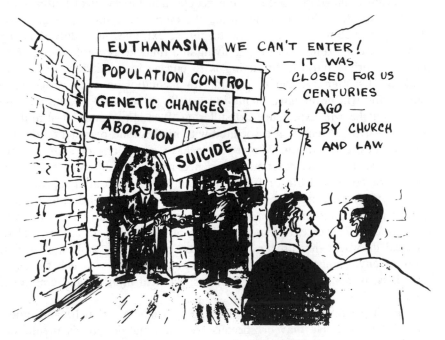

Fig. 1. Strong resistance has prevailed to changes in laws and religious policies permitting greater roles by man in influencing propagation and termination of life.

bad aspects, of course, but each needs to make modifications commensurate with current problems. This requirement is emphasized by the marked decrease in church attendance. A recent Gallup Poll in the United States revealed a decrease in church attendance from 49 percent in 1955 to 40 percent in 1971. In 1971, 57 percent of Catholics, 37 percent of Protestants, and 19 percent of Jews attended religious services. Attendance in the age group 21 to 29 had decreased to 28 percent. Ministers have also become discouraged. Indeed, among those below the age of 40 in the three major faiths, about 40 percent have seriously considered leaving the ministry (Gallup Poll). Ministers complained of being in a straitjacket of rules and regulations. Many local, national, and international schisms in various religious groups have arisen. There is a desire for less formal preaching about ancient events and for more extensive discussion of prominent current problems—for example, unnecessary discrimination (race, sex, age, pseudo-handicaps), war, population control, marriage, drug addiction and alcoholism, violence, careers, and current interpretation of body-spiritual relationships. Discussions should be interdenominational. With increased enlightenment there will undoubtedly be an increase in uniformity of religious policies and fewer arguments, for arguments often are exchanges of ignorance. The following statement by Einstein shows how good aspects of another's religion can be appreciated: "Christianity as Jesus taught it is the cure for all the social ills of humanity." It is distressing that certain top religious leaders have adopted and firmly enforced policies that have actually promoted extensive poverty, disease, crime, and suffering in many ways, yet have magnificently instituted other measures to help avoid these troubles and to generously assist the sick, poor, and distressed.

Laws in states and nations vary markedly. Frequently, there also are major differences in interpreting them. Some laws are so outdated that they are either forgotten or intentionally by-passed. Many major changes in laws and public traditions are needed, especially concerning: (a) methods for inhibiting excessive population increases, (b) liberalization of abortion restrictions, (c) euthanasia, (d) management of criminals, (e) welfare measures, and (f) treatment of psychopaths and health problems.

QUALITY AND QUANTITY OF POPULATION

Since health is the major determinant of happiness, great attention must be devoted to it. The first consideration concerns the quality and quantity of propagation. We do not have the capacity to generate life. Except for recent generation in the laboratory of life at a highly elementary level, all life was generated many centuries ago. We are able to influence markedly the quantity and quality of people propagated (Chapters 4–7), but have used these capacities relatively little. In some countries the population is increasing at an alarming rate. Such increases can present great problems of food supply, social adjustments, psychological stability, violence, war, and disease. Controlled experiments with animals have shown that when they exist in crowded conditions, mothers become frustrated and insufficiently suckle and rear their young. Anger, fighting, and homosexuality increase markedly—simulating the parental neglect, juvenile delinquency, homosexuality, and crime observed in man in overpopulated cities.

The quality of man's progeny can be improved significantly with better counseling and actions concerning marriages, the number and timing of pregnancies, the detection and abortion of diseased fetuses, improvement in genetic patterns, and improvement in nutritional and environmental influences. We have devoted tremendous time and money to improving the progeny of horses, beef, pigs, other animals, and plants, but relatively little to improving the progeny of man. Interest, cooperation, and action in these areas have increased in recent years. It is important that participation be extended to include everyone, especially those whose progeny would offer great problems for themselves, their families, and society.

CHILDHOOD AND ADOLESCENCE

Most of life's problems, including those in adolescence and those that develop in later life, are based upon abnormalities in genes or pregnancy, or environmental influences during the early years of life. I have been increasingly impressed by the strong impact on "young tender minds" of factors that seem only slightly upsetting.

During the last half century parents have been very ambitious for their children's attainment of high social, educational, professional, and financial status, and, consequently, competition in these areas has become great. Parents have plotted much of the course desired for their children before they have entered the first grade, often unaware of the importance of considering differences in their capabilities and desires and of not trying to make each of them fit the same mold. Instead, superconventionality has been applied. Parents have proceeded with the concept that there is a definite time and place to begin kindergarten, to learn to swim, dance, ski, and play tennis, to participate in the Cub Scout program, to start dating, and to indulge in an endless number of other activities. Competition has become strenuous, for example, in Little League baseball, football, and other sports, as well as in education. Great rewards are given to those who really excel, but many of those who do not excel feel disappointed and are inclined to turn away from some of the programs entirely. Competition among some parents and teachers to get their boys and girls admitted to one of a few prestigious schools is intense. With the constant pressure to attain ambitious goals, many children develop anxiety, fear, disappointment, frustration, resentment, and rebellion. These reactions make a child want to avoid his parents; he seeks others who are experiencing similar difficulties and to exchange empathy, comfort, respect, and love. While withdrawing from the parents in some ways, he also wants the parents' love, guidance, assurance, and attentive ears.

A few decades ago, along about the time the foregoing superambitions and superconventionalities were beginning to flower, child psychiatrists were emphasizing the great danger of inhibiting the activities of our children. "Freedom" was echoed strongly as the preferred course for children. Thereupon, extensive freedom was granted. Some of this freedom proved to be a delight for the children, but its magnitude became overwhelming and in itself provoked anxieties and other problems. Many major decisions were presented to children at times when they felt incapable of facing them. All these factors combined to encourage many to withdraw from reality to their own dream world created by marijuana and other drugs. Moreover, along with this went many dropouts from school and strong reactions to the entire Establishment. While still adolescents some of these youths have stated that they would have strongly preferred for their parents to have *made them* do many things rather than having left the decisions to them. Some opinions on this subject were revealed recently by the Campus Opinion Survey (Indiana University) of college students. About half stated that they would rear their children in a manner similar to their own upbringing. The large majority who preferred to be more permissive as parents indicated that their parents had been "either somewhat strict or very strict." Less than 5 percent indicated that they would rear their children in a very permissive manner.

In retrospect, it seems that some good lessons in child management can be found in salmon fishing, where we are taught to be constantly on the alert and to avoid letting the line get tight enough to break, but to watch for opportunities to wind up the catch. Meanwhile, patience must be exercised to permit a certain amount of roaming in various directions.

STUDENT RIOTS AND DEMANDS

Reactions against traditional ways of managing many problems in life have been frequent, and often vigorous, on university campuses. Protests have been directed against war, racial discrimination, social restrictions, and grading systems; they have also been aimed at improving health and welfare measures and general standards of living. Extremists, students and nonstudents, have participated in many of the disorders, some of which have resulted in personal injuries and property damage. At times revolution has seemed to greatly exceed evolution. However, with time other students have exerted a moderating influence, and significant net improve-

ments have occurred. Fig. 2 illustrates various sequences of reactions that
have developed.

Emerson has stated: "Every great and commanding movement in the
annals of the world is the triumph of some enthusiast." Enthusiasts can
either prompt great progress or hamper it, depending upon their goals and
the manner in which they proceed in attaining them. Not uncommonly,
the ultimate goals may be desirable, but some enthusiasts proceed somewhat ruthlessly and incite fear, antagonism, and counteractivities. To successfully implement major changes affecting the public, it usually is wise
to first condition the public with appropriate information. Interpreters between divergent groups that do not have sufficient mutual understanding
often play an important role. They can assist each group in appreciating
the merits and problems of the other, the solution of which can lead to
common good. Understanding frequently generates bonds of friendship and
peace. Whereas patience and a gentle approach promote relaxation—increasing the chances of careful consideration, understanding, and optimism—harsh words incite anger, resistance, and pessimism.

ACTIONS IN FACING LIFE PROBLEMS

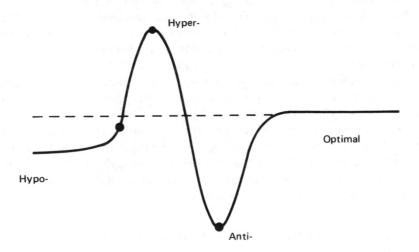

Fig. 2. This figure portrays four phases observed in many aspects of life: (a) Hypo-
activity is often applied in managing certain problems. (b) As the effects of undesirable consequences accumulate, certain individuals and groups initiate vigorous
and often dramatic campaigns for radical change, resulting in hyperactive responses.
(c) In time it becomes increasingly obvious that the changes have produced not
only distinct benefits but also major undesirable responses. This leads to strong
anti-actions. (d) A group of wise, patient, and considerate leaders carefully analyze
the entire situation systematically and institute plans and enlightenment that offer
optimal progress. Thereby they markedly decrease the hyperactions (apogee) and
the anti-actions (nadir).

CAREERS

The type of career chosen and the amount of success encountered in attaining career goals can greatly influence the health and happiness of many people (Chapter 15). The most rewarding careers tend to require long training as well as much hard work. It is important for a person to pursue a career in which he has the greatest interest and seemingly the best capacity. These elements are usually complementary, because man rejoices in his handiwork.

Many of the major leaders must apply originality and courage in exploring the unknown, being sufficiently aware of the past to avoid some of its pitfalls. Conditions and needs are changing constantly, so we must plot future courses realizing that some failures are scattered along the pathways leading to success. Selection of a career pattern that necessitates performance beyond a person's capacity has often led to much trouble. Indeed, failure in attaining a career goal has often led to anxiety and distress—sometimes to depression and suicide (Fig. 3). These and allied developments are discussed in succeeding sections.

ANXIETIES AND FEARS

Our bodies are provided with an "internal watchdog" that warns us of significant internal or external changes. Appraisal by the brain of various activities ranges from the unconscious to the highly conscious. The character of the interpretation and resulting responses depend upon previous experiences and conditioning of the individual. Past experiences of presumably similar type that have been associated with many ill-consequences can cause the person to respond with anxiety and fear—sometimes with panic, rage, and other such strong reactions. On the other hand, when the new experience is reminiscent of pleasant past activities it provokes new reactions of pleasure. Moreover, one can make great progress in conditioning himself to face tragic situations with relative calm and wisdom, along with appropriate empathy. As Milton states in *Paradise Lost,* "The mind is its own place, and in itself can make a heaven of hell, a hell of heaven."

The brain's alarm system commonly serves great benefits to the body, because it leads to a large number of protecting and rewarding reactions for the body. The system is involved in strong emotional reactions, some of which offer our greatest pleasures. The emotional reactions often spur vigorous determinations which eventually net great progress—be it in sports, art, music, literature, medicine, the ministry, or law. On the other hand, the frequent experiencing of alarm reactions with associated disappointing responses may drive a person down the road of failure (Fig. 3). As the impacts of failure grow strong, a person may become overwhelmed and surrender, ending it all by suicide, or he may ask for help. On the

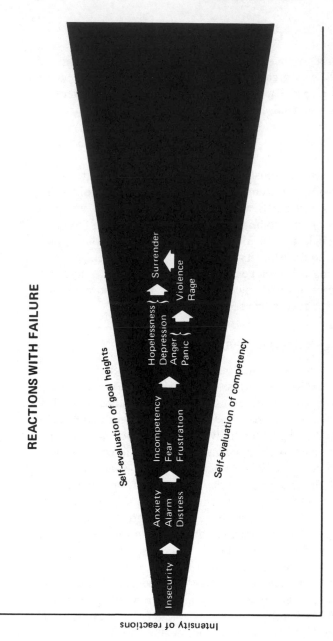

Fig. 3. A large number of problems in life result from sensations of incompetency in attaining a goal (or goals) that an individual has chosen or others have selected for him. Initially his reactions may consist chiefly of some doubts and feelings of insecurity. With time the intensity of the responses tends to increase in proportion to the gap between his estimation of his competency and the height of the goal. Moreover, even though the goal does not change, it frequently appears to him to rise as his estimate of his competency drops. As the gap increases the individual tends to experience anxiety, alarm, and distress. Fear, frustration, and conviction of incompetency increase. Sensations of hopelessness may become marked and be accompanied by so much depression that he surrenders, thereupon calling loudly for help or preferring to commit suicide. Others may develop anger and panic, accompanied by tirades of rage and violence, with destruction to objects, self, or other people.

other hand, certain individuals are incited to vigorous protest, manifesting violence. The violence may involve various destructive measures, including homicide and/or suicide. The capacities of the individual, as well as his previous conditioning, are highly important in promoting responses for good or bad. Body organs are responsive to certain messages from the brain, especially via the autonomic nervous system, and associated changes in the activities of the endocrine system. Individuals who repeatedly interpret certain confrontations with excessive anxiety, fear, and distress often experience abnormalities in body functions. The manifestations of these abnormalities include headache, "hay fever," loss of appetite, diarrhea, abdominal pains, pulse abnormalities, high blood pressure, skin rashes, muscle pains, impaired gonad function, excessive nervousness, insomnia, weakness, fatigue, and depression. Most psychoneuroses result in this manner. Moreover, the frequent vascular and other changes associated with hyperresponsiveness to stress promote an increased incidence of infection and other diseases. Most of the stress involves relationships between people; as population density increases, so does the stress. Man is especially concerned with how he fits in with others and how he is rated by them—he wants to be "well thought of." Some individuals have episodes of headache, skin rash, and so forth, only when exposed to certain people or other situations that produce excessive distress. Sudden major changes in environment that require major changes in the ways of life and in adapting to new situations are especially stressful to some persons.

DRUG USE AND ALCOHOLISM

The annual costs, directly and indirectly, resulting from the use of psychotomimetic drugs and alcohol are astronomical. A large proportion of automobile accidents, suicides, and crimes take place under their influence. Their excessive use often results from feelings of inferiority, rejection, depression, nervousness, and anxiety. Initial indulgence may come from a desire for adventure, but psychologic changes produced when using drugs and alcohol may cause their continued use. These changes depend upon the nature of the drug and the conditioning of the individual. However, there often is a change in sensations of reality, responsibilities, and duties, in one's evaluation of himself in his relation to others, and in the relative values of many phases of life. In some instances perceptions of time and space are altered. As the alcohol or drug habits grow, numerous biochemical and psychologic changes occur throughout the body. With continued use there develops a continuing "need" for certain compounds. Indeed, compulsion for them may become "a must at any cost," including thievery and destruction of people and things. With time the person tends to lose ambition, neglect his responsibilities, lose his self-respect and pride, and feel that he is a social outcast. Eventually he becomes depressed and antisocial and is unable to support himself financially. These personality characteristics prompt indulgence in crime. Some reports have indicated more than 80 percent of crimes are related to narcotics or excessive use of alcohol.

CRIME

Crime in the United States has become increasingly frequent and costly. It is produced by many factors and is very ineffectively managed. During 1968–1972 the number of women who are afraid to go out alone in their neighborhood has increased from 44 percent to 58 percent (Gallup Poll); for those older than 50 years it is 75 percent. Crime and lawlessness has recently been rated by the government as one of the public's two greatest concerns on the domestic front (the economic status is the other). The police force is understaffed, underpaid, undertrained in certain respects, and inadequately supported. Only a small proportion of crimes are detected or reported. Convictions result in relatively few instances, and many criminals are released soon, unrehabilitated. Most crimes are committed in one of the following categories: activities related directly or indirectly to drug or alcohol abuse, theft and embezzlement, sex deviation, assault, or homocide.

Crime is characterized by erroneous behavior. Indeed, it often results from abnormal thinking, which is due to an abnormal chemical status of the brain (Chapter 2). Numerous factors, internal or external, may produce the abnormalities. Among the causes are metabolic disorders, genetic alterations, tumors, infections, drugs, faulty nutrition, poisons, mechanical injuries, and various environmental factors. A good example of the effects of a compound on killing reactions is shown in Fig. 4. When a compound closely related in action to a normal brain hormone (acetylcholine) was injected into one specific area of the base of the brain (lateral hypothalamus) in rats, it caused 100 percent of the rats to kill mice. Some tumors found in this brain region of man have been associated with homicidal actions. Among a group of patients who sought medical aid because of violent behavior, or tendencies for such, one-third had abnormal electroencephalographic tracings. Also, about half of the prisoners in a medium-security penitentiary showed similar abnormalities.

Among environmental factors inducing crime are poverty, neglect, broken homes, crowded living conditions, social ostracism, persecution, and social injustices; other factors promoting disappointment and feelings of worthlessness, resentment, and hostility often develop. For example, some thievery is conditioned by socialist reactions. Since some governments forcefully seize money and property for division among the "have nots," seizure on an individual basis is often rationalized.

Management of prisoners now consists chiefly of confinement and

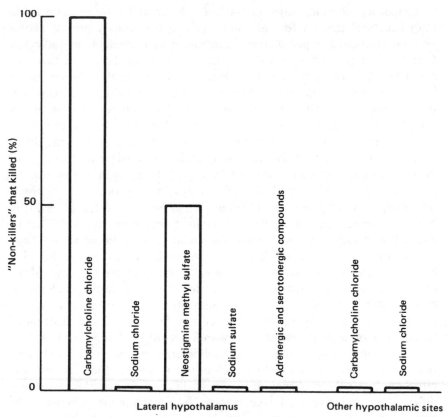

Fig. 4. Stimulus to kill is produced by injection of high concentrations of a compound similar to a major nerve hormone (acetylcholine) into the hypothalamus (at the base of the brain) of rats. (Smith et al., 1970, *Science,* **167**:900.)

punishment. About 95 percent of prison budgets goes for custodial care, chiefly to pay for walls, bars, and guards; only 5 percent is devoted to rehabilitation. Much abuse occurs between prisoners. Homicide, suicide, riots, and sex deviation occur. There certainly is extreme unhappiness. Many prisoners accumulate more psychological problems in prison than they had previously. All prisons in the United States combined have a total of only 60 full-time psychiatrists. All but 2 percent of criminals are returned to society. More than 50 percent commit additional crimes. A significant number of crimes are committed by people who were indicted but not convicted. Most criminal defense attorneys work vigorously toward only one goal—to gain freedom for their client—when in fact that freedom may be harmful for the client and for society.

Many criminals have psychiatric problems, and a large proportion of the others have emotional problems. These behavioral problems may be temporary, chronic, major or mild. To detect and manage these in the most beneficial manner for the offenders and for society, prisons should give each criminal a psychiatric examination and attention as indicated. Punishment and confinement should be used only to the extent that they are advantageous; both need not always be used together. Sometimes it is good to apply confinement with kind, tender, and loving care, indicating to the criminal that it is for his own protection and for that of others. Punishment is often given with the concept: "You have been mean to another, so we will punish (be mean to) you." In studies of "conditioned reflexes" where a rat always gets an electric shock when he travels path A but luxurious rat food when he travels path B, he soon learns to avoid path A and to follow path B. The same does or does not apply to prisoners, depending upon their conditioning. Some of them are so frustrated, confused, and hostile that punishment proves to have a deleterious effect. For example, one who is already greatly embittered about his many misfortunes and abuses in life becomes more hostile to the public while isolated in his cold, bleak, bare cell for many lonely nights and days. Moreover, some who have rallied somewhat for the good during confinement relapse after being released into a competitive environment, where they are rejected repeatedly in job applications, face inadequate sustenance, think often of their distressingly smeared record, and feel ostracized.

To manage prisons appropriately, different types of institutional facilities should be established so that each criminal receives the most effective attention. Since the problems of prisoners differ, their management should differ. Most criminals should be involved in rehabilitation programs, and many should receive continuing psychiatric care. Some should live in a dormitory with appropriate rehabilitation personnel and facilities, while making adjustments to "the outside world." Even after discharge from prison, periodic examinations and therapies should often be continued. Of course, this is a very expensive program—one that would involve construction of different types of buildings with pleasant surroundings and would necessitate staffing of many psychiatrists and other health personnel. However, it would produce much more effective rehabilitation and result in many more useful and self-supporting happy citizens than the present system, which is already very expensive.

Continuation of confinement and the amount of treatment should be correlated more with the intensity and persistence of the criminal's problems than with the magnitude of a given crime. However, no matter how extensive the treatment and rehabilitation programs, many criminals will not be cured. Indeed, some will always have major psychiatric problems. It seems more desirable that the criminal's life be terminated on the basis of the hopelessness of his cure rather than as a punishment for a major crime. Life's termination for a criminal offense should be regarded as euthanasia, exercised for the protection of the patient and others. In certain instances the patient could be offered the choice between euthanasia and permanent confinement necessitated by his mental sickness.

I wish to re-emphasize that the degrees of mental abnormality vary among many criminals and that they should be systematically, meticulously, and thoroughly dealt with accordingly. Very few criminals are "insane" in legal terms. Punishment has value in some instances, but it should be applied only when considered the most advantageous treatment of the offender, and then combined with other measures that net optimal improvement in behavior and performance.

EQUALIZATION OF PEOPLE

There are marked inequalities in the mental and physical status of people, initiated before birth and by a variety of influences through the years. These differences in capacities result in different levels of performance. Much unhappiness results from promulgating the concept that all people are equal, and that in instances where they are unequal we can equalize them. As emphasized in Chapter 15, certain individuals, when pressured to reach goals that are too high for them to attain, often suffer anxiety, fear, frustration, and great distress. Each person should attempt to achieve what he can do best and what makes him the happiest.

Significant assistance can be given in many ways to those who need it. "Unto whom much is given, of him shall much be required" (Luke xii:48) is a policy that is good and that is being pushed strongly today. However, this policy can be overextended and hamper net progress in society as a whole. Excessive extraction of various contributions from some individuals for others can hamper progress in general. Society is obligated to provide for individuals: (1) basic needs (food, clothing, shelter, and other comfortable living conditions); (2) protection from environmental harms (excessive pollution of air, water, food; crimes; various mental and physical abuses); (3) positive measures for happiness (opportunities for individual accomplishment, education, mental and physical development, and entertainment); (4) health care (all types); and (5) freedom, to an extent that it is not too damaging or costly (mental and physical) to others (this includes reproduction and hastening or delaying one's own death). *Each* individual owes something to society, and most persons should make determined efforts to make their appropriate contribution for the good of others. The status of society equals the total status of individuals.

I favor an all-out effort to help the needy as much as possible. We can do an enormous amount to prevent the frequency and amount of mental and physical abnormalities as well as economic, social, and other problems that are causing so much suffering for individuals and society today. Many applicable methods are discussed in this book.

PREJUDICE AND DISCRIMINATION

With marked increases in population density and intermingling of people with different backgrounds in religion, politics, color, race, social level, economic rank, and education, we must change laws and policies to permit more freedom of activity while protecting certain rights of individuals and of society. Some disfavor with segments of certain groups and resistance to them may have seemed justified, but many other discriminations have not. With conflicts between groups, those in the minority tend to be oppressed more than those in the majority, but often there are errors on each side. Discrimination naturally encourages members of a minority group to be group conscious, to cling together, and to concentrate upon furthering its progress. Any group that practices favoritism for its members and discrimination against others can expect counteroffenses. Such actions have propagated vicious circles. Extremists in each group make conciliation difficult, but continued honest, genuine, and considerate efforts of others net eventual progress (Fig. 2). Each group should study the needs and desires of those in the other groups and carefully consider making an increasing number of concessions. Each group should make genuine efforts not to reward its members at the expense of rejecting equally deserving members of other groups.

MARRIAGE

Marriage often has a highly important influence upon living and dying—when, why, and how. In some instances it is the grandest experience in life, nurturing rich pleasures, social success, and business success. At the other extreme it can cause enormous unhappiness and suffering, sometimes leading to failure in business and other activities, homicide, and suicide. The frequent discontent in marriage is evidenced by the present divorce rate in the United States of about 40 percent. Many couples remain married but have little respect or love for each; some chiefly "room and board" together and endure their suffering as best they can.

The three major objectives in marriage are: (a) reproduction and rearing of children, (b) sexual pleasures, and (c) companionship and collaboration in many of life's activities.

Many factors are important in establishing success in marriage. Some of the same principles apply to growing beautiful roses. Selection of genetic strain is very important. However, poor results are obtained with a prize-winning species when it is improperly nurtured, such as providing inappropriate soil, temperature, sunshine, and moisture. Growth of roses that excite great pride, admiration, and pleasure necessitates continuing careful attention. The same applies to marriage, and some of us believe that the rewards amply justify the efforts.

The selection of a marital partner has some analogies to a jigsaw puzzle in that even with many beautiful pieces, some fit together poorly while others fit beautifully, although no two pieces are alike. In recent years it has been common for a young couple, in their search for romance, "to go steady," beginning in high school or earlier. Unfortunately, many of the couples who have "gone steady" before marriage start going "unsteady" after marriage, and about 75 percent get divorced. It seems important for each person to experience a wide variety of associations and to mature sufficiently before selecting the most appropriate marital partner. Often, too much attention is given to immediate biological sex satiation and too little to personality traits and other factors.

It is best for a couple not to get married until they are fully convinced that the marriage is desirable. When getting married, a couple should do so with strong hope, faith, love, and expectations of a permanent bonding of satisfaction and pleasure. However, the couple must fully realize that the minister's ceremony does not magically produce a spontaneous flow of marital bliss and grandeur and that the results depend upon them. *For optimal happiness in marriage* genuine love is a necessity, and it should be accompanied by many things: appropriate sexual attraction and satiation, respect, admiration, appreciation, kindness, understanding, consideration, patience, helpfulness, generosity, humility, good temper, and sufficient intercommunication. At the time of marriage, a two-in-one concept is helpful. This concept regards the two people as becoming essentially one, with each person pooling mental and physical assets unreservedly for the good of both. Each should aim at doing somewhat more than his or her share. This helps to avoid negligence from overestimation of one's contributions and produces a good psychologic flavor.

Mistakes occur from spending too much or too little time together. A large amount of time together can cause monotony, boredom, and resentment of excessive repetition. Separation can rekindle a fresh longing and welcome. Separation also permits each to engage in some associations with other people and activities that may not offer great interest to the mate. Conversely, prolonged separation can cause excessive loneliness and feelings in the wife that she is chiefly a housekeeper and bedmate, and in the husband that he is needed chiefly to pay the bills; in each it may cause the sensation of insufficient interest and love.

Spouses can differ markedly in philosophies about many phases of life and yet have a highly successful marriage. This conclusion is based upon my observations of many couples and on the 30 years of great mutual happiness in my own marriage. In many instances where opinions differ, no conjoint action is required, and the consequences of these differences are not significant. When action is needed, each should desire to have the wishes of the other fulfilled and make concessions. This seems justified in exchange for marital happiness in general. Decisions involving the larger issues should be associated with calm discussions about the net advantages and disadvantages, with mutually satisfactory agreements. In making my own decisions concerning domestic (or professional) considerations I have found nothing makes me be more straightforward and honest than a realistic application of the Golden Rule. Many a marital failure has resulted from a failure to apply this rule.

In instances of marital discord, negligence, selfishness, and inconsiderateness have often prevailed. As the years of marriage go by, for example, there may be negligence in cleanliness, dress, grooming, industry, performance, and in other ways that influence the net image that one mate imparts to the other one. Along with these changes are decreasing manifestations of interest, attentiveness, consideration, kindness, and helpfulness devoted to the mate. Respect, admiration, and love decline, while criticism and nagging increase. The couple does not have enough calm and diplomatic discussions to correct some of the problems. Other people of the opposite sex may appear very interesting and alluring, providing a "ripe situation" for straying. As trouble mounts, anxiety and antagonisms accrue. Outside assistance in conciliation may be requested, but in many instances this occurs after loss of respect and love, which are hard to regain. On the other hand, when each mate continues to concentrate upon making the other one happy and enthusiastically persists in applying full-fledged love, the reward is often the grandest one in life.

EUTHANASIA

For centuries, laws, religious policies, and public traditions have forbidden euthanasia. However, with the present great array of drugs, mechanical devices, environmental protections, and other provisions for maintaining life, numerous patients are maintained in a state of suffering from mental and/or physical problems. The agonies outweigh the benefits derived by the patient, his family and friends, and society. Recently, there have been numerous heated debates throughout the world regarding permissibility for exercising euthanasia. The two extreme viewpoints are generally as follows. (a) *Opponents:* Euthanasia is directly opposed to the will of God, as indicated by the Fifth Commandment. It is murder. It is not in the best interests of the individual patient, his relatives and friends, or society. It is the wedge for extension of "murder" to an extreme degree. Those who would engage in such measures are grossly ungodly, immoral, unethical, stupid, unjust, selfish, and cowardly. (b) *Proponents:* Both negative euthanasia (withholding of treatment that will promote continued survival of the patient) and positive euthanasia (application of measures that will soon produce death of the patient) should be applied as often as seem justified, with approval by the patient and/or his family and his physician. Euthanasia is in keeping with the will of God, who is a very kind, considerate, compassionate, loving, and just God. It is for the benefit of the patient, his friends and relatives, and for society. Opponents of euthanasia are unwise, unjust, and cowardly.

Most people take a position between these extremes. For example, approximately 80 percent of physicians and laity whom I questioned favored negative euthanasia, but fewer favored positive euthanasia (Chapter 7). Many aspects of this subject are discussed in various parts of this book.

SUMMARY

In this chapter I have presented some major objectives and guidelines for living and dying. More attention and action are needed in dealing with the quality and quantity of people generated. The type of marital existence one experiences has frequently made a great difference in health, happiness, success, and the desire to live or die. The manner in which children are reared has a significant effect upon their motivation, the goals they set for themselves, their performance, and emotional status. Since people differ greatly in mental and physical capacities, the goals selected, type of training given, and rewards for performances should differ accordingly. Thus far, the patterns promoted for these have been too uniform and have caused much emotional and economic turmoil. Much anxiety, fear, frustration, and insecurity have developed and often prompted career failure, drug addiction, thievery, and destructive actions. Trouble has also been promoted by prejudice and unjustified discrimination.

CHAPTER 2

METABOLISM, MENTATION, AND BEHAVIOR*

ROBERT H. WILLIAMS

INTRODUCTION

The ultimate supreme function of the body is mentation, or thinking. Without mentation the body is of no significant use. Mentation plays the major role in all our pleasures and pains. The amounts and types of mental and physical behavior depend upon the body's metabolism. All abnormalities in mentation are associated with altered metabolism. Metabolic changes lead to psychic alterations and vice versa; often this sort of multicyclic relationship occurs in the same individual. Moreover, metabolic or psychic abnormalities can lead to changes in other parts of the body which further influence the metabolic and psychic states. The chemical and/or physical status of the brain can be altered by many influences. These include abnormalities within the brain itself, disorders in other parts of the body, and such influences from outside the body as social, climatic, and nutritional factors. There often is an interplay among these factors. For example, certain genetic enzyme abnormalities in the brain can tremendously alter behavior and, in turn, lead to adverse environmental conditions; contrariwise, abnormal environmental factors can markedly influence behavior. Even a total lack of sleep for a week can make a normal person have hallucinations. Each endocrine gland function can influence mentation; mentation can influence each endocrine and other metabolic function.

Since abnormal thinking (dysmentation) is common, causes enormous suffering, and is highly expensive, we must improve our methods for its prevention and correction. The primary biochemical defects in disordered thinking are being identified increasingly, with remarkable results.

Some Factors in Normal Mentation

The brain is the most important organ in the body. Its delicate structures are encased by a thick bone, the cranium. Intercommunication of

* Based on material presented as the presidential address before the Endocrine Society (JCEM **31:**461, 1970; reproduced by courtesy of the J. B. Lippincott Company). It should be consulted for further detail.

nerve fibers coordinates activities within the brain and throughout the body. The nerve fibers have the capacity to conduct bioelectrical impulses over long distances without loss of signal strength. The brain is constantly receiving and sending messages throughout the body. Since it demands a high level of metabolism at all times, an excellent circulation is required for the rapid delivery and removal of various constituents. There are numerous components in the plasma that can readily gain entrance to most of the other cells of the body but that cannot enter brain cells. A "blood-brain barrier" exists for carefully selecting needed constituents, many of which are of small molecular weight. The brain must receive the appropriate supply of water, minerals (especially calcium, magnesium, sodium, and potassium), vitamins, glucose, amino acids, oxygen, and other compounds. Marked changes in these can produce mental confusion, delirium, hallucinations, coma, and death. The brain has a high degree of independence for the synthesis of a large proportion of the chemicals it requires, including those for structure, energy, and transmission of messages. Glucose is a most important requirement, because it supplies most of the brain's energy and serves as a precursor for the synthesis of proteins, amino acids, and lipids, which compose about 90 percent of the brain's dry weight. Glucose is also the precursor for such important components as acetylcholine, glycine, prostaglandins, and glutamate. However, the brain must derive from the plasma three very important essential amino acids for the synthesis of three neurotransmitters: phenylalanine for catecholamines, tryptophan for serotonin, and histidine for histamine. Now a brief description is presented of some of the biochemical and other changes associated with neurotransmission, learning, memory, sleep, and coma. Some brief intricate scientific discussions seem justified so that we may illustrate the influences of certain factors in mentation, the body's primary function.

NEUROTRANSMITTERS

A large number of messages are rapidly transmitted through nerve fibers of the brain and elsewhere. The messengers, or neurotransmitters, include catecholamines (norepinephrine, dopamine), serotonin, acetylcholine, histamine, and certain amino acids. Since most of these compounds do not adequately permeate the blood-brain barrier, they are synthesized in the brain. Their precursors are carefully transported across the blood-brain barrier by catalytic mechanisms which are rapid, selective, and specific. Abnormalities in the amounts and types of monoamines in the brain produce clinical disorders such as phenylketonuria and histidinemia. Excesses of certain amino acids can be quite toxic to the brain. Leucine causes severe mental retardation. Tryptophan produces abnormal behavior; phenylalanine and leucine decrease serotonin but tryptophan increases it. Analogs of acetylcholine, norepinephrine, or serotonin may be hallucinogenic; they affect consciousness and perception. Some nerve fibers respond to some neurotransmitters but not to others. Transmission at most synapses (junctions of fibrous endings between two nerves) is produced by the release of small amounts of transmitter chemicals, which become bound to receptors on postsynaptic membranes of the effector cells. This results in transient alteration in membrane permeability, particularly to certain ions. Major alterations in sodium, potassium, magnesium, or calcium significantly influence brain function.

Since excesses of the neurotransmitters produce abnormal behavior, mechanisms are provided for rapid destruction of such excesses. Also, a number of neurotransmitters counteract effects of others. Various workers have demonstrated that during severe stress there is a focal and/or total decrease of one or more neurotransmitters in the brain. Stimulation of a specific area (amygdala) in the brain causes a rage response, whereas at other times it has no effect or causes sedation. The rage response is associated with a marked fall in norepinephrine in the telencephalon. When rage does not occur there is no change in the level of this hormone. Acetylcholine, norepinephrine, dopamine, and serotonin activate or inhibit particular cells at various places in the brain. Norepinephrine appears to suppress the stimulation caused by acetylcholine. Glutamate and a number of amino acids are predominantly excitatory.

Emotional reactions are associated with changes in the release and metabolism of neurotransmitters. A large number of drugs influence behavior by altering levels of activities of neurotransmitters. As little as 70 μg of LSD (lysergic acid diethylamide) can produce acute psychosis with hallucinations, delusions and other psychotic features, presumably by altering serotonin metabolism. Essentially all drugs with a fairly specific effect on mood in man affect the level of norepinephrine in the brain. The brain level of this hormone tends to be subnormal with depression and hypernormal with mania.

Acetylcholine.   The highest levels of acetylcholine in the brain tend to be found in the midbrain and in the base of the brain, especially in the hypothalamo-neurophyophyseal tracts.

When a nerve is stimulated, acetylcholine is rapidly released from the end of the nerve (presynapse) and is bound to specific receptor molecules in the adjacent nerve segment (postsynaptic membrane). Acetylcholine tends to be excitatory at the presynaptic terminals and inhibitory at the postsynaptic membrane. It presumably induces consciousness and a wakened state. Drugs that stimulate the central nervous system tend to increase acetylcholine levels. Some patients with disease in the vicinity of the hypothalamus have exhibited episodes of marked anger and rage. In rats that ordinarily do not kill mice, the injection of an acetylcholine-type compound (carbamylcholine) into the lateral hypothalamus caused 100 percent to become killers (Fig. 1, Chapter 1).

Catecholamines.   The main catecholamines found in the brain are norepinephrine and dopamine. They cannot be transferred from blood to brain readily because of a blood-brain barrier. Following manufacture in the brain, they are stored in granules in nerve endings. With nerve stimulation they are released and produce specific reactions. Immediately, there is an increase in the synthesis of the hormones.

Alterations in catecholamine metabolism produce abnormal behavior, including depression, mania, anxiety neurosis, and possibly schizophrenia.

Norepinephrine mediates alertness, wakefulness, pleasure, euphoria, anger, and fear. Dopamine and serotonin also affect these activities. The amount and type of reactions to norepinephrine depend upon the setting and past experiences of the individual. Norepinephrine and acetylcholine are important in memory, learning, and adaptation.

Serotonin.   Serotonin greatly influences behavior. It affects the emotional reactions and the level of intellectual performance. It depresses a number of activities, but over long intervals it facilitates the recruiting and synchronizing systems. A number of studies have suggested that an alteration in serotonin metabolism exists in schizophrenia. Virtually all of the brain contains some serotonin. Very little serotonin crosses the blood-brain barrier. The brain level of serotonin is dependent upon supply to the brain of an amino acid, tryptophan. Imipramine increases its actions. Chlorpromazine (Thorazine), imipramine (Tofranil), LSD, and lithium influence serotonin action. Compounds with structures similar to serotonin, such as LSD, produce a schizophrenic-type picture. These compounds may produce a variety of personality changes: hallucinations, pleasant sensations, excitement, agitation, and violence. With a decrease in serotonin levels in the brain, depression and insomnia tend to occur.

LEARNING AND MEMORY

Young rats exposed to a great many learning experiences have heavier and thicker cerebral cortices, more brain cells, greater enzymatic activity, and better blood supply than do their unexperienced siblings given the same food and kept under the same general physical conditions. With the increase in brain growth, there is an increase in synthesis of ribonucleic acid, protein, lipid, and other constituents. Such animals are also better at problem solving, learning, and other intellectual functions. These studies indicate that environmental influences are important in addition to the genetic status.

Numerous compounds affect learning and memory (e.g., acetylcholine and norepinephrine) and affect protein and RNA synthesis. Increases in acetylcholine in the synapses decrease synaptic transmission, which in turn can lead to amnesia. Short-term memory does not require protein and RNA synthesis; it is associated with electrical changes in the synapses.

With long-term memory, protein and RNA synthesis increase shortly after learning. Some soluble proteins, unique to the brain, are highly acidic, and they may influence DNA activity by combining with histones attached to DNA, thereby permitting more RNA and protein synthesis. The injection of brain extract or RNA from trained rats into untrained ones facilitates learning. The hippocampus is one of the structures involved in learning and short-term memory. The mammillary bodies, thalamic dorsomedial nucleus, and medical portion of the pulvinar are involved in long-term memory. Extensive lesions in the frontal lobe do not seem to influence this memory significantly. Relatively little is known regarding the coordinated storage and retrieval of knowledge.

SLEEP

Sleep is very much influenced by serotonin, catecholamines, adrenal steroids, and numerous other compounds as well as by nerve structure and many environmental factors. Moreover, there are distinct differences in the stages of sleep and in the influence of various factors upon these levels of sleep. Stages 1 and 2 consist of low-amplitude, fast-frequency electroencephalographic activity; stages 3 and 4 consist of high-amplitude, slow-frequency waves. Stage 1 is the lightest of the four stages. Stage 2 is deeper; the electroencephalogram has lower frequencies and higher amplitude than in stage 1. Stage 3 has waves of lower frequencies and higher amplitude than stage 2. The deepest sleep is stage 4, with a very slow cycle and waves of high amplitude. The rapid-eye-movement (REM) period occurs at the end of stage 1. REM sleep occurs only after prolonged non-REM sleep. During REM sleep, neuronal and metabolic activities and autonomic functions such as heart rate, respiration, and blood pressure are at increased levels, often comparable to the waking state. With the REM stage, there is a marked decrease in the tonus of head and neck muscles and the electroencephalographic waves are of low amplitude and high frequency. This is the period in which dreams are most common, including hallucinatory ones. Dream recall when the sleeper is awakened during this stage is reported in 80 percent but is infrequent during the other stages of sleep. The normal young adult dreams approximately one-fifth of his eight hour period of sleep. The REM periods occur periodically throughout the night at intervals of 90 ± minutes.

In normal sleep, all stages are present and occur during a similar percentage of time in chronological order. The percentage of REM sleep after infancy remains relatively stable through life, whereas total sleep and stage 4 sleep decrease progressively with age. Normally, the greatest amounts of stages 3 and 4 are in the first third of the night, and the greatest amounts of stage 1 and REM occur in the last third, whereas stage 2 is evenly distributed. On the average, the young adult spends 50 percent of his sleep in stage 2, the remainder being about evenly divided between stages 3 and 4, and stage 1 and REM. With abnormal sleep, all stages may be present, but their percentage distribution and sequence are not normal.

Most sedatives induce abnormal sleep, especially since they decrease the REM sleep. Upon withdrawal of sedatives, REM sleep occurs in excess, and there is an increased tendency to nightmares. Excess brain catecholamine decreases REM sleep, with a compensatory increase in non-REM sleep. Conversely subnormal brain catecholamine levels increase REM sleep and promote mental depression. Drugs which increase brain levels of serotonin increase sleep, whereas those that decrease serotonin may induce a state of permanent wakefulness.

Anxiety, agitation, and some drugs that prevent sleep may thereby produce psychotic changes. Numerous short periods of sleep deprivation, as well as long periods, tend to cause psychotic reactions. Persons who go without sleep for extended periods frequently exhibit disorders of thought and perception, sometimes indistinguishable from those seen in schizophrenia. Minor psychological changes are observed in subjects deprived of REM sleep. It appears that loss of REM sleep necessitates its makeup later. Hallucinations and delusions may appear after a week or more of total sleep deprivation.

Less total sleep and early morning awakening characterize depression; also, there is often a decrease in stage 4 sleep. In normal middle-aged and adolescent subjects, there tends to be a decrease in stage 4, but this level is very high in childhood. Schizophrenics have shown relatively few abnormalities of REM sleep.

COMA

Despite certain similarities between sleep and coma, there are major differences. One of these is in cerebral oxidation, which is decreased in coma but not in sleep. A high level of oxidation, chiefly involving glucose, is needed for the normal maintenance of electrical potentials across neuronal membranes and for the synthesis of numerous compounds. When the decrease in oxidation is not severe, there may be a decrease in alertness, orientation, perception, attention, memory, and affect. As the anoxia intensifies, coma occurs. With intensification and persistence of anoxia, the brain cells catabolize themselves, and permanent damage is produced. A severe deficiency of glucose in the brain produces many biochemical, anatomical, and clinical changes similar to those that occur with severe anoxia. In each instance a marked deficiency in oxidation occurs. Several types of coma are associated with increased levels of ammonia in the brain; by increasing the concentration of glutamic acid the ammonia and coma are reduced. The effect of such changes upon the thalamus is particularly important because it is the major site for maintenance of consciousness.

METABOLIC DISORDERS ASSOCIATED WITH
ABNORMAL MENTATION

A vast number of disorders cause abnormal mentation. For example, numerous cardiac, vascular, or pulmonary abnormalities impair mentation by failing to deliver sufficient oxygen, glucose, and other constituents, and/or by failing to remove certain chemicals which prove to be toxic. Likewise tumors and infections may impair mentation by compressing brain cells, usurping energy, or liberating toxic products. Extensive liver or kidney disease permits excess accumulation of products that damage brain function. Abnormal mentation results from excesses or deficiencies in water, electrolytes, or glucose. It results also from deficiencies of thiamine, nicotinamide, pantothenic acid, pyridoxine, vitamin B_{12}, and other items of diet. Of course, a vast number of plants or drugs cause marked mental changes. Some other examples of metabolic changes affecting mentation are now presented in detail.

Genetic Disorders. Abnormal mentation is associated with many different genetic disorders. Table I lists disorders with a high incidence of abnormal mentation, especially mental retardation. A marked defect in the activity of almost any enzyme involved in amino acid metabolism may be associated with mental retardation.

Table I. Etiologic Enzyme Deficiency in Some Genetic Disorders with Abnormal Mentation in More Than 75% of Patients

Disease	Etiologic Enzyme Deficiency
Fabry's disease	Ceramide trihexosidase
Galactosemia	Galactose-1-phosphate uridyl transferase
Gaucher's disease—infantile form	Glucocerebrosidase
Histidinemia	Histidase
Homocystinuria	Cystathionine synthetase
Lesch-Nyhan disease	Hypoxanthiane-guanine-phosphoribosyl-transferase
Niemann-Pick disease	Sphingomyelinase
Phenylketonuria	Phenylalanine hydroxylase

Hundreds of mutations may lead to various alterations in enzyme activity. However, intelligence is not decreased in all instances. For example, superior intelligence has been reported in association with retinoblastoma and hyperuricemia and in siblings of patients with phenylketonuria and parents of autistic children.

That an enzyme defect can lead to marked behavioral changes is well illustrated by the Lesch-Nyhan syndrome (Fig. 1). This genetic disorder

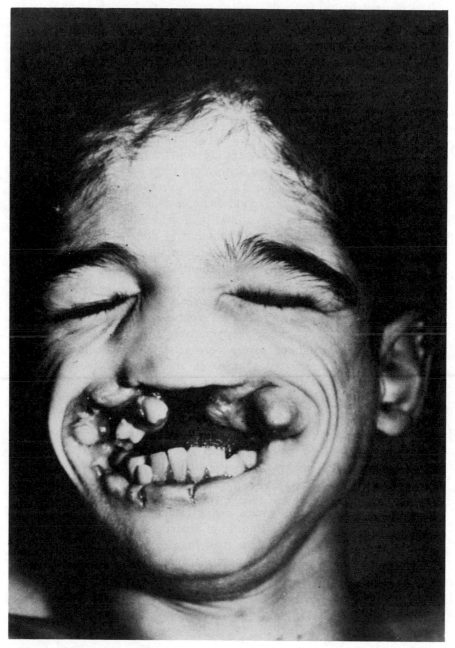

Fig. 1. Marked self-mutilation of lips, gums, and other structures in a boy with Lesch-Nyhan syndrome, at age 14 (from Nyhan).

of purine metabolism leads to marked mental retardation and aggressive-compulsive self-mutilative behavior, such as extensive chewing off of the lips, the fingers, and other areas; it also causes spastic cerebral palsy and choreic movements. In phenylketonuria there is an enzyme defect which promotes phenylalanine accumulation and causes marked mental abnormalities. Reductions in the dietary intake of this amino acid decrease progression of the disease. Likewise, in galactosemia, galactose can be removed from the diet with great benefit. In orotic aciduria, the feeding of cytidylic and uridylic acids offers distinct advantages.

Many of these genetic disorders are now being managed more effectively because they are diagnosed in the fetal stage by means of amniocentesis (removal of a small amount of fluid surrounding the fetus); often abortion is performed. A very good example is mongolism (Down's syndrome), which occurs in approximately 2 percent of the offspring of mothers who are older than 40. Thousands of amniocenteses have been performed with minimal maternal and fetal mortality.

Endocrine Disorders. Mental abnormalities frequently occur with certain endocrine disorders. Those producing marked changes in calcium levels frequently produce behavioral changes. For example, in 54 patients with hyperparathyroidism, not selected from a psychiatric point of view, Petersen found in 46 observed preoperatively that 9 percent were psychotic, 39 percent exhibited severe personality change, and 35 percent showed moderate personality change. In the majority, the personality change began with an affective disturbance characterized by loss of initiative, spontaneity, and interest. Many of the patients were listless and depressed. There was impaired memory in a few. Those with psychosis had disorientation, delirium, confusion, paranoia, and hallucinations. Those with acute psychosis had a violent onset, and an immediate operation was necessary. With the removal of the parathyroid tumors and the return of the serum calcium level to normal, most of the patients regained their former mental condition. The degree of psychiatric disorder tended to be proportionate to the serum excess in the calcium level. Acute psychoses were seen when the serum calcium level attained 16 mg percent. That the calcium level itself was more important than the increase in parathyroid hormone was demonstrated by the fact that mental changes subsided when the calcium level was lowered by peritoneal dialysis, despite persisting high levels of parathyroid hormone.

The following case abstract illustrates how one simple biochemical disorder can cause severe behavioral changes:

P. B. D., a boy aged 19, gave a long history of peculiar actions, social maladjustment, and other behavioral difficulties. Nine years previously, he had started to have seizures. Sometimes he would have as many as 20 in a day, but at other times he would go as long as one week without any. He had been seen by many excellent physicians, including neurologists and psychiatrists. The diagnoses were epilepsy, hysteria, and schizophrenia. He had had anticonvulsant therapy for three years, with some decrease in the frequency of seizures but not much change in his personality problems. During this time he spent more than one year in a mental hospital. We found his serum calcium level markedly subnormal (5 mg percent) and his phosphorus level was 7 mg percent, and diagnosed him as having hypoparathyroidism. Following treatment sufficient to return the calcium level to normal, the seizures and personality problems disappeared. He now is working regularly and is very happy.

Abnormal mentation was found (Denko) in 89 percent of 178 patients with primary hypoparathyroidism and in 98 percent of 111 with postoperative hypoparathyroidism (Fig. 2). The patients designated as having organic brain syndrome had major emotional disturbances with impaired intellect. In those with functional psychoses, some displayed schizoid changes. Other features were irritability, emotional alteration, impaired memory, and mental confusion; some had depression. The neurotic group showed such traits as obsessions and phobias. Calcium therapy markedly relieved the symptoms of individuals with hypoparathyroidism, but permanent abnormal mentation persisted in some. In conclusion, severe alteration in mentation occurs with either marked hypercalcemia or hypocalcemia. This is expected in view of the highly important role of calcium

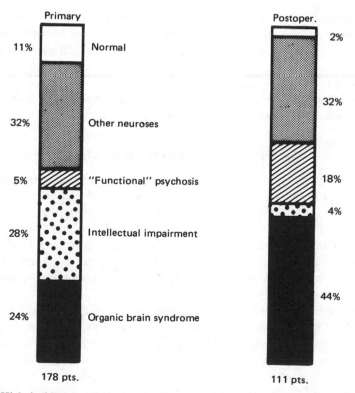

Fig. 2. High incidences of abnormal mentation are shown for hypoparathyroidism, primary and postoperative (Denko and Kaebling).

in cell membrane permeability, enzyme functions, nerve transmission, and other reactions.

With excess adrenal steroid secretion, as in Cushing's disease, some authors have reported moderate or severe mental changes in more than 50 percent. The commonest type of mental alteration is depression; schizoid manifestations are found in many. Although in some patients the mental symptoms diminish dramatically after adrenalectomy, in others they persist.

With severe adrenal insufficiency (Addison's disease) mental abnormalities have been found in more than 59 percent of the patients and have included a variety of neurotic traits, depression, and paranoid psychosis. In most patients there is dramatic improvement with corticosteroid therapy.

In an excellent study (Clinical Society of London Report), most of 109 unselected patients with myxedema were found to have alterations in mentation. Impairment of learning and memory was common; many experienced delusions and hallucinations; approximately one-third were designated as insane. Most of these features are reversed by thyroid hormone therapy.

Patients with insulin-producing tumors (insulinoma) usually have impairment of mentation at some time. With acute severe hypoglycemic episodes there may be anxiety and mental confusion, which may progress to coma, with or without permanent brain damage. For months or years some of these patients have periods of depression, bizarre behavior or various psychoneurotic manifestations; some have a schizophrenic pattern. These symptoms usually disappear after removal of the tumor tissue.

MENTAL DEPRESSION AND MANIA

A large variety of metabolic disorders are associated with mental depression, and often the depression is relieved after their correction. Excess adrenal steroid (e.g., hydrocortisone) often has caused depression; as the steroid level becomes normal the depression disappears. In depression there tend to be deficiencies of catecholamine and serotonin in the brain. Compounds that cause catecholamine deficiency produce depression (e.g., reserpine), while those that increase brain catecholamine relieve depression (e.g., Tofranil, Elavil).

In mania, there are increases in cerebral levels of norepinephrine and serotonin. Mania is benefited by drugs that lower the levels of these compounds. Lithium controls mania to a significant degree, and sometimes it benefits depression. In mania there tends to be excess cyclic AMP (adenosine 3'5'-phosphate), but there is a deficiency in depression. This compound is very important in mentation. Its levels are significantly influenced by catecholamine and serotonin.

SCHIZOPHRENIA

Schizophrenic reactions have been found in approximately 60 percent of patients in mental hospitals and in 50 percent of those admitted to some adult psychiatric clinics. Many studies have indicated that genetic factors play a prominent etiologic role. Monozygotic (identical) twins have concordance rates for schizophrenia four times greater than dizygotic (fraternal) twins. Among monozygotic twins with one member showing schizophrenia, the second one was found to be schizophrenic in 46 percent of the instances. Moreover, most of the remaining 54 percent were mentally abnormal; apparently all of them were schizoid. Only 13 percent were judged normal or near normal. When both parents are schizophrenic, an estimated 66 percent of their children have been found to be schizoid or schizophrenic. Among children born of schizophrenic mothers who were reared from the age of approximately one month in adoptive or foster homes, in comparison with similar adopted children born to normal parents, there was a several-fold higher incidence of schizophrenia, mental deficiency, antisocial personality, involvement in crime, and commitment to psychiatric institutions. About 45 percent of the siblings, parents, and children of schizophrenic patients are schizoid or schizophrenic. Many other reports show the high incidence of genetic transmission of schizophrenia. However, in many instances the genetic disorder combines with prenatal and/or postnatal environmental influences to bring about schizophrenia.

There have been many reports of neurochemical disorders in schizophrenia. Many of the psychomimetic compounds which do not upset consciousness are chemically related to norepinephrine, dopamine, and serotonin. Schizophrenic-type patterns have been produced by LSD, mescaline, hypoglycemia, adrenal disorders, and many other drugs and diseases. In the light of present information, it seems best to regard schizophrenia as a characteristic syndrome with many causes. The primary chemical abnormalities producing it may be exogenous, but presumably are more often endogenous. Environmental and other influences are also important in producing the syndrome.

SUMMARY

The ultimate supreme function of the body is mentation; all portions of the body are subservient to it. Abnormal mentation is very common, highly distressing, and enormously expensive. *All abnormalities in mentation are presumably associated with altered metabolism.* Abnormal metabolism causes abnormal mentation and vice versa. Altered cerebral metabolism is produced by primary or secondary cerebral disorders in the body, and by extracorporeal influences—abnormalities in diet, climate, social status, and numerous other environmental factors; frequently the inter-play of influences is most complicated. Abnormal mentation is found in many cerebral, vascular, pulmonary, hepatic, renal, and endocrine dis-orders. It also occurs in numerous other conditions that alter the chemical and/or physical status of the brain. Many neurotransmitters have been described, including especially acetylcholine, norepinephrine, dopamine, and serotonin. Abnormalities in the metabolism of one or more of these have been reported in various types of mental disorders. In depression and mania there are abnormalities in catecholamine metabolism, with lesser changes in serotonin. Certain observations have suggested abnormalities in serotonin metabolism in schizophrenia, but data remain inadequate. Hal-lucinations and other marked behavioral changes have accompanied al-tered serotonin metabolism and/or ingestion of serotonin-like compounds. Changes in brain acetylcholine levels have produced anger, rage, anxiety, and other altered behavioral states. Sleep seems to be associated with in-creased serotonin and decreased catecholamine levels; insomnia accom-panies the reverse. Learning and memory are influenced by the metabolism of protein, nucleotides, carbohydrate, fat, vitamins, minerals, and numer-ous other factors.

REFERENCES

Bloom, F. E., and N. J. Giarman. 1968. Physiologic and pharmacologic consid-erations of biogenic amines in the nervous system. *Ann. Rev. Pharmacol.* **8:**229–258.

Clinical Society of London Report on Myxedema. 1880. *In* Transactions of the Clinical Society of London. Vol. 21, suppl. London, Longmans, Green & Co.

Cooper, J. R., F. E. Bloom, and R. H. Roth. 1970. The Biochemical Basis of Neuropharmacology. New York-London-Toronto, Oxford University Press.

Curtis, D. R., and J. C. Watkins. 1965. The pharmacology of amino acids related to gamma-aminobutyric acid. *Pharmacol. Rev.* **17:**347–391.

Denko, J. D., and R. Kaebling. 1962. The psychiatric aspects of hypoparathy-roidism. *Acta Psychiat. Scand.* **38:**7–70.

Iversen, L. L. 1967. The Uptake and Storage of Noradrenaline in Sympathetic Nerves. Cambridge, Cambridge University Press. Page 30.

Jouvet, M. 1967. Neurophysiology of the States of Sleep. *In* The Neurosciences. G. C. Quarton, T. Melnechuk, and F. O. Schmitt, eds. New York, The Rockefeller University Press. Page 529.

Kety, S. S. 1967. Psychoendocrine Systems and Emotion: Biological Aspects. *In* Neurophysiology and Emotion. D. C. Glass, ed. New York, The Rocke-feller University Press and Russell Sage Foundation. Page 103.

Kety, S. S. 1967. The Central Physiological and Pharmacological Effects of the Biogenic Amines and Their Correlations with Behavior. *In* The Neurosciences. G. C. Quarton, T. Melnechuk, and F. O. Schmitt, eds. New York, The Rockefeller University Press. Page 444.

Koella, W. P. 1966. *In* Molecular Basis of Some Aspects of Mental Activity. O. Walaas, ed. London-New York, Academic Press. Page 431.

Kopin, I. J. 1967. The Adrenergic Synapse. *In* The Neurosciences. G. C. Quarton, T. Melnechuk, and F. O. Schmitt, eds. New York, The Rockefeller University Press. Page 427.

Kravitz, E. A. 1967. Acetylcholine, γ-Aminobutyric Acid, and Glutamic Acid: Physiological and Chemical Studies Related to Their Roles as Neurotransmitter Agents. *In* The Neurosciences. G. C. Quarton, T. Melnechuk, and F. O. Schmitt, eds. New York, The Rockefeller University Press. Page 433.

Nyhan, W. L. 1968. Clinical features of the Lesch-Nyhan Syndrome: Introduction—clinical and genetic features. *Fed. Proc.* **27:**1027–1033.

Page, I. H., and A. Carlsson. 1970. Serotonin. *In* Handbook of Neurochemistry. A. Lajtha, ed. Vol. 4. New York, Plenum Press. Page 251.

Pauling, L. 1968. Orthomolecular psychiatry. *Science.* **160:**265–271.

Petersen, P. J. 1968. Psychiatric disorders in primary hyperparathyroidism. *Clin. Endocr.* **28:**1491–1495.

Plum, F., and J. B. Posner. 1966. Diagnosis of Stupor and Coma. Philadelphia, F. A. Davis Co.

Potter, L. T. 1970. Acetylcholine, Choline Acetyltransferase and Acetylcholinesterase. *In* Handbook of Neurochemistry. A. Lajtha, ed. Vol. 4. New York, Plenum Press. Page 263.

Rupp, C., ed. 1968. Mind as a Tissue. New York-Evanston-London, Harper & Row.

Smith, D. E., M. B. King, and B. G. Hoebel. 1970. Lateral hypothalamic control of killing: evidence for a cholinoceptive mechanism. *Science.* **167:**900–901.

Tower, D. B. 1969. Neurochemical Mechanisms. *In* Basic Mechanisms of the Epilepsies. H. H. Jasper, A. A. Ward, Jr., and A. Pope, eds. Boston, Little, Brown and Co. Page 611.

Williams, R. H. 1970. Metabolism and mentation. *J. Clin. Endocr.* **31:**461–479.

Woolley, D. W. 1967. Involvement in the Hormone Serotonin in Emotion and Mind. *In* Neurophysiology and Emotion. D. C. Glass, ed. New York, The Rockefeller University Press and Russell Sage Foundation. Page 108.

CHAPTER 3

BODY, MIND, AND SOUL

ROBERT H. WILLIAMS

Some people maintain that the individual should not play a role in formulating morality because we must follow the words of God. However, we cannot actively follow God's words without interpreting those words, and the fact that there are hundreds of religions shows that many interpretations are possible. The words of God are generally considered to have been spoken centuries ago. Two questions are pertinent: (a) Has God stopped speaking? (b) Should interpretations cease? Whatever the answers, the fact is that, for better or worse, interpretations do continue to be made. Interpretations depend upon mentation, but our relations with God are considered to be mediated through the soul. Therefore, this chapter will discuss briefly the relationships of body, mind, and soul.

The preceding chapter discussed some important mind-body relations. Far from being a mysterious entity superimposed upon the body, the mind is a function of the psychobiologically integrated organism. Thus it is preferable to speak of mentation rather than of the mind. Mentation is the supreme function of the body. All other body organs subserve the brain, the heart acting as a pump, the kidneys as a filter, the liver as a chemical processing unit, the lungs as a gas exchanger, the gastrointestines as a processor of food and eliminator of waste, etc. Even the gonads ultimately contribute to mentation by producing other people. *Without mentation the body serves no important purpose.*

The preceding chapter mentioned many activities of the body that are necessary for normal mentation and showed that even diseases with only one basic biochemical defect can cause several behavioral abnormalities. To emphasize the effect of metabolism upon mentation, a renowned psychiatrist, Adolph Meyer, asked his students the following question: If it were possible to construct in the laboratory a cat that was atom for atom and molecule for molecule like a living cat, would it be alive and have memories and other thoughts like the living cat? Of course it would. In fact, some recent research has shown that the injection of brain extract or ribonucleic acid from trained rats into untrained ones gave the recipient some memories of the donor.

It seems likely that in the future the possibilities of extensive organ

32

transplantation will further highlight problems of body-mind-soul interrelations. Since the technical and immunological difficulties that now limit such operations will probably be overcome eventually, it is possible that one person could receive several transplanted organs, as for example brain, heart, liver, and kidneys (Fig. 1). The recipient, John Doe, would have origination of thoughts, perception, memories, correlation of ideas, and other mental activities like those of Rebecca Goldstein—at least as far as these activities are influenced by the brain's primary biochemical reactions. John Doe would have memories like Rebecca Goldstein's because they would be preserved by the previous deposition in certain areas of Rebecca Goldstein's brain of specific protein, RNA, and other chemical constituents. Even after transplantation, the design for the synthesis of more protein and other constituents of the brain would be controlled by DNA that had been synthesized in Rebecca Goldstein's brain. Moreover, the same type of DNA would continue to be formed after brain transplantation. Very significantly, in my judgment, the brain transplant would cause John Doe to lose his own patterns of mentation and thus to lose his soul. He would acquire the soul of the donor, Rebecca Goldstein. John Doe would have a personality like that of Rebecca Goldstein.

Considerations of the soul and its relationship to mind and body are important not only with regard to organ transplantation, but also in many other ways, including man's role in modifying the propagation and termination of life and the patterns of life.

The soul has been characterized in many ways. It has been considered to be the spirit, separate from the body; the moral component, contending with sin; the seat of emotions and sentiments; parts of the mind; the deepseated part of personality. Webster's New World Dictionary of the American Language (College Edition, 1959) includes these definitions:

1. "An entity which is regarded as being the immortal or spiritual part of the person and, though having no physical or material reality, is credited with the functions of thinking and willing, and hence, determining all behavior."
2. "The spirit of a dead person, thought of as separate from the body and leading an existence of its own."

Adolf Meyer taught that "the soul is an ultrabiological entity which is the postulate of faith. It is the emotionalistic and voluntaristic integrate and the resource of feeling."

I have been offering courses to medical students and physicians in the religious and philosophical aspects of medical care. Ministers of many faiths have participated in some of the sessions. Their concepts of the soul have differed greatly. Some believe that a soul resides in each form of animal life—dog, snake, worm, spermatozoon, ameba, etc.—but that there is none in plants. Some say that the soul enters man when the ovum is

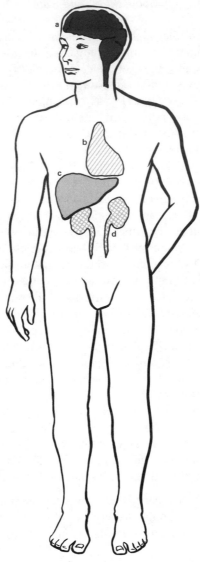

Fig. 1. This figure serves as a basis for considering possible future problems (ethical, moral, mental, and physical) presented by multiple organ transplantation. The recipient, John Doe, aged 32, had been normal and well until he had a severe accident a few days before receiving transplants of four normal organs obtained from donors, aged 30–35, as follows: (*a*) brain from Rebecca Goldstein, (*b*) heart from Moses Jones, (*c*) liver from Joe Murphy, and (*d*) kidney from Ho Chinn. After completion of these transplantations the following questions are presented: Who is he—John Doe or one or more of the donors? Does he have one soul or several? If one, whose? Are his memories and patterns of thinking more like those of John Doe or Rebecca Goldstein? These questions are answered in the text. (In the Epilogue are considered the effects of various organ transplants upon sex reactions, prejudices and discrimination, progeny, mentation, morals, crime, and the Hereafter.)

fertilized, whereas others believe it enters at the time of fetal "quickening," or at birth. "Quickening" is chiefly a manifestation of neuromuscular development. If activities of the soul are correlated with mentation, it is difficult to believe that the soul is active in the fetus, because there appears to be little or no fetal mentation. However, the most common view seems to be that the soul enters at conception. There is also disagreement as to when the soul leaves the body; most believe this occurs with the last heartbeat, with the last breath, or with terminal coma.

Of the many possible concepts of the soul that have been entertained, we will consider only four: (a) The soul is an entity (spiritual, ethereal) with existence and function totally unrelated to body composition or function. (b) The soul is independent of body composition and function but mediates its role through them in a manner that is not understood. (c) The soul constitutes a union of a specialized aspect of mentation and the Holy Spirit (God). (d) The soul is a specialized aspect of mentation. If the first proposal is correct, the soul would exist as a great mystery to us; we would not know when it appears or disappears, or when or how it functions. Since we could neither control nor modify the soul, it is difficult to picture it as an integral part of ourselves. However, a concept of the soul that embodies mysteries need not be abandoned because of the mysteries per se. In the second and third concepts, functioning of the soul is a conjoint activity of the Holy Spirit and mentation. In the second instance, the soul is conceived as an aspect of the Holy Spirit but is not individualized without mentation. In the third, the soul is an aspect of mentation serving as a special receptor for the Holy Spirit; in this instance there would be no soul when there was no mentation. In the fourth, the soul is manifested as a special phase of mentation and functions independent of a Holy Spirit.

With each of the last three concepts, the individual is seen to play an increasingly greater role and to hold increasing responsibility in moral activities. Any operation of the soul other than through mentation is passive for a person; it is not under our control and appears not to involve our participation. This concept that the soul is a special aspect of mentation—at least in terms of any active role we play in its function—is the most comprehensible. In keeping with this concept, a person born without a brain, and thus without mentation, would not manifest activities of the soul. He would never recognize any moral or religious principles. The Bible, sermons, and religious teachings would have no meaning to him. Some individuals commit horrible crimes, yet they do not remember them and experience no guilt; sometimes there are overwhelming compulsions to commit crime. However, after court trial and psychiatric examination, the edict is given: "He is not guilty by reason of insanity; he does not have the capacity to differentiate right and wrong."

When a person deals with moral issues, he commonly follows, to greater or lesser degree, interpretations and decisions that were made by others and passed on to him as religious policies, laws, traditions, etc. Many of the basic decisions in our culture were made centuries ago. Supposedly these decisions were based upon the words of God, but many bitter battles have been waged over two points: (a) What were the exact words of God and who has received them? (b) How are they interpreted best, particularly with respect to individual issues? The most important decisions on moral issues have been formulated, adopted, and enforced by churches and governments. However, the fact that there are so many religious groups with differing interpretations and policies, as well as the fact that laws and policies differ so markedly throughout the world, illustrates the great freedom that has been exercised in applying concepts of soul, mind, and body to moral issues. These facts also illustrate the lack of conformity in concepts.

Since the beginning of man, mentation has been used to formulate policies concerning man's role in the propagation, modification, and termination of life. Moreover, such decisions are still being made, but some of them do not best fit our needs. The scientific understanding of the present contrasts with the lack of understanding in the past. We must apply our own best thoughts to analyze our needs and to plan to meet them. We must consider that we have both the authority and responsibility for this planning. It seems reasonable to assume that our mentation is as good as it was centuries ago, and that we can use it as well as our forefathers did.

Since the activities of the soul appear to be related to specialized aspects of mentation, and since the amount and type of mentation depend upon numerous factors affecting the chemical and physical status of the brain, we can visualize that people would differ markedly in the quality and quantity of mentation and of the soul. Consequently, differences in capacities, behavior, goals, and accomplishments are to be expected. Such differences might be considered in dealing with an individual's philosophies, education, morals, career, and other phases of life. These differences are also important in making general and individual decisions regarding population expansion, abortion, euthanasia, and other measures affecting the propagation, modification, and termination of life. Plans in such areas should be based upon what appears best for mankind in general while protecting each individual as much as is feasible. Each person must make some sacrifices for the general good. Policies must be modified as the needs of society change.

CONCLUSIONS

Of all the ways that the soul has been characterized, the concept that the soul is a special aspect of mentation is the most comprehensible one;

certainly this concept seems to apply to any *active* role that we play in the function of the soul. Presumably, with no mentation there is no soul, no active communication with God, no personality, and no moral actions. It seems reasonable to assume that when there is definite, permanent, and total loss of mentation, only the body remains of the body-mind-soul triad, and it yields little benefit as such. With this concept, it appears that people vary in their capacities for both mentation and activities of the soul. Qualitative as well as quantitative abnormalities in function of the mind and soul exist. Mentation depends chiefly upon the physical and chemical aspects of the brain, which are influenced by a vast number of factors, many of which have acted over numerous centuries. Since mentation is the basis for our behavior, it is important that each of us apply it as best we can for the good of individuals, singly and collectively. This approach should be applied to laws, religious policies, public philosophies, and many other aspects which guide our lives, including our active role in the propagation and termination of life, and in our decisions as to when and how we live.

REFERENCE

Walker, J. L. 1971. Body and soul. Nashville, Abingdon Press.

CHAPTER 4

ON THE ORIGIN OF LIFE

EDMOND H. FISCHER

THE CONCEPT

Since the dawn of human civilization, man has been confronted with the mysteries of his origin and fate, and the nature of life itself. In the earliest accounts of Egyptian, Indian, Asian, and Greek cultures, we find a mixture of de facto acceptance of the continuous creation of life and some mythical description of man's own origin (Oparin).

Life is inherent in matter and therefore omnipresent; its spontaneous appearance is just a manifestation of this intrinsic property. It might have resulted from the proper interaction of the right kinds of elements, (e.g., moist mud and fire [Democritus]) but, until the writings of Plato, without "outside" interference. In modern language, life appeared according to the natural laws of chemistry and physics, and not with the help of some supernatural force or magical "life substance" (the immortal spirit of Psyche [Plato]).

The purpose of this chapter is to indicate how life might have emerged on the earth, not because of some divine intervention, but perhaps as an almost inescapable consequence of the physical and chemical conditions that prevailed in primordial times. We will show that hundreds of thousands of organic molecules were produced because nothing could have prevented their formation by chance collision. Furthermore, because of the very nature of the reproduction of genetic material as seen today in all living organisms, a similar cyclic process could have well been produced, setting in motion the first self-duplicating system. Finally, we shall try to answer the next crucial question: since life exists on this planet, what is the chance that it exists elsewhere in the universe; and if it has indeed emerged elsewhere, what is the probability that it has led to something resembling man?

THE SEARCH FOR AN ANSWER

Of course, during many periods of history, particularly since the advent of Christianity, it has been a perilous game to attempt to consider the origin of life apart from the mysticism attached to it by most religious philosophies, to exorcise this phenomenon from any of its "vitalistic" connotations. And many a scholar found himself suspected of heresy—more than one had a good whiff of smoke—for merely suggesting that life might have appeared as a predictable outcome of certain chemical interactions, however extraordinarily complex they might have been.

Interestingly enough, until a few hundred years ago, it was not heretical to assume that life was appearing spontaneously at all times, of course with divine help. Indeed, we are told that on the fifth day of creation, the Lord said, "Let the waters bring forth abundantly the moving creatures that hath life and fowl that may fly above the earth in the open firmament of heaven" (Genesis 1:20). At dawn of the third day, He had not *created* "grass and herb yielding seed" but, again, demanded "earth to bring them forth." This was done by executive order, a directive that had never been abrogated, and hence, there was no reason to believe that the process had ever ceased.

Actually, this made a lot of sense. Everybody could see that tadpoles and fish are produced from water, worms from mud, molds from rotting fruits, and maggots from rotting meat. In the 17th century, the Flemish physiologist J. B. Van Helmont even published a recipe for the spontaneous generation of mice: "Place in an attic a few wheat stalks, a dirty shirt, and do not disturb for twenty-one days." During that time, human perspiration emanating from the shirt would provide for the necessary "breath of life," and, sure enough, mice would be produced miraculously identical in all ways to those born by a mother mouse.

The real philosophical controversy exploded when a few clever experiments challenged the very dogma of spontaneous generation. In the first of these carried out three centuries ago, the Florentine physician Francesco Redi disproved the accepted opinion that maggots appear spontaneously from rotting flesh: by placing a piece of meat under a fine screen so that no fly could lay its eggs, he demonstrated that no maggot grew, but of course the meat did rot. The conclusion was that whereas one particular form of life did not indeed appear, many others did. The next step was taken in 1765 by the Italian priest Lazzaro Spallanzani who sealed some beef broth in a flask while it was still boiling, and showed that the broth failed to rot. His detractors contended that boiling had rendered the broth unfit to sustain life. Spallanzani easily disposed of this criticism: by opening the flask, the broth rapidly became infected. But he could never answer a further criticism, i.e., that heat had spoiled the surrounding atmosphere. It took another century for the French biologist Louis Pasteur to put to rest the theory of spontaneous generation. Pasteur repeated Spallanzani's experiment, but instead of sealing the flasks, he boiled the broth in vessels with elongated necks bent in the form of an "S." Whereas air could easily diffuse in and out, spores and germs could not get through and most flasks remained sterile. On the other hand, if at any time the vessels were tilted so that some broth touched the rim where particles of dust had evidently collected, microorganisms rapidly grew. Pasteur was of such undisputed reputation that the whole question appeared to be settled once and for all: only life creates life: *omne vivum ex vivo.*

But then, if life does not emerge incessantly from inanimate matter, either spontaneously or under some supernatural influence, how did it come about? Obviously, we do not now have nor will we ever have the exact answer. But we do know today much about the conditions that must have prevailed in primeval times, and many of the reactions that must have occurred, through which a self-duplicating system could have developed.

THE PAST

The earth was born ca. 4.5 billion years ago, apparently through the condensation of cold cosmic dust; gravitational compression transformed it into a mass of molten rocks and vapors and gasses. For more than a billion years it gradually cooled down, while mountains were disintegrating under the pull of gravity and the force of rain and wind, and continents slowly dissolved into the oceans. During all that time, more and more complex molecules began to be formed. Of course, this required some internal or external source of energy such as the ultraviolet and visible rays of the sun, heat from volcanic activity, corona (electric) discharges from pointed objects, radioactive decay, or cosmic rays (Miller and Urey).

From the work of Oparin, Urey, and others, we now know that the earth's atmosphere was "reducing," that is, that it contained a lot more hydrogen than it does today and essentially no oxygen. Almost all of the oxygen was reduced in the form of water, carbon in the form of methane with very little carbon monoxide and still less carbon dioxide, and nitrogen in the form of ammonia. Actually, only the outer crust of the earth is oxidized today; all its deeper layers are still reduced. In the last 20 years, mostly following the striking experiment by Urey and Miller, many reports have indicated that under such conditions innumerable organic compounds found today in living cells can be synthesized (Calvin; Lemmon). Miller and Urey showed that when an atmosphere consisting of hydrogen, methane, ammonia, and water vapor is subjected to an electric discharge, within a week more than 20 of the most common elements of living systems are not only produced, but produced in remarkably high quantities. Among these were α-amino acids and other amines, and intermediates of carbohydrate metabolism. Since then, the abiogenic synthesis of hundreds of compounds, simple building blocks of living matter, as well as highly complex polypeptides and nucleic acids, has been demonstrated under a variety of simulated prebiotic conditions (Calvin; Lemmon). Electric discharges, ultraviolet or ionizing radiations, and heat have all been used, all forms of energy which were available as the earth was born, each providing its own driving force and contributing to the formation of one organic molecule or the other. And this process went on and on until the accumulation of millions of these transformed every puddle, lake, or ocean into an immense culture broth. Since the earth was then in its most asceptic condition and there was no free oxygen, most of these compounds remained perfectly stable. Until one day one such extraordinarily complex system underwent an amazing autocatalytic process—that of self-replication.

SOME THERMODYNAMICS AND KINETICS

Here, there are two concepts that should be emphasized. First, it is not because a compound possesses a complicated structure that it cannot be formed spontaneously—that is, that its synthesis is thermodynamically disfavored. For example, let us consider the porphyrins: these are the complex molecules which, upon binding certain metal ions, form the red pigment in hemoglobin or the green pigment in chlorophyll. Porphyrins must have played a crucial role in the evolution of chemical and biological systems because they absorb visible light readily. Before their appearance, only a fraction of the energy emitted by the sun (e.g., its far-ultraviolet rays) could excite the very simple molecules that then existed; once they were formed, visible light could be absorbed as well and its energy efficiently utilized to drive hundreds of more complex reactions. The biological synthesis of porphyrins occurs through a multistep pathway catalyzed by many enzymes. However, only the first step (the synthesis of δ-aminolevulinic acid) is energy-requiring; once it has been performed, the others follow almost automatically because the porphyrins are strongly stabilized by resonance. In other words, whenever the first intermediate is formed, others will also be produced because the subsequent reactions are "downhill," that is, they are thermodynamically preferred. So much so that a spectral study has indicated the presence of magnesium porphyrin in interstellar space. If true, it would make it one of the most complex organic compounds so far detected in outer space, along with a dozen or so much simpler molecules.

This brings us to the second point that should be stressed. Any biologist will readily admit that the most complex compounds can be produced in a living organism because of an arsenal of enzymes acting as powerful and specific catalysts. However, physical chemistry tells us that enzymes can only increase the rate of a reaction, not change its final equilibrium. In other words, enzymes will allow reactions to proceed extremely rapidly, but only on the condition that they are thermodynamically permitted; they will not allow a reaction to take place that would not occur eventually by itself. However, in primeval times, time was no object. In the life of a cell, reactions must proceed within seconds to assure for the proper response to physiological stimuli, the right balance of metabolic processes, and the intricate mechanisms by which they are controlled. But in those times one could afford to wait for a year, for a hundred or a thousand years.

Of course, with a battery of enzymes to catalyze a series of reactions and the ability to modulate their concentration and activities, one can remove an unstable intermediate from the mainstream of reactions and divert it to an alternate pathway not otherwise favored. Nonetheless all reactions that are thermodynamically allowed will eventually occur, and if time is not limiting, the need for enzymes becomes much less imperative.

This is not to say that catalysts did not exist in primordial times. Many chemical compounds can catalyze one reaction or another. As the diversity of organic molecules increased through random synthesis, the variety and effectiveness of these catalysts also increased. This paved the way for a purely "chemical evolution" long before the onset of Darwinian evolution of living species (Calvin; Lemmon). Chemical evolution selects a particular pathway among several equally probable ones because, for one reason or another, one particular product can affect the reaction through which it was produced.

For instance, let us assume that compound A could be converted to B, C or D; if D (or one of its descendants, D_1, D_2, . . . etc.) happens to favor the $A \rightarrow D$ reaction, then this pathway will be selected among all equally probable ones. If the rate were increased, we would have an autocatalytic process; alternatively, if among all the reactants randomly produced, one would be more apt to further react, for instance, by better absorbing light, the flow of reactions would run in that direction.

SELF-REPLICATION

At this point then, during ca. 1.5 billion years, thousands of small molecules and tens of millions of high polymers of varying structures were formed and preserved; in fact, nothing could have prevented their accumulation. What then is the probability that among all these molecular species, certain specific interactions began to take place, slowly allowing one such system to replicate itself? This is the crucial point, since self-duplication from foreign material represents the most fundamental attribute of a living system.

There is, of course, an extraordinary diversity in living organisms, in their shape, metabolism, and behavior, but an equally remarkable unity in their basic molecular mechanisms. All living species presently known store their genetic information in the same kind of molecules (DNA mostly and some RNA); these are reproduced in essentially the same ways and the information they carry is further translated into the functional units of the cell (the proteins) by similar mechanisms. It is no coincidence that

DNA possesses a very unusual property: this linear polymer is made up of four kinds of building blocks called nucleotides, two of which have a preferential affinity for the two others. Whenever such "complementary" nucleotides occur on separate molecules, they will tend to associate with one another (base pairing). What this means is that if one DNA chain were produced (and this has been well documented under abiotic conditions [Lemmon]), it would preferentially interact with another chain of complementary structure. Furthermore, the thermal stability of the resulting double strand is maximum when the two chains are perfectly matched, that is, when each base is precisely paired with its correct counterpart. This might have provided for one of the early selective pressures: any chain randomly produced would tend to serve as a template for the formation of a complementary strand. Any set of reactions that brought about a separation of these chains would then lead to the formation of two new strands identical to the original ones, and, eventually, to a self-replicating system.

It is most likely that many intermediary steps were required to set in motion such an autocatalytic cycle, and that more than a single kind of molecule was involved (Monod; Eigen). Because of their chemical characteristics, polynucleotides react with certain polypeptides, and perhaps very early, specific interactions between the two species were taking place. The same dual relationship exists today between DNA and proteins in the expression of genetic inheritance: whereas our genetic past is inscribed in some specific sequence of DNA, it is only expressed through the synthesis of corresponding proteins. In turn, some of these will catalyze the replication of those same nucleic acids that directed their synthesis in the first place.

Of course, self-reproduction is only one of the attributes of a living structure; by itself, it could only yield a completely primitive and surely most inefficient form of life. For such a system to survive, it must become autonomous; that is, it must be able to isolate itself from its surroundings so that fuel can be taken in and waste eliminated (Oparin). This is why life is always packaged in the form of cells, and all metabolic processes take place within these entities.

In comparison to the self-replicating systems of those times, the simplest bacterial cell seen today is a world of complexity. Nonetheless, self-replication has endowed these early structures of two most essential properties, i.e., invariance in the faithful reproduction of the stored information, with the added possibility of modifying this genetic blueprint by chance mutation. Of course, under the laws of evolution, any mutation that makes an organism better adapted to its environment will be retained, any alteration that increases its chances of survival will survive. And so, through countless reproductive cycles, with their errors in duplication and rejections of what is of no advantage, one such self-replicating system has evolved into these extraordinarily complex and sophisticated organisms that surround us today.

EVOLUTION

Whereas it is conceivable that, if life exists elsewhere, some of the basic mechanisms for duplicating genetic information are similar to ours, the probability that it could follow the same evolutionary path we followed is essentially nil. It would have had to go through the same cosmic and planetary events that we went through at essentially the same time, and respond to all successive changes and accidents and selective pressures in precisely the same fashion. This would be just as improbable as two pinballs ending up in exactly the same point in space after trickling down for millions of years through a boundless pinball machine, with the added complication that each nail would be different from every other and each hit would modify the shape of the cascading ball.

The path that eventually led to man was not necessarily easy, just as the future was never assured, once the first faltering steps in self-replication had been taken. As Jacques Monod said, "Destiny is written as it occurs, not before." For instance, soon after their creation, living organisms had to face a major crisis—the slow poisoning of their atmosphere by oxygen. We said earlier that in prebiotic times the earth's atmosphere was reducing and contained essentially no oxygen. However, photosynthesis must have evolved early, providing the main pathway by which solar energy could be utilized for the synthesis of organic matter. At first, this occurred through the reduction of CO rather than CO_2, and plants that can do this today do it very efficiently; but for every carbon atom reduced and fixed, oxygen was produced, triggering a pollution problem of immense proportion. The danger lasted until the existing organisms learned to utilize oxygen for their own benefit, to such an extent that today, most organisms are aerobic and can derive much more energy from food than the rare obligate anaerobes. Incidentally, there is no way of knowing whether the latter are remnants from the past or the descendants of modern aerobic bacteria that have lost their ability to utilize oxygen; living now in the absence of oxygen, they have not felt the selective pressure to regain their lost function.

DOES LIFE EXIST ELSEWHERE?

Now comes the last question: since life has indeed appeared on the earth, on how many planets throughout the universe can one expect to find it? For some, the emergence of life was such an extraordinarily rare event that it must have occurred only once; for others, considering all pre-existing conditions, it was essentially unavoidable (Monod; Eigen; Wald).

Just how probable this phenomenon must have been, no one rightly knows. On the basis of our knowledge of molecular biology, the properties of nucleic acids and proteins and their interactions, Manfred Eigen has attempted to describe in kinetic and thermodynamic terms the fundamental laws of self-reproduction and evolution of biological macromolecules and to define their probability.

On the Earth, it has taken approximately 1.5 billion years for life to appear, and twice that long to fashion an intelligent species such as man. Had the mean temperature of the earth been 10°C cooler, we might still be a billion years behind in evolution, since chemical reactions are slowed by a factor of 2 for every such decrease in temperature. Actually, additional factors would intervene, making it possible that life wouldn't have emerged at all: with a temperature 10° lower, we would be in an "ice age" with much of the earth's water in the form of ice. On the other hand, had the mean temperature been warmer, we could be millions of years ahead—or have entirely disappeared—depending on how long one can expect any civilization that has mastered the secret of atomic energy to survive.

Nevertheless, based on our own history, we can assume that a planet would have had to exist for something like a billion years for life to appear. This would exclude planets orbiting around the younger stars which would have not resided on the main sequence for a sufficient period of time (Shklovskii and Sagan). Furthermore, during these billion years, the luminosity of the central star would have had to remain essentially constant; this is the case with our sun which hasn't varied in luminosity by more than 20 percent since the earth came into being. This requirement for constancy in radiation emitted would seem to exclude most planetary systems around multiple stars, or around older stars rapidly evolving toward the red giant state: the huge increase in luminosity and diameter would necessarily vaporize away the atmosphere and water of all but the most distant planets and burn to a crisp all their organic matter. Planets too close to their star are too hot to sustain life, those too distant are too cold to allow for its appearance. Too small planets cannot retain a proper atmosphere and, hence, lose all their water; too large ones have too dense an atmosphere that excludes all outside radiation; their surface might never solidify, and life could be visualized as existing only in a state of suspension in certain upper layers (Shklovskii and Sagan).

George Wald pointed out that if ammonia replaced water on the earth, probably no life would have appeared: ammonia is liquid at too low temperatures (between −77° and −30°C), and like most chemical compounds its solid state is denser than its liquid phase. That is, frozen ammonia sinks. If ice sank to the bottom of the oceans, it would never have had a chance to melt in the warmth of the sun, and would have held down the temperature of the earth like blocks of ice stored in a freezer.

Well, then, taking all these factors into consideration, on how many planets can one expect to find life? From what we know today of the nature and evolution of stars, at the very least 0.1 percent of them would have a planetary system with one planet satisfying the above requirements. Since there are 150 billion stars in the Milky Way, this makes 150 million planets suitable for life in our galaxy alone. And since there are approximately 100 million galaxies in the visible universe, we can assume that there are more than 100 million billion planets on which life could exist. From what we said above, the abiogenic synthesis of chemicals including macromolecules cannot be avoided, no more than can be prevented the collision of molecules in a liquid or gas. With millions of compounds produced, self-replication would have to be an extraordinarily rare event indeed to have occurred once only, on this planet alone among all those in the universe.

In our solar system, we might discover life even if it is "nonintelligent," i.e., unable to communicate with us. On the other hand, outside of our solar system and unless our technology in space exploration is way ahead of what we can even conceive, discovery of life will have to rely solely on communication between advanced beings. But the universe is huge, and even communication by electromagnetic means could take thousands if not millions of years. On this time scale, whatever civilizations we might one day contact would probably have nothing in common with those that initiated communication in the first place, and perhaps none of their original interests . . . assuming that they still existed. Because no life is permanent.

Just as stars are born, slowly go through their life cycle, and inexorably die, life that appears on their surrounding planets must inexorably disappear. Within six to eight billion years, the sun will have exhausted the hydrogen that fuels its thermonuclear reaction (Shklovskii and Sagan). Before cooling down into a dead black dwarf of fantastic density, it will evolve into a red giant: its temperature will be hundreds of times what it is today and its diameter, after overtaking Mercury and Venus, will approach the orbit of the earth. Unless man, if man still exists, learns how to travel at will through space, or transport the earth into the orbit of another star, nothing could prevent its ultimate annihilation.

REFERENCES

Calvin, M. 1969. Chemical Evolution. Oxford, Clarendon Press.
Eigen, M. 1971. Self-organization of matter and the evolution of biological macromolecules. *Naturwissenschaften.* **58**:465.
Lemmon, R. M. 1969. Chemical evolution. *Chem. Rev.* **70**:95.
Miller, S. L., and H. C. Urey. 1959. *Science.* **130**:245.

Monod, J. 1970. Le Hazard et La Necessite. Paris, Editions du Sevil.

Oparin, A. I. 1957. The Origin of Life on the Earth. New York, Academic Press.

Shklovskii, I. S., and C. Sagan. 1966. Intelligent Life in the Universe. San Francisco, Holden-Day, Inc.

Wald, G. 1964. The origins of life. *Proc. Natl. Acad. Sci. U.S.* **52:**595.

CHAPTER 5

GENETIC ENGINEERING: PRESENT AND FUTURE*

GILBERT S. OMENN

Basic understanding of genes and processes of reproduction has advanced rapidly in recent years and generated speculation about the potential manipulation of human genes and human reproduction. Both enthusiasts who seek to eliminate certain diseases or undesirable traits and doomsday soothsayers who predict political-social control of the right to have children and of the determination of which traits are desirable are writing in lay magazines. Scientists are motivated to understand the processes involved and to develop useful therapies for human disorders. Nevertheless, social and political philosophy may become important forces in the application of such knowledge, just as Einstein's "pure" formulation of the relationship between energy and mass led eventually to its application in atomic bombs. The potential bombshells of what is sometimes called "the biological revolution" include direct alteration of human physical or mental characteristics by "treatment" with genes and fertilization of human eggs in the test tube. We will discuss several current practices and certain futuristic possibilities, in the context of present knowledge and foreseeable developments in human genetics.

GENE ACTION: DNA → RNA → PROTEIN

A brief summary of the mechanisms of gene action is essential for understanding the following sections on treatment of genetic diseases and manipulation of the genes of man. In the nucleus of every cell are 23 pairs of chromosomes, each containing thousands of genes arranged along the length of the chromosome. One chromosome of each pair is derived from the egg and the other from the sperm. The genetic material in the chromosomes is DNA, which has a special code for translation of the inherited information into the structures of the proteins of the cell. When each cell divides, starting with the fertilized egg, the DNA must be replicated so

* This work is supported by Grant GM 15253 from the U.S. Public Health Service.

that every daughter cell gets a precise copy of the DNA, or genome, of that individual. Meanwhile, an enzyme in the nucleus transcribes the coded sequence in the DNA into a messenger RNA molecule that leaves the nucleus and goes out into the cytoplasm of the cell to be translated into a protein sequence. Proteins are the effector molecules of the cell—enzymes, hormones, antibodies, structural elements like collagen, hemoglobin, membrane units. Enzymes, for example, are responsible for carrying out the steps of metabolism, converting one compound into another, using foodstuffs to generate and store energy and to maintain cell structures.

Every cell is derived from the fertilized egg and has the same complement of DNA, the same genes. However, the processes of differentiation of the various tissues of the body lead to differential expression of the genetic information. The messenger RNA molecules made in different tissues include some messages in common, for basic functions of cells like energy production and protein synthesis, but many others that are specific to each tissue. The nature of such regulation of gene expression is complex and basic to the normal development and function of every individual.

If a change occurs in a particular gene (a "mutation"), the messenger RNA will carry that altered message to the protein-synthesizing sites in the cytoplasm and direct synthesis of an altered protein. The alteration in protein structure may cause an enzyme to lose its function, so that one compound (the substrate upon which the enzyme acts) cannot be converted to the product of the reaction. The substrate accumulates and may become toxic to certain tissues, while lack of its product makes the tissues deficient in an essential substance. Such biochemical considerations underlie inherited diseases. For important practical reasons geneticists distinguish diseases that are caused by single abnormal genes from those in which many genes seem to be involved. For example, sickle-cell anemia is due to a mutation in a gene for hemoglobin of the red blood cells. The pattern of inheritance is autosomal recessive, meaning that the mutant gene must be present in double dose, being passed on to the child by each parent. Each parent, however, has one normal and one mutant gene and is unaffected. In many recessive diseases there is evidence for abnormal or deficient enzyme function, pinpointing the biochemical defect and providing clues to effective therapy. In contrast, autosomal dominant disorders are those in which a single dose of the abnormal gene, received from either parent or arising as a brand new mutation, causes disease in the person even though the other chromosome of the pair carries a normal gene. Little is known of the biochemical mechanisms of dominant genetic disorders, so that treatment of the basic defect is not feasible. It is hoped that new methods of analysis of membranes and structural proteins and regulatory processes will unravel the lesions of these important diseases. In sex-linked recessive disorders like hemophilia the responsible gene is on the X chromosome, so that males (XY) are affected and females (XX) are carriers. Considerable progress can be anticipated in the biochemical characterization and prenatal diagnosis of these diseases.

The question is often asked "What proportion of patients have genetic diseases?" Crude estimates fall in the range of 5 to 25 percent, depending upon how severe a condition must be to be called a disease and depending upon criteria for genetic determination. In addition to thousands of rare diseases due to a single abnormal gene, genetic factors are known to be important in predisposing individuals to the development of such common diseases as coronary heart disease, diabetes, high blood pressure, epilepsy, schizophrenia, and depression through interaction with other factors in the diet or the interpersonal environment. Often it would seem to be easier to correct the environmental factors in these multifactorial disorders than to seek the gene(s) that may underlie the predisposition and try to alter them or their effects. For example, control of obesity, reduction of high blood pressure, cessation of cigarette smoking, and moderation of life stresses all decrease the risk of heart attacks, even in individuals who are genetically predisposed. For the optimal management of diseases, including genetic disorders, rational manipulation of behavioral and environmental as well as of metabolic and genetic factors is necessary.

PREVENTION OF THE BIRTH OF CHILDREN WITH GENETIC DEFECTS

Mutations

The most basic approach to preventing the birth of affected children is the prevention of mutations in the genes. Mutations occur at a low but significant frequency, which is increased by such agents as medical X-ray exposures, atomic radiation background, and various chemical compounds in the air and food. Obviously, it is important to minimize exposure to mutagenic agents. However, there is a long-range possibility of enhancing the ability of cells to "correct" mutations that occur. The clue comes from patients with a rare genetic disorder, xeroderma pigmentosum. Affected individuals have an inherited defect in the enzymatic repair of minor changes in the DNA caused by ultraviolet radiation, so that ordinary exposure to the sun produces destruction of skin cells and development of malignant skin cancers. Perhaps a way will be found to enhance the corresponding enzymatic function of normal cells to correct similar mutagenic changes in the DNA that lead to disease or cancer. To prevent genetic defects in offspring, mutations must be corrected in the germ cells, not just in somatic cells.

Gross accidents in the normal process of distribution of one of each pair of chromosomes to each egg or sperm can cause one too many or one too few chromosomes or a rearranged chromosome to be transmitted in the egg or sperm. If fertilization occurs and proceeds to birth, the child is likely to be abnormal. Fortunately, the vast majority of chromosome aberrations of this kind lead to spontaneous miscarriages—nature's way of dealing with such abnormalities. Parents who have had radiation exposure and older mothers have an increased risk of bearing children with chromosomal abnormalities (with mongolism, for example).

Genetic Counseling

After the birth of a child with some specific disorder, the parents may seek genetic counseling to learn whether the disorder is, in fact, genetic and what the chance is that it will recur in subsequent children. The risks range from 5 to 25 to 50 percent for multifactorial, recessive, and dominant conditions, respectively. If the risk seems too high, many couples try to have no more children, on a voluntary basis. But what is too high for some couples is interpreted differently by others. For example, some couples note that a risk of 25 percent means that three-fourths of the children would be unaffected. They are optimists! At present, genetic counselors explain the inheritance and severity of the disease to the parents and leave the decision about child-bearing to them. Of course, should they have another affected child, medical and social responsibility for the child's care may eventually fall to society as a whole, raising the possibility that society may not continue to rely upon the judgment or whims of individual couples. Society has already made rules to prevent child-bearing by the intellectually retarded or by prisoners, at least while they are in institutions. There is even an occasional cry that such inmates be sterilized. Nature has its own way of preventing child-bearing, through infertility. Many genetic disorders are characterized by what is technically called "decreased biologic fitness," meaning decreased survival to reproductive age and/or decreased fertility. For example, all adult males with cystic fibrosis are infertile. Many intellectually retarded and some psychopathic individuals are infertile. Many severe conditions do not allow survival to adulthood.

Couples who fear the recurrence of a genetic disorder, should they have their own children, have two options: adoption and artificial insemination. By adoption, they avoid passing on the abnormal gene altogether. If they are both carriers for the same rare recessive gene, they can avoid having an affected child if they mate with someone else who is not a carrier. Sometimes, unfortunately, this realization leads to the dissolution of a marriage. Occasionally, the couple may choose to have the wife's egg fertilized by sperm from an anonymous sperm bank, by artificial insemination. If the disease is transmitted from parent to child as an autosomal dominant, artificial insemination is appropriate only if the affected parent is the father. If the mother is the affected parent, adoption is the only option. However, women with genetic diseases that reduce their life expectancy or impair health may have difficulty in convincing adoption agencies to help them. The decreased availability of babies for adoption has contributed to interest in artificial insemination, but many husbands find the subject unthinkable. Outside of the genetic context, many people interested in population control are now considering artificial insemination as an important "loophole," such that the husband can donate his own sperm to a sperm bank, undergo sterilization by vasectomy, and have the assurance that he could later "have his own children" should circumstances lead him to change his decision. There is always a risk that something might happen to sperm in the "bank" to damage their function or to lead to genetic changes in the offspring. Thus far, there are no scientific or social controls over the burgeoning business of sperm banks.

Intrauterine Diagnosis and Selective Abortion

The technique of amniocentesis, puncturing the abdominal and uterine walls with a needle to withdraw a little amniotic fluid containing fetal cells during pregnancy, has allowed a dramatic advance in genetic counseling. Now it is possible to establish definitively whether the developing fetus is affected or is not affected with certain specific genetic and chromosomal defects. Couples who previously felt the statistical recurrence risk was too high to have children can cautiously proceed with a pregnancy and have the pregnancy monitored to determine the status of the fetus. The time at which amniocentesis is first carried out (14th week of pregnancy) is a compromise. The more advanced the pregnancy, the greater likelihood of obtaining an adequate sample of fluid for study. On the other hand, amniocentesis must be carried out early enough so that complicated laboratory studies can be completed and abortion be done safely (and legally), if termination of the pregnancy is necessary. Several hundred amniocenteses have been performed without serious immediate complications, such as bleeding, infection, uterine rupture, induced miscarriage, congenital malformations, or puncture wounds. However, the effects, if any, of disturbing the amniotic fluid are unknown. For this reason, amniocentesis is not recommended in pregnancies with less than 1 percent recurrence risk for a given disease. Depending how abhorrent the disorder is, the parents may agree to forego amniocentesis and take their chances or they may elect to terminate the pregnancy when the risk is below 1 percent.

Indications for Intrauterine Diagnosis

There are three types of disorders suitable for intrauterine diagnosis: (1) chromosomal disorders; (2) autosomal or X-linked recessive diseases due to deficiency of a specific enzyme that is normally present in cultured amniotic cells; and (3) X-linked recessive conditions for which no biochemical lesion can be detected in amniotic fluid cells, but for which determination of fetal sex will distinguish between girls, who will be unaffected, and boys who have a high risk of being affected. These disorders are discussed further below.

Chromosomal Disorders. The most common indication for intrauterine diagnosis is Down's syndrome or mongolism, characterized by mental retardation, particular physical features, and the presence of an extra chromosome (trisomy 21). The incidence is 1 per 660 births in the general population, a frequency that surprises most people. The incidence rises with age of the mother, from less than 1 in 2000 births at age 20, to 1 in 500 births at age 35, to 1 in 40 births at age 45. If a couple has already had a child with Down's syndrome, the risk of having a second affected child will be 1 to 2 percent and possibly much higher, depending on the precise chromosomal abnormality. Half of the cases of Down's syndrome could be prevented if women over age 35 simply did not have children. Will we come to a time when society will require amniocentesis for all pregnant women over 35, as well as for those with a previously affected child, and require abortion of fetuses with trisomy 21 or other severe chromosomal defects? What if the parents refuse?

Enzyme Deficiencies. Among the dozen biochemical defects that have been diagnosed thus far in utero, the most suitable for genetic counseling is Tay-Sachs disease, a neurological disorder that causes blindness, progressive motor and mental disability, and death, by age 2 years. The gene for this disease is more common among Ashkenazic Jews than among others, for unknown reasons. The chance that both parents will be carriers and have affected children is 100 times higher in this high-risk population. If a couple has already had an affected child, subsequent pregnancies can be monitored effectively. In addition, carriers can be distinguished from normal individuals by a serum enzyme test. Therefore, large-scale screening programs have been initiated in the Baltimore-Washington area to identify couples who are both carriers, so that they can avoid having an affected child. It is hoped that this screening will be extended to teenagers, so that they may use the information in deciding upon their mates.

Another autosomal recessive condition with a high-risk population is sickle-cell anemia among blacks. The sickle hemoglobin in the red blood cells leads to damage of many organs as the result of severe anemia and blockage of small blood vessels. Intrauterine diagnosis is not yet feasible, since red blood cells must be obtained to examine the hemoglobin, but techniques to do so are expected to be developed soon. At present, counseling is limited to testing blacks to identify carriers (6 to 10 percent of the population) and explaining to couples who are both carriers that they have a 25 percent risk of bearing affected children. It is hoped that normal carriers of the genes for Tay-Sachs disease or sickle-cell anemia will voluntarily utilize the genetic information in choosing a mate or in family planning.

X-Chromosome Diseases.   Hemophilia is an example of an
X-linked disorder, affecting boys but not girls, for which biochemical diagnosis is not yet possible in utero. By examining the chromosomes of the
fetal cells cultured from the amniotic fluid, however, it is easy to determine
whether the fetus is male or female. If the couple, for example, want two
healthy children, they can be assured of having two normal girls, though
they must have an abortion for any male fetus. Their daughters do have
a 50 percent chance of being carriers for hemophilia, as did their mother.

The long-term effects of selective abortion on gene frequency and on
frequency of genetic diseases have been calculated for programs in which
only affected fetuses or affected plus carrier fetuses would be aborted.
Maximal case reduction requires detection of high-risk mothers before
pregnancy and heterozygous carriers before marriage. However, even very
aggressive programs of intrauterine diagnosis and abortion will have only
minor effects on the frequencies of abnormal genes (Motulsky, Fraser, and
Felsenstein, 1971).

Determination of the Sex of the Baby

Probably throughout the history of man parents have had preferences
about the sex of their child. There are no known methods to influence
the sex at the time of conception; even with artificial insemination, there
are no methods to separate sperm carrying an X chromosome from sperm
carrying a Y chromosome. Now, however, establishing the sex of the fetus
is quite feasible, by checking the chromosomes of amniotic cells. It should
be emphasized that reliable sex determination requires the cultivation of
amniotic fluid cells, to be certain that fetal cells and not maternal cells
are studied, and full karyotype, not just staining for a condensed X or
a fluorescent Y chromosome as indications of the sex. Given the potential
hazards of amniocentesis, the long delay into mid-pregnancy before the
test can be done, the possibility that the mother will "feel life" before the
results are available, and the definite hazards to the mother of second-tri-
mester abortions, most couples wisely proceed without any test. But some
couples who have several children of one sex and are determined to have
one of their choice have demanded the test. They pose a difficult dilemma
for the physician: he finds no medical indication for a procedure with
possible risks to normal fetuses, yet he may be moved by the psychological
ferment the couple has developed; he knows that some states now allow
abortion "on demand," yet he does not want his facilities or his institution
to be abused for what he and segments of the public may consider a frivolous indication for abortion. After all, genetic counselors consider the approach of intrauterine diagnosis and selective abortion of affected fetuses,
in pregnancies with high risk for a genetic disorder, to be *life saving* for
the *normal* fetus, since most couples seek abortion if there is no test to
distinguish the affected from the unaffected fetus.

Artificial Fertilization

A futuristic approach to control of the genome of the offspring is artificial fertilization. The research of R. G. Edwards in Cambridge on in vitro maturation of oocytes, fertilization of the eggs with sperm, growth of the embryo in "test tubes," and implantation of the blastocyst into the mother's uterus has generated as violent a controversy in England as have Jensen's studies on the genetic factors in IQ in this country. Investigations of artificial fertilization have tremendous potential for unraveling some of the physiological mysteries of the conception of human life. And some patients with suitable causes of infertility desperately desire their own children. But critics fear that "monsters" may result from the unnatural conditions, or that the whole process of conception and child-bearing might be dehumanized. The method can be summarized as follows: The woman receives hormones to stimulate the ovary to ovulate. An instrument is introduced through the abdominal wall, through which oocytes can be "collected" from the visualized ovarian surface. Washed ejaculated sperm are capable of penetrating the membranes of the egg and achieving fertilization in quite simple culture media in the laboratory. Then different culture conditions support successive divisions of the egg and development of the blastocyst, with 100 or more cells. Now, the work has approached the most controversial stage: the implantation of such a laboratory-reared blastocyst into the hormone-stimulated uterus of the (donor) woman. In fact, one can imagine implanting blastocysts derived from eggs from one woman, fertilized with sperm from one or various men, into many hormonally prepared women. The notion of growing the embryo to "full-term" in an artificial womb is a more remote possibility. The risk that something will go wrong in this exceedingly complex and delicate process seems very high. The fact that many natural pregnancies lead to miscarriages or stillborns or defective children certainly does not provide much reassurance.

Cloning

Another popular fantasy, based upon experiments in tadpoles, is nuclear cloning. Nuclei from some accessible tissue, like skin or intestine, may be surgically placed into an unfertilized egg, whose nucleus has been removed. Viable tadpoles have developed. In such a way whole organisms might be developed with precisely the features of the adult from which the nuclei were obtained. The differences between frogs and humans lead to great technical, as well as moral, difficulties. Furthermore, when we realize that even identical twins have personality differences and different diseases, it seems preposterous to expect that nuclei taken from some "much admired" individual could reliably give rise to a multitude of people in his (or her) image!

THERAPY OF GENETIC DISEASES WITHOUT CHANGING THE ABNORMAL GENE

An impressive number of genetic conditions can be treated by correcting biochemical abnormalities in the tissues or blood, even though we have no way to alter the abnormal gene itself. Table I presents some examples of these treatment approaches.

Table I. Therapy of Genetic Diseases by Conventional Means

Treatment Approach	Examples
1. Add missing substance (product)	Thyroid hormone, cortisol, insulin, anti-hemophilic globulin, gamma globulin, blood cells, vitamin B_{12}
2. Prevent accumulation of toxic precursor (substrate)	Phenylalanine in PKU; galactose-1-phosphate in galactosemia
3. Replace the defective enzyme	Plasma pseudocholinesterase deficiency; Fabry's; metachromatic leukodystrophy
4. Use drug therapy (inhibit enzymes)	Allopurinol to prevent gout
5. Induce enzyme by drug	Phenobarbital for jaundice in newborn
6. Remove toxic substance	Metal-removing drugs for copper (Wilson's disease) or iron (hemochromatosis)
7. Surgically remove organ	Colon in congenital polyposis; spleen in spherocytosis; lens with cataracts
8. Transplant	Kidney (polycystic kidneys, cystinosis); bone marrow (thalassemia); cornea.
9. Use artificial aids	Eyeglasses; hearing aids; kidney machine
10. Block physiological (immune) response	Rhogam treatment of Rh-negative mothers who deliver Rh-positive babies

Disorders due to a defective enzyme may be treated effectively in several different ways. First, the deficient product may be administered. When there is a block in the synthesis of thyroid hormone or adrenal hormone, the patient is given pills containing those hormones. Other products replaced are clotting factors in bleeding disorders, insulin in diabetes, gamma globulin in antibody-deficiency syndromes, and red blood cells in certain types of anemia. Second, the accumulation of unconverted substrate may be prevented by reducing the amount of substrate that gets into the body. For example, the mental retardation that results from accumulation of phenylalanine in phenylketonuria, or from galactose-1-phosphate in galactosemia, can be prevented by reducing the amount of phenylalanine in the infant's diet or eliminating milk (containing galactose). A more basic approach is the replacement of the defective enzyme itself. Infusion of enzyme has given transient effects in several cases, but the enzyme is rapidly degraded in the blood and antibodies may be made. Techniques that protect the enzyme in some type of capsule may make this approach more successful.

Certain drugs may be used to affect enzymes that are directly or indirectly involved in particular genetic disorders. Drugs that are enzyme inhibitors can prevent over-production of uric acid, which causes gout. Other drugs, like phenobarbital, increase enzyme activity in combating jaundice in newborns. Still other drugs combine with potentially toxic substances, as in the removal of excess copper or iron in certain diseases of mineral metabolism.

In a number of conditions, effective therapy is available even without knowledge of biochemical abnormalities. The organ most affected by a life-threatening genetic disease may be removed surgically or be replaced by transplantation from a suitable donor. Of course, artificial aids may be utilized, including eyeglasses, hearing aids, or kidney machines. Finally, a physiological response may be blocked, as in the treatment of Rh-negative mothers with Rhogam, to block her from making antibodies against the Rh factor of the red blood cells of her Rh-positive child after delivery. In all of these examples, "conventional" medical therapies are utilized. Nevertheless, drastic alteration of the diet of an apparently normal newborn child with a single abnormal blood test (high phenylalanine) and treatment with an artificial kidney or by transplantation were not conventional methods a few years ago.

Almost all the treatable diseases listed in Table I are determined by a single gene. Only diabetes mellitus is an example of a polygenic genetic disease, and insulin therapy fails to counteract the long-term complications of diabetes, suggesting that the basic defect is not being corrected. When we turn to behavioral disorders, we have even less knowledge of the ways in which genetic factors operate. Genetic factors are known to be important in intellectual function, personality, epilepsy, schizophrenia, and manic-depressive psychosis. Genetic factors may operate in different ways in different patients, of course, as we have learned from the myriad of specific causes of mental retardation, each requiring specific therapeutic approaches. Behavior-modifying treatments are widely applied, on an empirical basis, including drugs to induce or prevent sleep, combat anxiety, and alleviate depression, mania, or schizophrenia, surgery to improve Parkinson's disease or to prevent violent behavior, and psychoanalysis. Conventional therapies distress some people because individuals who are "less fit" survive to pass on their deleterious genes to future generations. However, fitness must be redefined as environment and culture change, so that a disease that can be successfully prevented by taking medicines, or by special diets in infancy, or by some intrauterine technique will not reduce the person's fitness, so long as the culture is maintained.

When we discuss treatment with selected or genetically modified germ cells, however, we are embarking upon quite a different journey into the unknown. The desirable and adverse effects of such approaches will be felt by the patient and be passed on to his descendants to affect indirectly all with whom they come into contact. Because man has the capacity to contemplate the consequences of his actions, research into the complexities of genetic and especially behavioral manipulation properly generates great curiosity and great fear. It is hoped that informed attitudes of people and their leaders will influence the application of technological advances.

GENE REPLACEMENT WITH NORMAL DNA: TRUE "GENETIC ENGINEERING"

Permanent genetic modification of human cells with DNA requires four successive steps: (1) preparation of the DNA containing the desired gene(s); (2) efficient and selective insertion of the DNA into the cells of the recipient; (3) stabilization of the exogenous DNA by insertion into a chromosome in the recipient cell; and (4) expression of the new gene in the cell, with synthesis of the needed protein product in normal amounts. This process is presented schematically in Fig. 1 and will be discussed sequentially.

Preparation of the DNA for Gene Replacement

Genetically normal cells grown in tissue culture can provide bulk cellular DNA. However, the gene needed to correct a particular defect constitutes only a tiny fraction of all the DNA in the cell, on the order of one part per 10 million. Even in culture medium the uptake of large amounts of DNA is unpredictable, and most of the DNA is degraded by enzymes in the cell. Thus, methods of restricting the DNA to copies of the desired gene and then assuring its uptake into cells are crucial to successful gene replacement. With bacteria and bacterial viruses, great progress has been made in the isolation of specific genes and in chemical synthesis of one particular gene. These techniques may not be applicable to human cells. However, the enzymatic synthesis of certain genes in vitro from the particular messenger RNA isolated from normal cells is feasible. For example, young red blood cells, called reticulocytes, very actively produce hemoglobin and relatively large amounts of the messenger RNA for the chains of hemoglobin. This approach uses a remarkable enzyme found first in tumor viruses which have no DNA, but instead have an enzyme that converts the information in their RNA into DNA in a host cell. This RNA-dependent DNA polymerase produces a significant amount of DNA specific for the messenger RNA template, overcoming the problem of the low specificity of isolated DNA. Of course, hemoglobin is a special case,

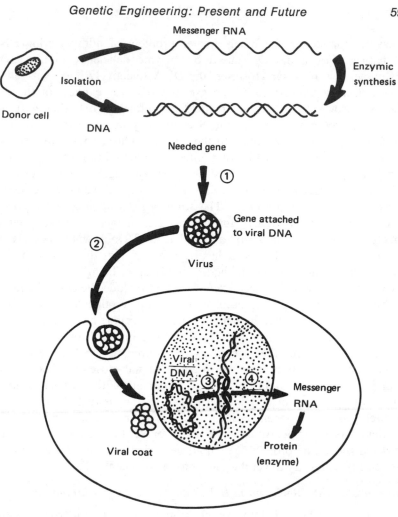

Fig. 1. Scheme depicts genetic modification of a human somatic cell or germ cell. The stepwise process includes (1) isolation or synthesis of DNA carrying specific genes and attachment of this DNA to the DNA of a virus; (2) infection of the cell in vitro or in the patient by the virus; (3) stable insertion of the specific DNA (and viral DNA) into a chromosome in the nucleus of the cell; and (4) expression of the gene by synthesis of the missing protein, such as a specific enzyme.

in which reticulocytes make large amounts of a particular protein. The isolation of specific messenger RNA for various enzymes involved in genetic disorders may be much more difficult.

Insertion of the DNA into Recipient Cells

The difficulty of getting DNA into cells bathed in a solution containing DNA in culture medium and of stabilizing the DNA against cellular enzymes foreshadows a much greater problem of administering DNA to a patient. For a disease caused by enzyme deficiency in the liver, for example, it is necessary to insert the DNA selectively into liver cells. The main strategy appears to be the use of viruses as carriers of the desired DNA. Viruses have certain practical advantages. First, they carry DNA within a protective protein coat. Second, they are able to get inside cells and deliver their DNA intact to the nucleus. Third, some viruses have remarkable specificity, so that they infect primarily brain cells or liver cells or kidney cells. Fourth, at least some viruses can definitely direct their DNA to be inserted into the DNA of the host cell, some place along one or more of the chromosomes. The strategy rests upon the ability to make the appropriate virus carry the desired human gene. Viruses that infect bacteria sometimes "pick up" a little bacterial DNA when they are reproduced in the bacterial cells. It has been hoped that the same can be done with human cells, but the method depends upon being able to select those very, very rare viral-host cell exchanges that include the desired gene. Even a bacterial gene might be used, if its enzyme product performs the same function as the defective human enzyme. One report has already been published in which a bacterial gene for galactose metabolism was "picked up" by a bacterial virus that served as the source of DNA for treatment of cells in tissue culture from a patient with galactosemia. The DNA was not in a form that could be given to a patient. With a chemical approach infectious particles of certain viruses can be reconstructed from DNA and protein coat components. Such "pseudovirions" might contain specific human DNA segments, either isolated or synthesized to be rich in the desired gene. The protein coat could be varied to provide the cell or tissue specificity necessary to get the gene into the deficient cells.

Integration of the Replacement DNA into the Host Cell Chromosome

Once the DNA is into the cell, it must be protected from degradation by host cell enzymes and it must be incorporated into a stable nuclear chromosomal site so that it may function. Cells in culture treated with naked DNA have occasionally exhibited a change in properties, suggesting that the DNA was taken up and was functional. However, such experiments have been extremely difficult to reproduce, presumably because of the low specificity of the DNA that has been available and because of the very low efficiency of integration of such DNA pieces. If the DNA is not integrated and replicated as part of the chromosome when the cells divide, the exogenous DNA will become "diluted," or lost, with each division into two daughter cells. Simply putting human DNA segments into a viral coat would not circumvent the problems that arise within the cell. But connecting the human gene to the DNA of a virus that is able to integrate its normal DNA into the chromosomes of the host cell offers much promise. It must be remembered, however, that this integrating function may be special to oncogenic viruses—those that may cause cancerous changes in cells. No one would wish to cause a malignancy in the process of experimenting with an attempt to replace a gene, so methods must be devised to maintain the integrating function while eliminating the oncogenic effects. Integration into any chromosome might be sufficient to protect the DNA from degradation, but it may be necessary for the DNA to be inserted in just the precise place where that gene normally occurs in human cells in order for the exogenous gene to function properly.

Expression of the New Gene in the Cell

As we noted in the beginning of this chapter, the action of a gene is mediated by several successive steps, regulated to fit the metabolic needs of the cell. The DNA genetic code is transcribed in the nucleus into a messenger RNA, which then is translated on the polyribosomes in the cytoplasm into polypeptide chains that make up the enzymes, structural proteins, antibodies, hormones, and complex membrane macromolecules of the cell. Somehow the structural gene that codes for the protein product is regulated in the amount of messenger RNA produced and the amount of protein synthesized, according to the varying needs of the cell. Just how such regulation is carried out is not known for mammalian cells. Enormous difficulties may be anticipated at this stage, even if specific genes can be synthesized, coupled to viruses with nononcogenic integrating functions, and inserted into the host genome.

Potential Applications

Specific gene-mediated therapy depends upon knowing the gene responsible for the clinical condition, not just knowing that it is an inherited disorder. In addition, it is essential that the defect cause production of an abnormal protein, which can be replaced by the action of a normally functioning gene that is inserted. If the defect were in the regulation of synthesis of a structurally normal protein, the insertion of a gene coding for that protein structure might have no benefit. The list of conditions for which specific enzyme deficiency is known will continue to grow, so that the potential applications will be more numerous. Most discouraging, however, is the fact that our knowledge is greatest for the rarer disorders and most limited for the common diseases in which genetic factors are certainly involved but act through unspecified polygenic mechanisms. As discussed earlier, coronary heart disease, high blood pressure, schizophrenia, depression, and diabetes all have significant genetic determinants, but the mechanisms are unknown. Thus, there are no clues as to which genes would need to be replaced. For the foreseeable future, genetic control of these common diseases will rest on control of child-bearing, rather than molecular intervention.

Pitfalls

Even if technological advances were to allow the orderly construction of pseudoviral particles containing both a coat that will attach selectively to the cells that need gene replacement and the desired gene for an increasing list of specific genetic disorders, certain scientific and social concerns remain to be considered. The safety of the treated individual must be guaranteed against an oncogenic carrier virus or contamination by other, unwanted viruses. In fact, such contamination occurred a few years ago in the preparation of one batch of Salk polio virus on monkey kidney cells in culture, although, fortunately, no untoward consequences have been recognized. The inserted DNA must function under normal control within the cell; otherwise, all sorts of metabolic imbalance might result, possibly damaging the tissue and patient even more than the original disease. Any such experiment must be limited to patients who will be seriously affected if untreated and for whom no simpler and safer treatment is available. The natural history of the disease must be well established, so that the effect of the gene therapy can be evaluated as unequivocally as possible. It must be remembered that different genetic mechanisms may lead to similar clinical abnormalities in different patients, so that the precise nature of the genetic and enzymatic defect must be established before attempting therapy. Presumably, this requirement would hold for any medical treatment, but the restrictions on success of gene therapy are more stringent than the manipulation of the clinical state with diet or drugs or other measures (see above). The inserted gene may function less well than the normal gene in normal chromosomal position. The treated patient may be incompletely well or may be unable to function effectively in society. It will be desirable to start treatment before the disorder results in irreversible damage to tissues. Thus, diagnosis must be made early, hopefully early in pregnancy. Informed consent from the treated individual is impossible, and even consent obtained from the parents may have certain legal complications.

There are possible long-term effects to be evaluated also. Changes in the genes and in chromosome structure may result in altered germ cell function that does not become manifest until children of the affected child are examined. Deliberate genetic modification of germ cells introduces many more complicated scientific and ethical concerns than does the genetic treatment of an affected individual.

Finally, there is the matter of societal priorities. Lederberg has drawn an analogy to the technological potential to build a land bridge from San Francisco to Honolulu; presumably other challenges would compete successfully for the energies and resources, even if "merely technical obstacles" were overcome! Research into the functioning of genes and the control of gene action when genes are inserted into chromosomes will provide important knowledge about the functioning of human cells. But will society invest in applications of such research for a relatively few individuals with specific single-gene inherited disorders? Or will priorities demand that applications, although less esoteric, be directed toward control of risk factors for common disorders, leaving prevention or treatment of the rarer conditions to the conventional methods discussed in the earlier sections? If population pressures lead to limitation of family size, will parents want guarantees against malformed or retarded children? The human brain has evolved the capacity to consider such weighty questions. Let us hope that ethical and moral values will be served as technological skills grow.

REFERENCES

Edwards, R. G. 1971. Problems of artificial fertilization. *Nature.* **233:**23–25 (1971).

Fleming, D. 1969. On living in a biological revolution. *The Atlantic Monthly* **223**(2):64–69.

Friedmann, T., and R. Roblin. 1972. Gene therapy for human genetic disease? *Science.* **175:**949–955.

Kass, L. R. 1971. Babies by means of in vitro fertilization: unethical experiments on the unborn? *New Engl. J. Med.* **285:**1174–1179.

Lederberg, J. 1971. Genetic engineering, or the amelioration of genetic defect. *The Pharos* **34:**9–12.

Milunsky, A., J. W. Littlefield, J. N. Kanfer, E. H. Kolodny, V. E. Shih, and L. Atkins. 1970. Prenatal genetic diagnosis. *New Engl. J. Med.* **283:**1370–1381, 1441–1447, 1498–1504.

Motulsky, A. G., G. R. Fraser, and J. Felsenstein. 1971. Public health and long-term genetic implications of intrauterine diagnosis and selective abortion. *In* Symposium on Intrauterine Diagnosis. D. Bergsma and A. G. Motulsky, eds. *Birth Defects Original Article Series* **7:**22–32.

Omenn, G. S., and A. G. Motulsky. 1972. Intra-uterine diagnosis and genetic counseling: implications for psychiatry in the future. *In* American Handbook of Psychiatry, vol. 6, 3rd ed. D. A. Hamburg and H. K. H. Brodie, eds. New York, Basic Books.

Time Magazine Cover Story: The Promise and Peril of the New Genetics. April 19, 1971.

Torrey, E. F. 1968. Ethical Issues in Medicine. Boston, Little Brown and Co.

Watson, J. D. 1970. Molecular Biology of the Gene. 2nd ed. New York, W. A. Benjamin.

CHAPTER 6

THE CLIMAX OF WORLD POPULATION GROWTH*

KINGSLEY DAVIS

In subsequent history the twentieth century may be called either the century of world wars or the century of the population plague. In 1900 the world's people numbered approximately 1.65 billion. Now, 70 years later, the number is almost twice as large and, by the end of the century, it may be almost four times as large. Correspondingly, the first two world

Table I. Major Periods of Human
Population Growth

	Estimated Population	Average Increase Per Century
	000's	%
400,000 B.C.	50	
8,000 B.C.	5,000	0.1
A.D. 1	300,000	5.3
A.D. 1750	791,000	5.7
A.D. 1970	3,632,000	99.9

The first figure is speculative; the next three are from John D. Durand, "The Modern Expansion of World Population," *Proceedings of the American Philosophical Society*, Vol. 111 (June 1967), p. 137. The last estimate is from the United Nations, *Demographic Yearbook, 1970*, p. 105. The rate is the exponential ratio of increase.

wars involved more casualties than any wars before, and the third one—due any moment now—will doubtless top both of these.

To understand man's demographic plight in the present century, one must realize that a climax of population growth has been reached. This can be seen, first of all, in the rate of increase. People often think of the main rise in the rate as having occurred recently, but as Table I indicates,

* This is a modified and expanded version of a paper first published in *California Medicine,* Vol. 113 (Nov. 1970), pp. 33–39.

the rate of growth after the Neolithic Revolution (the introduction of agriculture and animal husbandry around 8000 B.C.) may have been some 50 times greater than it was, on the average, during the long period before that. Once the agricultural revolution occurred, the rate seems to have gained little until the Industrial Revolution began, after which there was appoximately an 18-fold increase in the average rate. Within the period since the Industrial Revolution there has been, as Table II illustrates, a further rise in the rate—the main jump occurring after World War II; but this rise was smaller than the previous two major shifts.

Table II. Growth of World Population, 1750–1970, With and Without China

	World as a Whole		World Without China	
	Population	Increase Per Decade in Prior Period	Population	Increase Per Decade in Prior Period
	millions	%	*millions*	%
1750	791		591	
1800	978	4.3	655	2.1
1850	1,262	5.2	832	4.9
1900	1,650	5.5	1,214	7.8
1950	2,486	8.5	1,953	10.0
1970	3,632	20.9	2,872	21.3

Estimates from 1750 to 1900 are from Durand, *op. cit.*, p. 137. The 1950 and 1970 estimates are from United Nations, *Demographic Yearbook, 1970*, pp. 105, 128.

The climactic character of the world's population is clearer when absolute gains rather than rates are analyzed. Between 1900 and 1920 the world added about 210 million people, but between 1950 and 1970 it added 1,146 million. The difference in rate was 3.6 to 1, but the difference in actual increase was 5.5 to 1. If in 1950–70 the starting population had been the same as in 1900, the gain would have been 761 million instead of 1,146 million. Nearly half of the difference in population growth, as between the two periods, was due to the change of base rather than the change of rate. The more widely separated the periods, the greater is the role of the absolute base. For instance, the gain in population in *20* years from 1950 to 1970 exceeds the gain made in *70* years between 1750 and 1920, and it exceeds the gain made in some *400,000* years prior to 1820. Given the existing population, a mere continuation of the recent rate of increase would give the world approximately 165 billion people (some 45 times the present population) in only 200 years.

The conclusion seems inescapable that the earth's human multiplication has reached a climactic point and that a change of trend, probably in this century, is inevitable. The question at issue, then, is when and how this change will occur. Will it occur soon? Will it occur as a result of solicitude for collective welfare or as an unplanned and undesired consequence of the pursuit of individual goals? One should avoid the assumption that population trends, like earthquakes or sunspots, are automatic and uncontrollable. The growth of the human population is due to human actions and decisions. If it remains unregulated, this is not due to "natural" forces but to man's unwillingness to control himself.

The cause of the expansion of human numbers is the unusual capacity of the species to limit its mortality. As is well known, human beings are slow-breeding animals, but because of various cultural restrictions, they do not fulfill even their limited reproductive potential. The peculiar feature of the species, then, is its ability to keep the death rate below a singularly low birth rate. This is seen clearly in the modern period, because the rise in the rate of population increase since 1750 has come overwhelmingly from a drop in death rates rather than from a rise in birth rates. The United Nations estimates the world's birth rate in 1965–70 to be 34 per 1,000 and the death rate 14 per 1,000.[1] In 1800, if we had even an estimate, the world's birth rate probably would not have been much higher, if any, than it is in underdeveloped countries today—namely, 46 in Africa, 39 in Latin America, and 38 in Asia. The death rate, however, would have been almost equal to the birth rate, or some three times what it is now.

Man's low mortality is not a product of genetic adaptation to the natural environment, as has occurred in some other slow-breeding species. Rather, it is a result of technological alteration of the environment itself. Viewed in this light, the human species is climbing farther and faster onto an evolutionary limb. Increasingly, human survival is achieved by means that release us from rather than intensify genetic selection. The only environment to which "adaptation" is being made is the artificial one created by an ever more complex technology. The genius of this technology is that it makes biological adaptation unnecessary, because every demand made of the organism by the artificial environment is met, not by a genetic change suitable to satisfy that demand, but by a new alteration of the artificial environment. For example, one might think that the achievement of advanced civilization in providing nourishment and thus increasing diabetes would be met by evolutionary adaptation of the human organism to tolerate mass ingestion of sugars. On the contrary, diabetes is treated in such a way as to keep diabetics alive and reproducing, thus lowering rather than raising the pancreatic capacity of the population. At the very least one might think that life in a sociocultural environment would place a premium on the ability to learn, thus evolving a more intelligent animal over time; but technology rises to this demand in another way, by using the produc-

[1] United Nations, *Demographic Yearbook, 1970,* p. 105.

tion of the intelligent to support the unintelligent. As long as one in a million individuals has creative capacity, the process of improving the technological environment, thus releasing the evolutionary pressure on the organism, can continue.

Clearly, as the long period of man's slow population growth indicates (as shown in Table 1), the role of culture and technology in relieving selective pressure on human evolution is recent. Before the Neolithic Revolution, and to some extent even after that, it could be said that man's culture had virtually as much effect in producing a high mortality as it had in producing a low one. The reason for this was doubtless the fact that the supernatural beliefs, magical practices, and group conflicts engendered by cultural transmission tended to increase deaths, especially in childhood, thus canceling the beneficial effects of productive technology. Even so, of course, the selection tended to be not only in terms of the natural environment but also in terms of the crazy elements in human culture. Those human organisms tended to survive most abundantly who could best withstand the deprivations, hardships, infections, and lethal judgments imposed by the traditional prescriptions for child rearing and social interaction. Fortunately, the cultural elements had to have live carriers if they (the cultural elements) were themselves to survive. There were therefore limits to the cultural determination of genetic selection through mortality, but, as the record demonstrates, these limits throughout most of human history were quite wide.

If, then, the release of selective pressure by sociocultural means is mainly recent, we have to ask what has happened to give this result. An answer requires that two relevant aspects of the technological system be distinguished. Throughout most of human history, it was the expanding ability to augment the physical means of subsistence—food, shelter, clothing, warmth—that kept mortality down. Although therapeutic and preventive medicine was always attempted, it accomplished little. Since most of it was magical, it probably increased rather than reduced the death rate. Very late in human history, however, with the scientific and industrial revolution, medicine was *added* to economic development as a basis for lowering mortality, and in recent years it has become to some extent a *substitute* for economic development.

Neither of these mechanisms (productive technology and scientific medicine) by which the death rate was lowered would have been effective unless it moved faster than genetic evolution; otherwise, the organism would have adapted to the release of selective pressure as fast as the pressure was released, and the net long-run gain would have been nil. Beginning with the Neolithic Revolution, economic development moved much faster than genetic change could move. Still, for infectious diseases, it was an indirect and clumsy means of control. It acted by nourishing and protecting the organism, thus improving the body's capacity to fight off disease agents, but it multiplied human contacts and hence exposure to infection, and it could not cope with genetic and congenital defects, endocrine disturbances, and other noninfectious diseases. Accordingly, when scientific medicine and public health began to be effective in the latter half of the nineteenth century, the stage was set for the most dramatic reduction in mortality that ever occurred—a reduction that came both from continued economic development and from the added factor of public health and therapeutic medicine. This impetus gave the world its modern acceleration of population growth. The race between technological adaptation and genetic degeneration was a runaway one in favor of technology.

As long as economic development rather than public health effort was the main avenue to low mortality, the nations that had the most rapid population growth were those that were economically the most successful. For this reason, after 1750, the fastest growth occurred in the nations experiencing the Industrial Revolution. Despite the reduction of birth rates that eventually got under way in these countries, they maintained a greater human increase until World War I. After that, as Table III shows, the industrial nations lost out to the less developed countries. The main reason for the shift was that the techniques of public health and scientific medicine, which were invented and diffused slowly in the industrial countries during the nineteenth and early twentieth centuries, could later (after World War I) be transmitted overnight to less developed peoples, regardless of whether these peoples were developing economically. To an increasing degree, especially after World War II, public health became both more effective and more worldwide.

In the recent period most underdeveloped countries have exhibited both an economic and a medical gain. It is usually considered that these two trends reinforce each other, but this idea arises from thinking of the effect of lower morbidity and longer life on the product per worker, *other things being equal*. Such thinking ignores the fact that when mortality is reduced faster than fertility, the rate of population growth is increased, and that, as a consequence, the ratio of resources to population (bearing in mind quality as well as quantity of resources) may be seriously lowered. When the population growth effect is included, one can see that the rapid medical gains have begun to exert a net negative effect on economic progress. Not only has economic improvement been less rapid than it would have been had rapid betterment of mortality (with its consequent population growth) not occurred, but in a few less-developed countries a rapid expansion of life expectancy has occurred simultaneously with worsening economic conditions. In Mauritius, for example, between 1952 and 1962, life expectancy at birth rose from 51.1 years to 60.3—a remarkable improvement in 10 years; but income per capita fell approximately 15 percent. Other countries have shown a similar experience, but it is hard to document the facts because of the scarcity of life tables for underdeveloped countries. If we fall back on the crude death rate as an indicator of mortality change, here are a few cases of recent mortality improvement with declining per capita income:

| | | Percent Change in | | |
Country	Period	Death Rate	Income*	Population
Ceylon	1963–69	− 9.2	−10.4	+14.9
El Salvador	1958–69	−26.7	− 7.4	+46.1
Guyana	1958–68	−16.7	− 1.9	+35.8
India	1963–68	**	−17.7	+59.3
Mauritius	1958–67	−28.0	− 9.6	+25.4
Morocco	1958–69	**	− 7.6	+36.9

* Gross domestic product in constant U.S. dollars.
** Not available.

Such cases are simply extreme examples of an imbalance now found in most of the less-developed world. Up-to-date health technology has been deployed widely and effectively, but the productive technology, plagued by an increasing number of workers and an even greater increase in dependents in ratio to resources, has not been able to compensate fully for the deleterious effects of medical improvement. In most countries per capita product has simply grown more slowly than national product, but in some per capita product has declined.

The deployment of medical technology in less-developed regions has been accomplished with minimum interference with traditional social structure, out of deference to the "value systems" of the people. This hands-off attitude has meant that the institutional supports for high fertility have remained relatively untouched. Birth rates have thus continued at a high level or have even risen slightly (depending on where the country was in the process of development). The resulting population growth, wholly unprecedented in relative rate of gain and in absolute size, has depressed the capacity of the nations in question to improve the productive skills of their citizens. Thus, not only has the gain from improvements in productive technology been diluted by the necessity of dividing it among ever more consumers, but the modernization of productive technology itself has been hindered.

It should be noted that the shift of priority in population growth from the wealthy to the poor nations did not occur because of a slowing down of the rate in the wealthy countries. On the contrary, as Table III makes clear, the advanced nations had a more rapid population growth between 1950 and 1970 than they had at any time in the previous half century. This fact casts doubt on the claim that as people go through the urban-

Table III. Population Growth: Developed vs. Underdeveloped
Portions of the World, 1900–1970

	Population		Growth
	At Start	At End	% Per Decade
	millions		
1900–1920			
Developed	251	309	11.0
Underdeveloped	1,399	1,551	5.3
1920–1930			
Developed	317	349	10.1
Underdeveloped	1,543	1,721	11.5
1930–1940			
Developed	528	565	7.0
Underdeveloped	1,542	1,730	12.2
1940–1950			
Developed	649	674	3.9
Underdeveloped	1,646	1,843	12.0
1950–1960			
Developed	741	847	14.3
Underdeveloped	1,776	2,158	21.5
1960–1970			
Developed	957	1,074	12.3
Underdeveloped	2,048	2,558	24.9

For each period shown, the countries in either category are constant;
but between one period and the next, they change from "underdeveloped"
to "developed" if their economies justify it. Added later: Hungary, 1920–30;
Soviet Union, 1930–40; Czechoslovakia and Japan, 1940–50; Argentina,
Israel, Italy, and Uruquay, 1950–60; Chile, Poland, South Africa, Spain,
Venezuela, and Yugoslavia, 1960–70. Data are chiefly from Durand, *op.
cit.*, for 1900, and for this and later dates from United Nations, *Demographic
Yearbook*, 1960, 1962, 1968, and 1970, and *Population and Vital Statistics
Report*, January 1, 1970.

industrial transition, they voluntarily "adjust" their reproductive behavior
to the new conditions and thus escape population problems. In 10 years,
between 1960 and 1970, the United States *added* 24.7 million people to
its population. This exceeds the entire present population of Canada (22
million) and is three times the population of Sweden. The entire decade
during which this population growth was occurring was characterized by
a declining birth rate, and this trend led many people to believe that the
country had no particular population problem. By 1971, with the birth
rate down to 17.3 per 1,000 population and the general fertility rate down
to 82.3 births per 1,000 women 15 to 44 years of age, the journalists were
writing sensational articles about America's baby shortage. What they
failed to mention was that, even in 1971, the birth rate was still nearly

twice as high as the death rate, and that the population increase for the year was 1.11 percent (two-thirds from the excess of births over deaths and one-third from net immigration). Of course, both vital rates were influenced by the age structure, but the truth is that the population was actually growing at a pace that, if continued, would double the number in 63 years.[2]

The history of birth rates in industrial countries since World War I is one of fluctuation. All of these nations reached a very low point in the 1930's, but had a rise after that, reaching a postwar peak in the birth rate in 1946. The 1946 peak was followed by a decline, and this in turn was followed by a second postwar peak occurring sometime in the years 1957 to 1962, after which another decline began. Such fluctuation suggests that if the birth rate is low at any given time, this is a good sign that it will be higher later on.

Another characteristic of the industrialized nations is that they are nearly all adding to their populations by international migration. The net gain is often difficult to determine, because statistics on people who leave are rare. However, the following data give some idea of the extent to which industrialized countries are gaining inhabitants through international movement:

Country	Period	Net Number of Long-Term Migrants, 1962–69*
Belgium	1963–69	183,718
Denmark	1962–69	5,200
Germany (West)	1962–69	1,536,767
Sweden	1962–68	116,364
Australia	1962–69	813,362
New Zealand	1962–69	81,948
U.S.A.	1962–69	3,246,000

* For all except the U.S.A., the figures are derived from United Nations, *Demographic Yearbook, 1970,* Tables 25–26. For the United States, the figure is from *Statistical Abstract of the United States,* 1970, p. 6.

With both a substantial natural increase and a strong current of net immigration, the industrial countries as a class are maintaining a surprising rate of population growth.

[2] To eliminate the effect of the age structure, a net reproduction rate is sometimes calculated; but the NRR had no relevance to the U.S. situation in 1971, because it is a statistical concept that only says what would happen *if* the age-specific fertility and mortality rates of the year in question were to remain constant until the age-structure of the population normalized itself in terms of those rates. Since it would take at least three generations for the age-structure to normalize itself, one can see that the net reproduction rate is an extremely abstract and unrealistic measure of what is currently happening in a population. One can be absolutely certain that the age-specific fertility and mortality rates will *not* remain constant.

If the sole purpose of human endeavor were to maximize the level of living, one could say that the industrial nations have no problem, because their level of living is satisfactory by comparison with either their own past history or with present-day nonindustrial countries. However, the purpose of human existence is by no means to maximize the level of living at all costs. Indeed, in these advanced societies it is becoming ever more apparent that a high level of living is a part of the population problem, not its solution. With a high level of living, an increase in the population means not only more people but also disproportionately more goods. In other words, these societies are plagued by a double multiplier—more people and more goods per person. This double multiplier creates more pollution, congestion, and waste than the same population growth in less-developed countries would create.

An illustration is again provided by the United States. As noted above, the population in this country increased by 24.7 million between 1960 and 1970. During the same period the country added approximately 34.4 million cars and trucks to its number of motor vehicles in use. Some of this rise in motor vehicles was due to an increase in the number of people, but some of it was also due to a rise in the per capita usage of motor vehicles. Had the population remained fixed but the per capita usage of motor vehicles risen as it actually did, the number of cars added would have been 21.8 million instead of 34.4 million. On the other hand, if the population had risen as it actually did but the per capita consumption remained at the 1960 level, the number of cars added would have been 9.8 million. If, finally, neither the population nor auto consumption had risen, there would have been no gain in the number of automobiles and trucks during the decade: the United States would have had 34.4 million fewer of these vehicles in 1970 than it actually had, and this would have made a tremendous difference in air pollution.

IS WORLD POPULATION GROWTH SLOWING DOWN?

If the rate of population growth exhibited by the world between 1950 and 1970 is unprecedented, and if it cannot long continue in the future, it has obviously reached a climax. The question, then, is not *if* the rate of increase will slacken, but how it will do so.

A possible hypothesis is that birth rates will start gradually declining and eventually bring population increase to zero or near it. Most of those concerned with population problems doubt that this will occur automatically, but many believe that it will occur *if* deliberate policies are instituted to make it happen. With this position there can be no argument, because there are undoubtedly policies that, *if* put into effect, would reduce fertility sharply; in fact, some satellite communist regimes of Eastern Europe have unintentionally reduced the birth rate to a point scarcely above the death rate. The question therefore is whether effective antinatalist policies will in fact be adopted on a sufficiently wide basis to halt world increase. Unfortunately, a sober and responsible answer to this question must be that, as yet, there is no evidence that such effective policies are being, or will be, adopted.

Such an answer may seem strange, or perhaps even objectionable, to those who know that many countries are inaugurating family planning programs; but a "family planning" program, which so far is virtually the only population measure being pursued, is not a fertility control program. The idea that population can be controlled by a family planning program rests, basically, on the assumption that high birth rates are caused by unwanted births and that distribution of a 100 percent effective contraceptive will eliminate such births and thus "solve" the population problem. Typical is the Declaration on Social Progress and Development promulgated by the General Assembly of the United Nations on December 11, 1969. It calls for "the formation and establishment . . . of programs in the field of population." Then, under the impression that it is implementing this admonition, it stresses giving families "the knowledge and means necessary to enable them to exercise their right to determine freely and responsibly the number and spacing of their children." The number of children couples want, however, unless it is influenced by deliberate policy, is not likely to be the number that a society should have. Uncontrolled private goals seldom bring collective welfare. Traffic congestion is not avoided by letting each person drive as he pleases, air pollution by letting each individual burn as he wishes, or drug addiction by letting each person deal in narcotics as he wants. Analogously, excessive reproduction will hardly be stopped by letting each person multiply as he desires.

Apart from its sociological naiveté, the idea that family planning will bring population control fails to fit the facts. The reduction in the birth rate of industrial countries during the late nineteenth and early twentieth centuries—in some cases below replacement level—was hardly a consequence of a contraceptive program. It was accomplished by individual couples using simple devices in the face of official opposition. Nor was the subsequent postwar baby boom in the same countries caused by a deterioration in contraceptive technology or services. It was caused by a resurgence of employment and economic security, which gave people the feeling they could marry and have almost as many children as they desired. Again, the spectacular decline in Japanese fertility from 1920 to 1955 was not achieved primarily by the use of contraception, much less by a government contraceptive program or a "scientific" device.

Further back in history, the high birth rates of preindustrial societies were not the result of unwanted births, but just the opposite: here was intense desire to have many births in order to beat the high infant mortality and thus have a few living children. The institutional supports for this de-

sire are not altered by offering to insert a new-fangled device inside women
or give them a dangerous new pill that mysteriously makes them sterile.
Our notion of unwanted births is culture bound. In our prosperous society,
where the average woman wants about 3.3 children, we feel that the im-
poverished women of Pakistan, who have over six births, *must* not want
nearly that many. Actually, in a realistic sense, they do not want *any* births
as such; they go through the pain and inconvenience of pregnancy only
for the purpose of having children. In Pakistan it is a woman's mission
in life to have children, and the institutional structure is such as to reward
her for that role; but due to public health efforts the same number of births
women used to have will now produce more living children than it ever
did before. Therefore, her old reproductive behavior is counterproductive
for the national economy, but as yet she has been given no alternative
role. Indeed, the "family planning" program, although it offers new contraceptive devices, is traditionally familistic in its ideology. The United Nations Declaration already quoted, in further elaboration of U.N. population
policy, says, "The family as a basic unit of society . . . should be assisted
and protected. . . . Parents have the exclusive right to determine freely
and responsibly the number and spacing of their children." The declaration calls for "development and coordination of policies designed to
strengthen the essential functions of the family as a basic unit of society; . . . ." This conservative attitude suggests that the great emphasis
on contraceptive technology and services in so-called population control
programs is a way of avoiding the painful social reforms that would be
necessary to reduce the number of children that people want. A family
is obviously more of a family if there are three, four, or five children in
it; the two-child family is a risky and slender group by comparison. Any
system that could motivate a substantial fraction of the population to have
no children at all would of course allow those who do have families to
have from three to five offspring; but such a system would represent a
fairly drastic reorganization of our present institutional structure. Currently
the proportion of women in the American population who ever have children (about 90.4 percent) is higher than it has been at any time in our
statistically recorded history.

Of course, from a population point of view, there is nothing wrong
with giving people the means of birth control. Once motivated to reduce
their reproduction, couples will find the means anyway. But if their effort
is facilitated, they may accomplish it more quickly. Curiously, however,
family planning programs have in several ways tended to discourage birth
control. They have done this by making war on abortion (a policy now
abandoned in the United States but still prevalent in Latin America), by
being lukewarm toward sterilization, and, above all, by over-medicalizing
contraception itself. By proclaiming the necessity of a virtually 100 percent
efficient contraceptive, by emphasizing methods that require medical atten-

tion (such as the IUD and the pill), by thinking in terms of "clinics" and treating healthy women who want to stop having babies as "patients," the family planning movement has made the control of fertility by couples depend on an extremely scarce resource, medical personnel. The low fertility of European countries at certain times in their history was achieved by such homespun methods as withdrawal, the condom, nonvaginal intercourse, douches, and backup abortion. None of these, except the last, is any more a medical matter than chewing gum or mouthwash. In fact, a 100 percent efficient birth control device has long existed; it is any reasonably good contraceptive, such as the condom, plus legal abortion. Although abortions require medical service, they do not, when legalized and used as a backup measure, require so much of it as exclusive reliance on the IUD or the "pill." Family planning programs seem to convey the philosophy, so long prevalent in public health, that people are sheep who have to "visit a clinic" and "be told by the doctor" before they can figure out even such an elementary thing as how not to have children. The damaging effect of the medical mystique is particularly noticeable in underdeveloped countries, where medical personnel are not only scarce but are concentrated in the cities where people tend to control their fertility anyway.

With or without government programs, the people of the underdeveloped countries will lower their birth rates as their societies continue to urbanize and develop. This is already occurring in many of the more advanced of the less industrial nations. For instance, in 10 marginal countries—marginal in the sense that they can now be classified as either developed or underdeveloped—the average crude birth rate changed as follows:

Birth Rate			Percent Change	
1951	1960	1969	1951–60	1960–69
36.4	32.1	23.4	−13.4	−37.2

A part of this drop was due to a changing age structure, but most of it represented falling fertility as well. The fact that the drop was greater in the second period suggests that as these countries modernized, the effect on reproductive behavior accelerated. The limit of such change is probably the reproductive level of industrial nations. In these nations, where family planning has been prevalent for more than a century, there is no sign that the birth rate is declining to a point that will even come near matching the low mortality. As mentioned already, *the industrial nations experienced a more rapid population growth between 1950 and 1970 than the underdeveloped countries did at any time previous to that.* This continued growth is all the more remarkable when the extreme urbanization and already large population base are taken into account. For example, as Table IV

Table IV. Natural Increase and Population Growth in
Two 17-Year Periods of United States History

	1909–25	1946–62
Average Rates (‰)		
Birth rate	28.2	24.6
Death rate	13.4	9.6
Natural increase rate	14.9	15.0
Absolute Numbers (000's)		
Births	49,225	67,799
Deaths	23,255	26,360
Natural increase	25,970	41,438

shows, the rate of increase in the United States between 1946 and 1962
was the same as it was during an equal period from 1909 to 1925. Since
the base population was greater, the same rate of increase meant a much
greater absolute increment—41.4 million as against 26.0 million.

Obviously, urban-industrial success and the use of effective birth control devices do not bring a birth rate low enough to stop rapid human
multiplication. Furthermore, in countries such as Taiwan, Costa Rica,
South Korea, and Puerto Rico, the shift from a pre-industrial to an industrial birth rate is coming at a time when the death rate is already much
lower than it was at a similar birth rate level in the history of the advanced
nations. Now, in fact, the death rate is dropping at such an unprecedented
speed that population growth is not being reduced commensurately with
the birth rate decline. For instance, Taiwan, widely touted as a country
where a family planning program is helping to "solve" the population problem,[3] had a drop in the crude birth rate from 39.0 in 1960–64 to 31.5
in 1965–69. This may look impressive, but a birth rate of 30 per 1,000
is high for a country as urban and industrial as Taiwan already is; and
the crude death rate is extremely low and is also dropping, with the result
that the population grew during 1965–69 at a rate of 2.6 percent per year.
This growth was occurring in a country that was already one of the most
densely settled in the world. In 1965 Taiwan's average density (in an area
about the size of Massachusetts and Connecticut combined) was 896 per
square mile, compared with Japan's density of 686. This was over 16 times
the average density in the United States. Nevertheless, in five years from
1965 to 1970, Taiwan added over two million people (or 16.5 percent)
to its population, raising its density to 1,044 per square mile. The number

[3] See Population Council, *Country Profiles*, February 1970. "From 1964 to
1968 Taiwan has demonstrated that a family planning program can help accelerate
a wide-scale fertility decline in a developing Asian area. . . ." (p. 14).

of people *added during five years* was equal to 148 persons for every square mile in the nation—a figure 2.7 times the average density in the United States.[4] Although the people in Taiwan are controlling their individual fertility, they are not controlling the island's population, because they want families so large as to give the nation a rapid increase. Taiwan is therefore no shining example of modern population control.

One factor leading to lower crude birth rates in many of the underdeveloped countries has nothing to do with fertility per se. It is a more youthful age structure created by the rapid decline in mortality (because the main saving of lives is in the young ages). In Costa Rica, between 1950 and 1963, life expectancy rose from 55.5 years to 63.6 years, and the proportion of the population under 20 rose from 53.4 percent to 57.1 percent. In the same period the crude birth rate went down slightly, and this might lead one to think that fertility declined. Actually, however, births per 1,000 females in the reproductive ages *climbed* by 17 percent.

	Births Per 1,000 Population	Births Per 1,000 Women Aged 20–44
1950	46.5	275
1963	45.3	322
Change (%)	−2.6	+17.2

In Costa Rica the peak fertility was reached about 1961. From that year to 1968 the drop in the total fertility rate (the births a woman would have if she lived through the reproductive period and bore children at the age-specific rates shown by women in the population) fell from 7.4 children in 1961 to 5.5 in 1968—a drop of 26 percent.[5] However, during the same period, life expectancy continued to improve. In 1968 the excess of births over deaths in Costa Rica was 50,443; in 1961 it was 50,193. A shift toward an industrial level of fertility does not bring much demographic relief to underdeveloped countries today.

THE ALTERNATIVE POSSIBILITIES

The plight of the industrial and nonindustrial nations in the face of continuing gains in population will hardly be remedied by current family

[4] For further analysis of Taiwan as a case of "successful" population control, see the writer's paper, "Population Policy: Will Current Programs Succeed?" *Science,* Vol. 158 (Nov. 10, 1967), pp. 734–736.

[5] Ricardo Jimenez J., *Estadisticas Demograficas Bisicas de Costa Rica, 1970* (San Jose, Costa Rica: Associacion Demografica Costarricense, 1970), p. 11.

planning programs. Instead, the delusion that these programs are adequate—a delusion fostered by the powerful family planning lobby throughout the world—tends to delay the adoption of effective measures. If effective measures of controlling the level of fertility are not adopted, this method of controlling population will not be the one that actually controls it.

To anticipate what may actually happen, we therefore have to turn to the other way in which population increase may be halted. Earlier I pointed out that the low mortality responsible for the population upsurge has been achieved by technological rather than genetic adaptation. There is presumably a limit to this type of adaptation. As the species degenerates from lack of selective pressure, and as the technology itself becomes ever more complex, a time must be reached when the individuals capable of making technological innovations of an ever more complex kind become too few. This eventuality, which must be considered the ultimate limit on population growth, could be reached sooner than one might think, because it involves the meeting of two mutually approaching forces, the speed being the sum of the two velocities. Although genetic decline is relatively slow, technological complication is now quite fast.

Long before the ultimate, or theoretical, limit is reached, however, other limits will doubtless intervene to drive up mortality. One such possibility lies in the capacity of the technological system for destructiveness. As the species becomes more dependent on technology for survival, a worldwide disruption will have increasingly disastrous consequences. Furthermore, the technology itself becomes potentially more lethal and destructive, and as population and congestion increase, the occasions for conflict multiply. A third world war, or perhaps a fourth or a fifth, could thus be the occasion when the demographic books are balanced—when a major share of the abnormally swollen human population is written off. Perhaps a new beginning could then be made, if there were left a sufficient number of healthy people to reproduce another generation.

The prospect is not a happy one, but we cannot appraise the importance of an effective fertility control policy unless we understand what will happen with an ineffective one. Before the industrial age, the normal condition in human society was one in which, in each local region, the death rate fluctuated sharply and the birth rate remained rather steady. Most of the time the birth rate exceeded the death rate, but every few years or so there would come a flood, hard winter, famine, fire, epidemic, war, or combination of these calamities that would quickly write off most if not all of the population gain during the previous "normal" period. Population growth naturally came to be associated with "good times"—that is, times when there was no calamity and people were prosperous. Population decline, on the other hand, came to be associated with disaster. In modern times, since the onset of the industrial age (especially during the last five decades of it), there has been remarkable success in keeping the death rate below the birth rate for virtually the entire human population and for an unprecedented length of time. In other words, the world has become much more a single entity, and its situation has become exceptionally "normal." The result, of course, has been a long-term rapid increase in human numbers which nobody anticipated or intended.

To avoid further increases by deliberate and humane measures calls for a substantial reduction in the world's birth rate. This however, requires a reversal of all the built-in institutional rewards and penalties in the social order of all peoples around the world; because the traditional systems have been structured so as to motivate people to reproduce abundantly and to associate population growth with normality, prosperity, and group power. Under the old standards, women who had many children were regarded as contributing a service to society. Now we have to regard them as committing an offense *against* society. A region that had a rapidly growing population was regarded as one that was "developing" economically; now we have to regard it as one that is suffering from congestion, pollution, and impoverishment of the individual. A nation that was fast increasing the number of its citizens was regarded as gaining in political power; now we have to view it as losing its relative technological capability and hence moving down in the international scale. A candid view of the short-run future finds little evidence that such an about-face in attitudes and behavior will occur. A rise in the world's death rate seems more probable. After that, the remnant of the human population that is left may have learned to discipline itself sufficiently to control its population growth by controlling the level of fertility.

CHAPTER 7

PROPAGATION, MODIFICATION, AND TERMINATION OF LIFE: CONTRACEPTION, ABORTION, SUICIDE, EUTHANASIA*

ROBERT H. WILLIAMS

One of the greatest problems we face is the rapid increase in population. With the new drugs, life-sustaining apparatuses, and organ replacements being used to preserve and prolong life come many moral, philosophic, psychologic, social, economic, medical, and legal problems. This chapter discusses these problems with particular reference to genetic bioengineering, contraceptive and fertility measures, abortion, gerontology, suicide, euthanasia, and organ transplantation.

QUANTITY AND QUALITY OF PROPAGATION

The world's population is increasing at an alarming rate. The time required to double the earth's population is now 37 years. At the present rate, in nine centuries there will be 6 quatrillion people, 100 per square yard, land and sea. Problems of clothing, food, jobs, and housing will multiply rapidly. Violence and wars will also increase. Even now, food production in some regions cannot keep pace with the increasing population. It is estimated that 3.5 million people, most of them children, will die of starvation this year. It is for man to choose whether the population will be controlled rationally or violently.

Methods of Population Control

Many methods are used to control population, including spermicidal action and suppression of ovulation by hormones given orally or by injection, intrauterine devices, vaginal diaphragms, spermicidal agents inserted

* Based on a presidential address given by the author at the annual meeting of the Association of American Physicians (Arch. Int. Med. **124**:215, 1969). It should be consulted for more complete references.

80

intravaginally, castration, and ligation of the fallopian tubes or the vas deferens. Extensive research has been initiated in a search for new approaches and improvements in present methods. One new method being tested consists of producing antibodies to one or more hormones that are required for a fertile state. In addition, more effort is being directed toward developing contraceptive methods for males—drugs, operations, or other measures; this might be a much more effective and efficient approach than depending upon contraceptive methods in females. Each current common method leaves much to be desired. Oral contraceptives—"the pill"—have the widest application at present, and it appears that this method and others will be greatly improved in the future.

In a recent survey[1] a group of physicians and a group of college-educated lay persons were asked whether they favored having the U.S. government provide, free of charge, a relatively safe contraceptive drug to all married women and single women over 21 who requested it. Approximately 75 percent of each group favored this proposal for married women, and almost as many included single women as well. Since many women would neglect using an antifertility drug even if it were highly effective and free, the survey asked if a cash incentive should be offered with a regular antifertility injection to certain individuals with psychiatric, physical, social, or economic problems. About half of the respondents favored this proposal. Although some individuals and groups strongly oppose this approach, their opposition should subside with increased appreciation of the benefits to individuals and society.

Sterilization and Castration.   Sterilization and castration are the most dependable contraceptive measures; in both males and females they are essentially 100 percent successful. Cutting and tying off the fallopian tubes or the vas deferens generally cause permanent sterility, although progress has been made in developing operations that would permit fertility to be restored through another operation. Castration, which involves removal of the ovaries or testes, usually is not performed for contraception per se because it causes more physical and emotional changes than simple sterilization, yet provides no more protection against pregnancy—at least when the tubal ligation or vasectomy is properly performed. In some sex criminals castration is used both for decreasing the libido and for contraception.

Sterilization should be performed with the consent of the patient or of his parents, guardian, or other responsible person(s). Sometimes the patient and his relatives are not in a position to make the most appropriate decision for the patient and the public; in this instance a special group

---

[1] In soliciting the opinion of others on various subjects discussed in this chapter, I submitted a questionnaire to each member of two distinguished medical associations and to 1954 and 1955 graduates of the University of Washington. (Detailed analyses of the questionnaires are found in *Arch. Int. Med.* **124**:215–237, 1969, and *Northwest Medicine* **69**:493–501, 1970.)

should be designated for this responsibility. Occasionally, a similar problem occurs with castration, usually involving a patient with psychosis, mental retardation, or some other major mental disorder. The procedure should be regarded not as punishment but as therapy and protection of the patient and others. Such patients are mentally ill and need major treatment. In some, adequate improvement is not achieved by castration because of such factors as the type and extent of mental abnormality, economic problems, lack of cooperation, or unavailability of appropriate treatment; sometimes curative therapy is nonexistent. Constant confinement of such patients will protect the public from further offenses, but for various reasons most offenders are not confined. Almost half of the states have compulsory eugenic sterilization laws chiefly involving subjects with mental disorders. Castration is applied especially to mentally disordered individuals who are repeatedly involved in rape, child molestation, and other sex crimes. It is to be emphasized that in most cases castration is not curative, but it may offer some benefits. Each case must be considered individually and thoroughly.

Abortion.   Until recently, the laws on abortion in the United States have been so restrictive that abortion has been used relatively little for population control, even when continued pregnancy presented major mental, physical, social, or economic hazards. Several other countries, however, have used abortion extensively. Japan, for example, has used abortion as one of the main methods for reducing its birth rate to one of the lowest in the world. Britain, Sweden, and other countries have liberalized their abortion laws to distinct advantage. Fortunately, restrictions concerning employment of abortion have been markedly eased in certain areas in the United States, but wiser policies should be developed throughout the nation concerning the frequency, methods, and financing of abortions. Although we have a long way to go, what progress we have made in the last three years is commendable.

Various procedures are used for abortion; one of the simple and relatively safe ones is the instillation into the uterus of a hypertonic solution. Experience shows that there is almost no mortality and very little morbidity when abortions are performed by competent physicians in licensed hospitals. This is one of the main reasons that a physician who has performed an abortion in a licensed hospital has never been convicted of illegal abortion, even though many abortions are performed for reasons beyond those indicated by laws.

The survey mentioned earlier included a question about whether the criminal abortion laws should be made inapplicable to licensed physicians and to women under the care of a physician. Approximately 80 percent of both physicians and laymen voted yes. A majority of Catholics also favored the proposal, but not as much as others. Laws and religious policies concerning abortion are rapidly being changed throughout this nation.

The new policies must consider the present and future mental and physical status of the mother and child, and the effect of abortion on social, economic, and other conditions affecting both the family and society.

Amniocentesis. Amniocentesis, or the withdrawal of some amniotic fluid during pregnancy, is rapidly becoming an important procedure in the management of certain pregnancies, especially when there is the possibility of a genetically abnormal fetus. This procedure is best performed at about the 16th week. The amniotic fluid is examined for various chemical or cellular abnormalities, and in many instances cell cultures are made. At present, there is relatively little morbidity and mortality. Various conditions such as mongolism, galactosemia, cystic fibrosis, phenylketonuria, muscular dystrophy, and hemophilia can be diagnosed in this manner. If certain diseases, such as cystic fibrosis (probably the most common fatal genetic disease of childhood), are found, abortion is recommended. In other cases, treatment of the mother can minimize damage to the fetus. Sometimes merely omitting a specific item from the diet, such as galactose in galactosemia, or adding a specific item can prevent symptoms. In many instances, genetic counseling and other advisory approaches can be of great help.

Better Control of the Quantity and Quality of Propagation

Great mental and physical suffering results from our failure to control the quantity and quality of reproduction wisely. The major reasons for these inadequacies are (a) persistence of inappropriate religious policies, laws, and public philosophies, and (b) too little research and education and too few means for correcting the problems. As research and education in these areas are extended, public support will increase until laws and religious policies are changed.

Certain religious groups restrict abortion, chiefly because of the Sixth Commandment, "Thou shalt not kill." Abortion has been controversial for many centuries. Some condone it when performed before "life begins" or before "the soul enters the body"; some groups select "quickening" as the time the soul enters. However, quickening consists merely of kicking and other body movements by the fetus; there is no reason to equate it with activities of the soul or of the mind. Lower animals experience quickening, too; indeed, in their physical movements they far surpass the human fetus.

Some individuals erroneously maintain that life begins with fertilization of the ovum by a spermatozoon. A famous example to the contrary is Jesus Christ, who supposedly developed by parthenogenesis. As discussed in Chapter 8, life was created many centuries ago; therefore, fertilization of the egg by the spermatozoon does not initiate life but expands (propagates) it. In using antifertility measures we are applying a degree of negative euthanasia and/or positive euthanasia. (Negative euthanasia is the planned omission of actions to maintain life; positive euthasia is the taking of actions to induce death.) Abstinence from intercourse or use of the "rhythm" plan is negative euthanasia. Use of anovulatory drugs or spermicidal agents is positive euthanasia. A spermatozoon or an ovum is tiny compared with a child or adult, but so is a fertilized ovum. A fetus that is one, two, or three months of age is much further developed than the fertilized ovum, yet it has progressed relatively little on the long journey to full development. Many of its organs are not functioning, and indeed there are indications that these fetuses have no thoughts and experience no pain. Therefore, although life can be terminated in a fertilized or in an unfertilized ovum, in a fetus or in a man, there are great differences in the development of life in these groups. Depending upon the stage of life and many other factors, there are marked differences in the desire and need to perpetuate life, from the point of view of both the individual and others. At times we even justify taking the life of an adult, as, for example, in wars and by capital punishment. In the early history of man, relatively few people reached adulthood, and fewer still reached old age. Malnutrition, infections, destruction by animals, weather conditions, and other factors took a high toll. Therefore, efforts to increase propagation and survival have long been traditional. Now, however, we have much less need to promote propagation or prolongation of life. Prevention of pregnancy is far preferable to abortion for population control, but failure of the former should be corrected by the latter.

Untold suffering could be prevented if more attention were given to the mental and physical status of couples before and after marriage. Often there are incompatibilities which would not occur with other pairings. Couples must realize more than ever the obligations of parenthood. Too often conception is unplanned, a passing fancy. Such a birth may cause psychologic, economic, and social problems to the parents, agonies to the child, and various difficulties for society. Even the carefully planned pregnancy may be ill advised. Married couples traditionally wish to conceive children. If, as happens sometimes, the initial pleasure of parenthood is far overbalanced by the problems that the child, the parents, and society will face, then conception is unwise and selfish. If, too, there is the possibility of a genetic disorder that can bring mental or physical suffering, having children can perpetuate the trouble into further generations. Some genetic disorders are manifested in more than 75 percent of the offspring. Even when there is no significant genetic problem, mental or physical disorders can be produced during pregnancy by nutritional abnormalities, drugs, alcohol, irradiation, infections, trauma, and other factors. Many of these can be avoided or corrected more readily than in the past. Therefore, the likely disadvantages should be compared with the advantages before pregnancies are initiated or continued. Too much compassion by society for one generation can produce oppression for the next. World wide, there are few government restrictions with regard to reproduction. Children can be produced by parents as young as 10, by the very elderly, by unwed couples, by parents who cannot support them, or by parents who are insane or afflicted with a disease that may bring great suffering. Ordinarily, it is assumed that each individual has the freedom and right to reproduce whenever and wherever he chooses. Every effort should be made to change public opinion through enlightenment, tradition, pleas, and various incentive plans. However, we must be prepared to use legal measures if necessary.

Promoting Reproduction in Some Instances

Although we should prevent excess population both locally and internationally, some couples should be helped to reproduce. Many childless couples would probably produce healthy children if fertilization were possible. Failures can be due to psychologic, anatomic, nutritional, endocrinologic, environmental, and pharmacologic factors. Sometimes the problem is solved quickly; at other times many factors must be explored. When these efforts are unsuccessful, artificial insemination or adoption should be considered.

Artificial insemination should be used much more often than in the past. More than 10 percent of the people of the United States are considered to be involuntarily sterile, and among them are many couples who have a great desire for children. The number of healthy children available for adoption has become limited, as social and economic conditions have generally improved and contraceptives and abortions have been more extensively used. In many situations artificial insemination offers advantages over adoption. The mother and especially the donor tend to be of better health, and the child will be reared by his natural mother. Moreover, if the donor semen is mixed with that of the legal father there is a remote possibility that one of the father's spermatozoa will be the one that fertilizes the ovum. We do not really know why so many spermatozoa are necessary for fertilization even though only one actually does the fertilizing, but whatever aid they supply might benefit the father's hypospermia. Even the remote possibility that the one effective spermatozoon was the father's can be a comfort to both parents, especially the father. Of course, the physician must go over all the psychologic and physical considerations with the prospective parents.

Modification of Genetic Patterns

Genetics, which has been used extensively to improve the quality of plants and animals, has been used little in man. Many policies and laws must be changed for progress in eugenics. Fascinating experiments have been conducted in euphenics, described by Lederberg as "the reprogramming of somatic cells and the modification of development." Nirenberg has indicated that simple genetic messages can be synthesized chemically;

genes can be prepared from one strain of bacteria and inserted into another with the resulting cells and progeny programmed according to the messages and yielding respective responses. Man may be able to program himself with synthetic information in the future. Three experimental lines are of particular interest: use of viruses as carriers of genetic material, transplantation of cell nuclei, and hybridization of cells from the same or different species. Since both RNA and DNA viruses have been replicated in vitro, it is conceivable that either after replication or de novo synthesis of certain nucleotides the product may be complexed with certain select viruses for introduction into mammalian cells, leading to a reprogramming of the cells' activities. For example, the nucleic acid sequence bearing the code for phenylalanine hydroxylase synthesis might be attached to the virus and this complex could possibly be used as a vaccine for treating phenylketonuria. Cancer, certain birth defects, brain abnormalities, and organ transplantation may also be dealt with in a similar fashion.

The nucleus of a fertilized egg might be replaced by the nucleus of a cultured cell, and the resulting cell would have reprogrammed activity. It has been demonstrated that human cells which have been exposed to SV-40 virus can be fused with mouse cells, and the human-mouse cell hybrid, with its changed program, has been cultured for many generations.

Technological progress may permit application of some of these phenomena to problems of man before we are prepared to deal with social, psychologic, philosophic, moral, and other aspects. These problems exist also in the gross transplantation of different genetic material and in organ transplantation.

Genetic manipulation is also discussed in Chapter 5.

Organ Transplantation

Four major problems in organ transplantation are immunology, technology, organ supply, and philosophy. Suppression of the immune bodies makes the patient vulnerable to infection and other difficulties. However, the immunological problems can probably be controlled eventually. The surgeons have demonstrated that they can deal with the technical problems, particularly those of the heart and kidneys.

When these problems are solved, sufficient organs can be supplied only by use of post-morten tissue. Since the organ should be acquired from the donor while it is still viable, a number of problems are involved, particularly in obtaining hearts. Death has usually been considered to have occurred when the heart has stopped for several minutes. In such instances, the brain soon dies, and then other tissues. To acquire a viable heart, individuals whose brains die before their hearts are used. Obviously, a number of legal, psychological, moral, ethical, and social problems arise when the heart is removed while it is still beating; therefore, criteria have been formulated to establish brain death. Prominent among these criteria are deep and irreversible coma, the persistence of an isolectric electroencephalogram, no respiration after artificial respiration has been stopped, and no elicitable reflexes. Better methods for the earlier diagnosis of brain death, probably including neurochemical analyses, will become available.

Significant progress is promised by the Uniform Anatomical Gift Act, now adopted by almost all states, which authorizes donation by individuals 18 years of age or older before death, and donation by next of kin after death, of all or any part of the human body to a hospital, a physician or dentist, an educational or research institution, a storage bank, or some other such unit. It seems desirable to have a law that would permit routine autopsy and organ removal for medical purposes unless the subject or next of kin has indicated an objection. This places the responsibility upon the patient and his next of kin to object, rather than on the physician to seek permission routinely. The plan would cause less mental trauma and presumably give better results. In many ways this proposal was favored by 71 percent of the physicians and 57 percent of the lay persons surveyed by the author.

In the future, when many transplantation problems are conquered, one person may receive several organs. In the example shown in Fig. 1 of Chapter 3, a person has received organs from four donors. Now, has the recipient been changed to another person? The kidney is largely a filter, the heart chiefly a pump, and the liver a multiple servant, but the brain performs the major function of the body, mentation. All of the organs are subservient to mentation. The brain recipient presumably would have aspects of mentation possessed by the donor, including origination of thoughts, perception, memory, and correlation, at least as far as they are influenced by the brain's inherent chemical reactions. Compounds released by nonbrain structures, if they penetrate the blood-brain barrier, also influence mentation. Such compounds could be abnormal in either amount or type.

Termination of Life

The aged are involved more than others in the problems of suicide and euthanasia. As a group they are inappropriately handled in many ways; our medical school leaders are partly responsible for this negligence. Progress in the interesting subject of gerontology, with the cooperation and active participation of many specialists, is long overdue. Although each medical school has long had a department of pediatrics, until the last 10 years there have been less than a dozen with a department or division of gerontology.

We all know of individuals who have worked hard all of their lives, have amassed fame, fortune, and many honors, and have dreamed of the

millennium which presumably will blossom on retirement. Then there will
be plenty of time for rich pleasures, recreation, sweet memories; time to
bask in the glory of their handiwork. Even when this dream is realized,
later years may turn the dream sour. Mental and physical discomforts
mount; the future looms dark. Then the aged feel lonely and useless; they
feel they are a burden to relatives, friends, and society. Other individuals
may have these reactions after a lifetime of distressing social, economic,
mental, and physical problems. In either case, the aged person may eventually wish for the day when all troubles will cease. Such a wish, frequently
shared by the family, is often shattered by therapies given by a physician
who has only one consideration—*to prolong life, no matter what else is
involved.* Our goal should not be to prolong every life as long as possible
by the extensive use of drugs, operations, organ transplantation, artificial
organs, respirators, hemodialyzers, cross-circulation and pacemakers (Fig.
1). We must consider whether such prolongation leads to happiness or
to great physical or mental suffering for the patient and others. We must
also consider social, economic, and other concerns of society, including
the imminent problem of overpopulation.

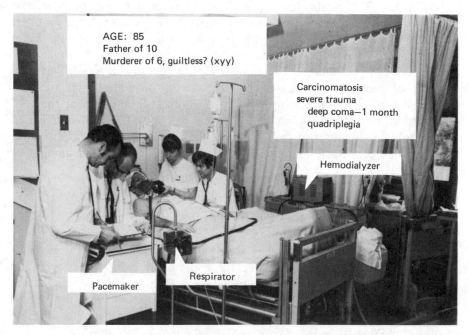

Fig. 1. An 85-year-old man with probably irreversible coma, quadriplegia, chronically
and severely damaged kidneys, and advanced heart disease. The patient would
most likely die if artificial respiration, hemodialysis, or the use of the pacemaker
were discontinued. Why prolong "life" when the next of kin prefer not to?

Suicide

There are no accurate figures for the incidence of suicide; certainly all reports are marked underestimates. A much larger number attempt suicide, and a still larger number seriously consider it. In males the incidence increases with age (Fig. 2). Physicians are among the leading groups. The Bible does not specifically condemn suicide, but some religions regard it as "the most fatal of sins." Certain laws label it a felony. Some members of society consider suicide victims to be cowards and weaklings; a horrible stigma prevails for them and their families. With so many punitive implications and castigations, with the lack of understanding and sympathy, many potential suicide victims contend with their problems alone, at least until they have reached a state of severe depression, anxiety, agitation, or frustration. Because of their great distress and exhaustion, many cannot analyze their problems satisfactorily and, in desperation, commit suicide. The extent of their suffering is emphasized by the horrible means of death some select, such as jumping into a fire, leaping in front of a train or a car or from a building, cutting wrists or throats, or shooting oneself. Certain chemical abnormalities and patterns of mentation drive them to the act. It is easy for those who are not experiencing the same agony to advocate calmness and clear thinking. This is like telling a person who is sitting on a red-hot burner to sit calmly and remain cool; his natural

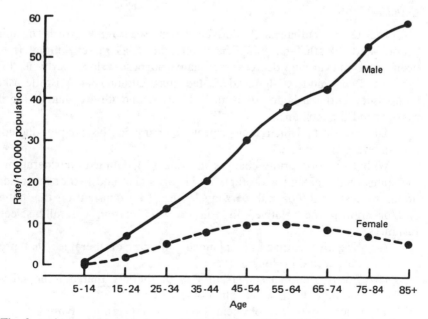

Fig. 2. Incidence of suicide in the United States, 1950–1964. The incidence is much higher in whites than in nonwhites and in males than in females.

defense mechanisms spur action. If all elements of society had a better approach to suicide, potential victims would seek aid sooner and be treated more effectively. Many depressions tend to be limited in duration and are eased by rest, relaxation, assurance, psychotherapy, and drug treatment, but we must acknowledge that we have many failures. Many psychiatrists are aware of this; some of them reveal a pessimistic view of their ability to deal with their own problems, since psychiatrists have one of the highest rates of suicide.

If the potential suicide victim is still in great agony even after he has received expert attention for a suitable period of time, should euthanasia be considered? Euthanasia, with appropriate approval, seems more desirable than suicide. Since we make a great effort to keep a patient alive when he desires it, should we give more attention to his wishes when he desires euthanasia? If the patient knows that euthanasia can be applied when the physician feels the situation is bad enough, some of his anxieties may be alleviated and suicide may be prevented. Some potential victims have carefully weighed the pros and cons and decided that what they will gain and contribute to others by continuing to live does not justify the severe mental and physical agony they are experiencing. In some instances, the decision is wise. On the other hand, many individuals would endure these agonies if they felt that their survival would benefit others or themselves sufficiently. Especially among professionals, many potential victims have shown much drive and have been excellent leaders.

Euthanasia

The term "euthanasia," derived from two Greek words meaning "good" and "death," has often been thought of as mercy killing. It has been used in varying degrees for many purposes since early history: Plutarch, Plato, and Aristotle advocated quasi-euthanasia; Aristotle asked compulsory euthanasia for deformed children; and Greeks had it for the aged, as did the Romans.

The survey to which I have been referring in this chapter included the following questions:

With (1) appropriate changes in laws, (2) detailed consideration of the status of the patient and others by his physician and two or more additional professional hospital personnel, and (3) consent of the patient and/or appropriate relative, do you favor in certain carefully selected instances:

    (a) Negative euthanasia (planned omission of therapies that probably would prolong life)?

    (b) Positive euthanasia (institution of therapy that it is hoped will promote death sooner than otherwise)?

About 80 percent of the physicians and the lay group favored negative euthanasia. Eighty percent of the physicians stated that they had practiced negative euthanasia. About 18 percent of the physicians and 35 percent of the lay group favored positive euthanasia. In a survey by Laws et al., 46 percent of the medical students believed that they would practice positive euthanasia if given the appropriate opportunity.

Negative Euthanasia.   Negative euthanasia has been applied much too infrequently, even though most physicians and members of the public clearly favor it in certain instances. A vast number of patients, as well as their families and friends, experience far more physical and mental suffering than they should. While we make a great effort to consider the wishes of the patient and members of the family in many situations, when it comes to euthanasia we do little to learn their wishes or to accommodate them. Many patients lead a vegetative existence for months or years; heart-lung perfusion and other subsidiary functions continue, but the prime function, mentation, has gone (Fig. 1).

The following patient was recently under my care in the hospital:

> A 68-year-old man had marked generalized atherosclerosis, myocardial infarction, and a ruptured aorta replaced by a graft. For three weeks he had had anuria associated with acute kidney necrosis and had been maintained on a regimen of repeated hemodialysis. There was extensive hepatic necrosis with intense jaundice, thrombosis of the inferior vena cava, pulmonary embolism, thrombosis of the right femoral artery, and gangrene of the legs. He had recently had a gastrostomy, vagotomy, and pyloroplasty, and was suffering from generalized peritonitis. He also had carcinoma of the prostate. When I first saw him there were tubes in all orifices, and various materials were being infused into many different blood vessels. The patient was in deep coma. It was clear that death was inevitable.

Why should such an elaborate array of useless and very expensive therapies be continued, especially when its use is very much against the wishes of his family and friends? Even in such a clearly hopeless situation there are people who maintain that there is a very remote chance that a miracle will happen and the patient will get better, but this possibility is overridden by essential certainty that other troubles will accrue, prolonging his vegetative existence and prolonging his agony if consciousness should be regained. Situations of this type put us at a major crossroad where we must choose between decisions based on wise reasoning and sound judgment and those based on flighty and poorly based emotionalism.

The medical profession in general has been taught to prolong life as long as possible, irrespective of other consequences. The Hippocratic Oath stresses the importance of relieving suffering and of prolonging and protecting life. Sometimes these two are in conflict. The patient may suffer so much that a compassionate relative or friend will commit positive euthanasia and, because he fears the consequences, commit suicide, thus causing two deaths. The custom of perpetuating life as long as possible, irrespective of the results, is continued chiefly because of certain religious policies, laws, traditions, and fear of death. Much more effort should be made to reduce fears of death; I myself have been almost entirely through the "pearly gates" and did not find it so bad.

The Lord intended for us all to die eventually, and He set up a genetic pattern that assures death. The Bible states that there is a time to die. Some have stated that it is for God to decide at what moment life should cease and that suffering is part of the divine plan for the good of man. Extending such reasoning, one might ask why we should interfere with the progress of diseases that may lead to death? Why should we use anesthesia for operations, or, indeed, why should we even operate?

Under law, a physician who withholds therapy that probably would prolong life faces prosecution for criminal negligence, but he is almost never prosecuted. Some say that legal approval of euthanasia would "weaken our moral fiber." However, I believe that our fiber must be weak to permit certain instances of prolonged suffering without instituting euthanasia.

Positive Euthanasia. The opposition to positive euthanasia is based upon highly restrictive existing laws, policies of certain religious groups, and philosophies of society. A major deterrent has been the biblical statement, "Thou shalt not kill" (Exodus 20:13); also "He who kills a man should be put to death" (Leviticus 24:17). However, the Bible has statements that can be interpreted as permitting killing under certain conditions: There is "a time to be born and a time to die—a time to kill and a time to heal" (Eccl. 3:2–3); God gave man dominion "over every living thing that moveth upon the earth" (Gen. 1:28). Legally, if a physician gives a fatal injection with the intention of killing a patient, the physician is considered a murderer. However, some laws qualify this by stating, "unless it is excusable and justified." Relatively few physicians have been prosecuted for positive euthanasia.

We recognize that homicide is justifiable in self-defense. Over 50 million people were killed in World War II and 9 million in the Korean War. We long have exercised capital punishment. We hold guiltless "murderers of unsound mind." Often, in medicine and surgery, we bring life to an end in our efforts to prolong it. We feel justified in terminating life with abortion, with sterilization, with spermicidal agents, and in other ways. Why should we not justify terminating life when there is severe and hopeless suffering, along with major problems for the relatives, friends, and society? Explosives and various other traumatic injuries can have mutilating results. Certain individuals with severe psychiatric disorders experience tortures worse than hell and do not obtain adequate relief despite our best efforts.

The mere fact that in some instances there is a remote possibility of recovery does not justify so much suffering by so many people. Although this is of subsidiary consideration, some thought should be given to the imminent problems of overpopulation discussed earlier. Euthanasia is a deplorable method for population control, but with overpopulation in the offing and with the patient, his family, his physician, and others concluding it is best not to prolong the agony, why engage in formidable procedures to gain some extra days? Some individuals favor the principle of euthanasia but fear the "wedge principle" (namely, that once started, euthanasia might be applied excessively), and are bothered by the difficulties of making decisions in various situations. While there would be many difficult decisions, fear of them does not justify the mental and physical suffering resulting from our failure to act. Appropriate changes in laws and policies should be made, after extensive consideration by many segments of society—physicians, religious leaders, legislators, sociologists, psychologists, and others. We then should have appropriate committees and consultants to deal with special problems that arise. Britain has been considering a proposed law that would allow physicians to end the lives of some incurably ill patients who request it (see Chapter 9). However, there must be a waiting period of at least 30 days after the request. Similar proposals have been made in other countries and in some parts of the United States.

Discussion of Euthanasia.   Now that numerous methods are available to prolong life, we must reformulate our thinking about when and to what extent these methods are to be applied in individual cases, bearing in mind the advantages and disadvantages to the patient, his family, and society. Continuing efforts to maintain life as long as possible and in as many people as possible does not serve many advantages to society or to some individuals. Today, in comparison with the past, the end of life may be associated with more agony or less agony, depending upon the approach of the physicians and others. If we are to change policies on euthanasia, we must deal with the attitudes of (a) religion, (b) law, (c) society, (d) the physician, and (e) the patient and his family.

(a) Religion.   Some groups maintain that it is a sin for man to terminate life, because it is God's right to end life by natural means. Others, however, state that a physician sins if in certain situations he does not hasten death. Still others declare that it is God's will that man should suffer. Logically, then, we should not use anesthetics, analgesics, antibiotics, operations, or many of the procedures now used in medicine. God gave man genetic and metabolic patterns that always eventually lead to death. Euthanasia in certain situations can be interpreted as a manifestation of God's love and compassion. As Thielicke (see Vaux) states, God's command to subdue the earth does not mean that we must play a passive role in such matters.

(b) Laws.   The laws of many countries have condemned euthanasia. Indeed, a physician can be held criminally and civilly liable for negative or positive euthanasia. Williams (see Downing) states: "If the doctor honestly and sincerely believes that the best service he can perform for his suffering patient is to accede to his request for euthanasia, it is a grave thing that the law should forbid him to do so." Many leading attorneys state that almost never is a physician convicted for euthanasia; they prefer that physicians apply their best judgment in these cases. However, with no changes in the law, this is unfair to the physician and to society. Lawmakers find it difficult to formulate satisfactory limitations in a law permitting euthanasia. It seems important to compose some major guidelines to be followed by the patient, his family, his physician, theologians, psychologists, attorneys, and others to be involved in such decisions.

(c) **Traditions of Society.**   Through the centuries it has been traditional to help each person to live as long as possible, because in ancient times relatively few survived until 70 years of age. Moreover, there were no good drugs for relieving terminal suffering. Therefore, the thought of death and the thereafter was associated with fear and anxiety. Now, many facilities permit us to prolong life, but sometimes we create more suffering than we alleviate. We must help the public realize that death is an inevitable process that need not be associated with significant suffering. Indeed, it often appears as a welcome relief.

(d) **Physician's Role.**   As mentioned earlier, responses to my questionnaires indicated that approximately 80 percent of the physicians and the lay persons favored negative euthanasia under certain conditions. About twice as many of the lay group and medical students favored positive euthanasia as did physicians. Although about 80 percent of the physicians had practiced negative euthanasia, they did so infrequently, chiefly owing to long-standing opposition from religious groups, laws, and social traditions. Moreover, physicians are strongly oriented toward giving essentially all treatments that will keep each patient alive as long as possible, regardless of the prognosis, expense, and mental and physical suffering that this may cause the patient and his relatives. Often, the patient and relatives would oppose some of the measures used if they were presented with a true picture of the probable course of the disease with and without special treatment. It is common for physicians to tell the patient chiefly the hopeful aspects of the diagnosis, treatment, and course, thereby often misleading him. Patients with an obviously poor prognosis are told that some miracle may happen or some wonder drug may be discovered. By similar logic, surgery with a 50 percent mortality should be replaced by anticipation of a miracle that would save all patients. However, this logic is not wise. When we weigh the probable advantages of continued living against the probable disadvantages, postponement of dying is often unjustified. Moreover, such a postponement may change the patient's reactions toward his physician from admiration to criticism. In some situations the physician can best express his love, compassion, and medical skill by helping the patient to die. I have often seen patients and their families become very angry with a physician who has falsely tried to raise their hopes (for example, when a correct diagnosis of a rapidly advancing malignancy has been made earlier by another physician and the patient and his family have made appropriate preparations for death—psychologically, socially, financially, and otherwise—and then attempts are made to have them believe [erroneously] that great improvement will probably result from a wide array of tests and therapies).

Leadership on the part of the physician often makes negative euthanasia possible when otherwise it would not be, as illustrated by the following case report.

> J. W., a 60-year-old woman from Boston, had a rapidly growing cancer with extensive metastases. The cancer produced excess hormone, which in turn caused a marked excess of calcium in the blood and resulting psychosis. The psychosis disappeared time and time again by adjustment of the blood calcium level, but the cancer continued to rampage. The chief physician frankly explained the entire situation to the patient (when she was mentally clear) and her husband, and told them that he and his colleagues could continue vigorous palliative treatments or they could eliminate some of this and concentrate chiefly on *comfort*. The patient and her husband readily chose comfort as the main goal. Nurses, interns, residents, and other physicians all agreed that this was the best course. However, it is so traditional for interns and residents to give extensive palliative therapy that they did not omit much of the treatment. The patient's (and her husband's) suffering continued much too long. One day the husband came to the chief physician's office, crying and very upset, and said: "My wife has faced so much agony because of the continuing treatment that I wish you would tell those doctors emphatically that they should not go on with therapy." At this time good cooperation was obtained from everyone. After the patient had died a few days later, the husband expressed great gratitude and added that it was too bad that we make humans endure suffering that we would not permit in animals.

(e) The Role of the Patient and His Family.   All too often the physician fails to give the patient a clear picture of his terminal illness, including the nature and extent of his disease, the diagnostic tests, the therapies, and the prognosis. Comments about prognosis are too optimistic because we assume, erroneously, that the truth would unduly upset the patient. Death should be explained to him as a natural phenomenon that may relieve much suffering. With proper attention, death itself need not be associated with major discomfort. The needs of the patient should be reviewed with him and his family. In many other phases of medicine the patient must give his "informed consent" before he can be treated. In protracted terminal illnesses, however, "informed consent" is rarely obtained from the patient, nor is he free to choose the time or the manner of his death. He and his family are often subjected unnecessarily and unwisely to prolonged suffering, expense, and inconvenience. This has increased the rate of suicide. It has also increased the frequency with which arrangements are made for the terminal patient to die in a nursing home, his own home, or a small hospital where the barrage of tests and treatments that would occur in an active large hospital will be avoided. Too often the patient, in a deep and irreversible coma, with widespread gross pathology, lingers indefinitely as a perfused protoplasmic mass, all thought processes and the soul having already departed. As Gresham (in Downing) states:

"It is surely the dignity, wisdom, and achievement of man that should concern us, and not mere existence or survival." With certain severe and incurable illnesses the patient and his family should be given a description of some aspects of the process and permitted to choose the most appropriate course, including euthanasia. If the patient is permanently incompetent, the next of kin, the physician, and other consultants, as indicated, should decide about negative euthanasia. Once the necessary legal changes have been made, positive euthanasia should be permitted in some cases upon approval of the physician and other members of a special committee, the patient, and his next of kin. If the patient is mentally incompetent, the decision could be made by the legally responsible person(s).

Conclusions

There are great differences in the quality and quantity of life and in its importance to individuals and society. Life exists in spermatozoa, ova, fetuses, infants, children, adults, and the aged. Certain stages of life are of far greater importance to the individual, his family, and society than are others. Man has been granted the opportunity to influence the propagation, modification, and termination of life, but there are great inequities in the manner and extent to which man has faced his responsibilities in these spheres. There has been far too much casual and unplanned propagation, and far too much restriction and lack of wise planning concerning the termination of life. Society, laws, and religious policies have greatly restricted the role of the individual in electing the time and manner of his death, but have granted him undue freedom regarding propagation. Traditionally, we anticipate death with too much anxiety and dread. Too often life is prolonged unduly through excessive use of drugs, machinery, and other facilities.

The problems of overpopulation are increasing. We must reduce population through education, counseling, extensive provision of contraceptives, and development of simple and effective methods for abortion. With progress in eugenics and euphenics, and with wiser selections concerning fertilization, the quality of the population will improve. The use of amniocentesis should be extended, and significantly defective fetuses should be aborted.

Many of the immunologic and technical aspects of organ transplantation will probably be surmounted soon, but this progress will raise important philosophic considerations. With transplantation as with other life-saving procedures, life should not necessarily be prolonged just because it can be; there may be more disadvantages than advantages to the recipient, his family, and society. The major function of the body is mentation; without it, the body does not serve a useful purpose. It appears that even the soul is a specialized aspect of mentation (Chapter 3). We have been negligent in our dealings with the aged, some of whom had to endure more distress than they should. For some people, young or old, mental or physical agonies become so unendurable that they commit suicide. We can help such people in many ways—one of which is to remove the religious and legal stigmata of suicide. We can also help by giving the potential victims much kindlier consideration and help of various types. However, we must admit that there are people whose suffering is so great and their prognosis so hopeless that negative euthanasia should be a legally and morally acceptable choice. We should also initiate the legal changes that would make positive euthanasia possible under appropriate conditions and precautions, although this should be delayed until more progress has been made in applying negative euthanasia.

Finally, I wish to emphasize that the topics discussed trigger strong emotional reactions—indeed, reactions that often stifle both reason and progress. Our present policies create many unnecessary mental, physical, social, economic, and other problems. If we are to bring about changes, long hard work will be required by many people—physicians, theologians, psychologists, attorneys, sociologists, and others. It is hoped that we will increase our activities immediately in population control, selective abortions, problems of mentation, aging, suicide, and negative euthanasia. At present, it appears that we will have to wait longer for significant application of genetic bioengineering, organ transplantation, and positive euthanasia. I hope we will have the courage, determination, and dedication to attain our goals.

REFERENCES

Downing, A. B. 1969. Euthanasia and the Right to Death. London, Peter Owen.

Ehrlich, P. R. 1968. The Population Bomb. New York, Ballantine Books, Inc.

Fletcher, J. F. 1954. Euthanasia, our right to die. *In* Morals and Medicine. New Jersey, Princeton University Press.

Laws, E. H., R. J. Bulger, T. R. Boyce, D. J. Thompson, and N. K. Brown. 1971. Views on euthanasia. *J. Med. Ed.* **46**:540.

Lederberg, J. 1967. Dangers of reprogramming cells. *Science.* **158**:313.

Meyers, D. W. 1970. The Human Body and the Law. Chicago, Aldine Publishing Company.

Nadler, H. L. 1969. Prenatal detection of genetic defects. *J. Ped.* **74**:132.

Nirenberg, M. W. 1967. Will society be prepared? *Science.* **157**:633.

Vaux, K. 1970. Who Shall Live? Philadelphia, Fortress Press.

Williams, G. 1957. The Sanctity of Life and the Criminal Law. New York, Alfred A. Knopf.

Williams, R. H. 1969. Our role in the generation, modification and termination of life. *Arch. Int. Med.* **124**:215.

Williams, R. H. 1970. Metabolism and mentation. *J. Clin. Endo.* **31**:461.

CHAPTER 8

AN ALTERNATIVE TO THE ETHIC OF EUTHANASIA

ARTHUR J. DYCK

Contemporary society and modern medicine face difficult policy decisions. This is illustrated most recently in the Voluntary Euthanasia Act of 1969, submitted for consideration in the British Parliament. The purpose of that act is to provide for "the administration of euthanasia to persons who request it and who are suffering from an irremediable condition" (Downing, 1971) and to enable such persons to make such a request in advance. For the purposes of that act, euthanasia means "the painless inducement of death" to be administered by a physician, i.e., "a registered medical practitioner."

The declaration that one signs under this act, should one become incurably ill and wish to have euthanasia administered, reads as follows:

> If I should at any time suffer from a serious physical illness or impairment reasonably thought in my case to be incurable and expected to cause me severe distress or render me incapable of rational existence, I request the administration of euthanasia at a time or in circumstances to be indicated or specified by me or, if it is apparent that I have become incapable of giving directions, at the discretion of the physician in charge of my case.
> In the event of my suffering from any of the conditions specified above, I request that no active steps should be taken . . . to prolong my life or restore me to consciousness.
> This declaration is to remain in force unless I revoke it, which I may do at any time. . . .
> I wish it to be understood that I have confidence in the good faith of my relatives and physicians, and fear degeneration and indignity far more than I fear premature death.

The ethic by which one justifies making such a declaration has been eloquently expressed by Joseph Fletcher. He speaks of "the right of spiritual beings to use intelligent control over physical nature rather than to submit beastlike to its blind workings." For Fletcher, "Death control, like birth control, is a matter of human dignity. Without it persons become puppets. To perceive this is to grasp the error lurking in the notion—widespread in medical circles—that life as such is the highest good."

Within our society today there are those who agree with the ethic of Joseph Fletcher. They agree also that an ethic that places a supreme value upon life is dominant in the medical profession. In a candid editorial (Cal. Med.), the traditional Western ethic with its affirmation of "the intrinsic worth and equal value of every human life regardless of its stage or condition" and with its roots in the Judaic and Christian heritage, is declared to be the basis for most of our laws and much of our social policy. What is more, the editorial says, "the reverence for each and every human life" is "a keystone of Western medicine and is the ethic which has caused physicians to try to preserve, protect, repair, prolong and enhance every human life which comes under their surveillance." Although this medical editor sees this traditional ethic as still clearly dominant, he is convinced that it is being eroded and that it is being replaced by a new ethic that he believes medicine should accept and applaud. This editor sees the beginning of the new ethic in the increasing acceptance of abortion, the general practice of which is in direct defiance of an ethic that affirms the "intrinsic and equal value for every human life regardless of its stage, condition, or status." For, in the opinion of this editor, human life begins at conception, and abortion is killing. Such killing is to be condoned and embraced by the new ethic.

In the above editorial a case is made for what is called "the quality of life." To increase the quality of life, it is assumed that the traditional Western ethic will necessarily have to be revised or even totally replaced. This, it is argued, is because it "will become necessary and acceptable to place relative rather than absolute values on such things as human lives, the use of scarce resources and the various elements which are to make up the quality of life or of living which is to be sought." On such a view, the new ethic aids medicine in improving the quality of life; the ethic designated as the old ethic, rooted in Judaism and Christianity, is treated as an impediment to medicine's efforts to improve the quality of life. What kind of ethic should guide contemporary decisions regarding sterilization, abortion, and euthanasia—decisions as to who shall live and who shall die? Given the limits of this chapter, we shall discuss and assess the ethic (moral policy) of those who favor a policy of voluntary euthanasia and the ethic (moral policy) of those who oppose it. (Abortion and sterilization are large topics I have discussed in some detail elsewhere [Dyck, 1971].) The term "euthanasia" is used here, exactly as in the Voluntary Euthanasia Act of 1969, to mean "the painless inducement of death."

THE ETHIC OF EUTHANASIA

What then is the ethic that guides those who support legislation like the Voluntary Euthanasia Act of 1969 and its Declaration? The arguments for euthanasia focus upon two humane and significant concerns: compassion for those who are painfully and terminally ill; and concern for the human dignity associated with freedom of choice. Compassion and freedom are values that sustain and enhance the common good. The question here, however, is how these values affect our behavior toward the dying.

The argument for compassion usually occurs in the form of attacking the inhumanity of keeping dying people alive when they are in great pain or when they have lost almost all of their usual functions, particularly when they have lost the ability or will to communicate with others. Thus, someone like Joseph Fletcher cites examples of people who are kept alive in a hopelessly debilitated state by means of the latest medical techniques, whether these be respirators, intravenous feeding, or the like. Often when Fletcher and others are arguing for the legalization of decisions not to intervene in these ways, the point is made that physicians already make decisions to turn off respirators or in other ways fail to use every means to prolong life. It is this allegedly compassionate behavior that the law would seek to condone and encourage.

The argument for compassion is supplemented by an argument for greater freedom for a patient to choose how and when he or she will die. For one thing, the patient should not be subjected to medical treatment to which that patient does not consent. Those who argue for voluntary euthanasia extend this notion by arguing that the choice to withhold techniques that would prolong life is a choice to shorten life. Hence, if one can choose to shorten one's life, why cannot one ask a physician by a simple and direct act of intervention to put an end to one's life? Here it is often argued that physicians already curtail life by means of painkilling drugs, which in the doses administered, will hasten death. Why should not the law recognize and sanction a simple and direct hastening of death, should the patient wish it?

How do the proponents of euthanasia view the general prohibition against killing? First of all, they maintain that we are dealing here with people who will surely die regardless of the intervention of medicine. They advocate the termination of suffering and the lawful foreshortening of the dying process. Secondly, although the patient is committing suicide, and the physician is an accomplice in such a suicide, both acts are morally justifiable to cut short the suffering of one who is dying.

It is important to be very clear about the precise moral reasoning by which advocates of voluntary euthanasia justify suicide and assisting a suicide. They make no moral distinction between those instances when a patient or a physician chooses to have life shortened by failing to accept or use life-prolonging techniques and those instances when a patient or a physician shorten life by employing a death-dealing chemical or instrument. They make no moral distinction between a drug given to kill pain, which also shortens life, and a substance given precisely to shorten life and for no other reason. Presumably these distinctions are not honored, because regardless of the stratagem employed—regardless of whether one is permitting to die or killing directly—the result is the same, the patient's life is shortened. Hence, it is maintained that, if you can justify one kind of act that shortens the life of the dying, you can justify any act that shortens the life of the dying when this act is seen to be willed by the one who is dying. Moral reasoning of this sort is strictly utilitarian; it focuses solely on the consequences of acts, not on their intent.

Even though the reasoning on the issue of compassion is so strictly utilitarian, one is puzzled about the failure to raise certain kinds of questions. A strict utilitarian might inquire about the effect of the medical practice of promoting or even encouraging direct acts on the part of physicians to shorten the lives of their patients. And, in the same vein, a utilitarian might also be very concerned about whether the loosening of constraints on physicians may not loosen the constraints on killing generally. There are two reasons these questions are either not raised or are dealt with rather summarily. First, it is alleged that there is no evidence that untoward consequences would result. And second, the value of freedom is invoked, so that the question of killing becomes a question of suicide and assistance in a suicide.

The appeal to freedom is not strictly a utilitarian argument, at least not for some proponents of voluntary euthanasia. Joseph Fletcher, for example, complains about the foolishness of nature in bringing about situations in which dying is a prolonged process of suffering. He feels strongly that the failure to permit or encourage euthanasia demeans the dignity of persons. Fletcher has two themes here: On the one hand, the more people are able to control the process of nature, the more dignity and freedom they have; on the other hand, people have dignity only insofar as they are able to choose when, how, and why they are to live or to die. For physicians this means also choices as to who is to die, because presumably one cannot assist in the suicide of just any patient who claims to be suffering, or who thinks he or she is dying.

The ethic that defends suicide as a matter of individual conscience and as an expression of human dignity is a very old ethic. Both the Stoics and the Epicureans considered the choice of one's own death as the ultimate expression of human freedom and as an essential component of the dignity that attaches to rational personhood. This willingness to take one's life is an aspect of Stoic courage (Tillich, 1952). A true Stoic could not be manipulated by those who threatened death. When death seemed inevitable, they chose it before someone could inflict it upon them. Human freedom for the Stoics was not complete unless one could also choose death and not compromise oneself for fear of it. All the "heroes" in literature exhibit this kind of Stoic courage in the face of death.

A euthanasia ethic, as exemplified already in ancient Stoicism, contains the following essential presuppositions or beliefs:

1) That an individual's life belongs to that individual to dispose of entirely as he or she wishes;
2) That the dignity that attaches to personhood by reason of the freedom to make moral choices demands also the freedom to take one's own life;
3) That there is such a thing as a life not worth living, whether by reason of distress, illness, physical or mental handicaps, or even sheer despair for whatever reason;
4) That what is sacred or supreme in value is the "human dignity" that resides in man's own rational capacity to choose and control life and death.

This commitment to the free exercise of the human capacity to control life and death takes on a distinct religious aura. Speaking of the death control that amniocentesis makes possible, Robert S. Morrison declares that, "the birth of babies with gross physical and mental handicaps will no longer be left entirely to God, to chance, or to the forces of nature."

AN ETHIC OF BENEMORTASIA

From our account of the ethic of euthanasia, those who oppose voluntary euthanasia would seem to lack compassion for the dying and the courage to affirm human freedom. They appear incompassionate because they oppose what has come to be regarded as synonymous with a good death—namely, a painless and deliberately foreshortened process of dying. The term euthanasia originally meant a painless and happy death with no reference to whether such a death was induced. Although this definition still appears in modern dictionaries, a second meaning of the term has come to prevail: euthanasia now generally means "an act or method of causing death painlessly so as to end suffering" (Webster's New World Dictionary, 1962). In short, it would appear that the advocates of euthanasia, i.e., of *causing* death, are the advocates of a good death, and the advocates of voluntary euthanasia seek for all of us the freedom to have a good death.

Because of this loss of a merely descriptive term for a happy death, it is necessary to invent a term for a happy or good death—namely, benemortasia. The familiar derivatives for this new term are *bene* (good) and *mors* (death). The meaning of "bene" in "benemortasia" is deliberately unspecified so that it does not necessarily imply that a death must be painless and/or induced in order to be good. What constitutes a good or happy death is a disputable matter of moral policy. How then should one view the arguments for voluntary euthanasia? And, if an ethic of euthanasia is unacceptable, what is an acceptable ethic of benemortasia?

An ethic of benemortasia does not stand in opposition to the values of compassion and human freedom. It differs, however, from the ethic of euthanasia in its understanding of how these values are best realized. In particular, certain constraints upon human freedom are recognized and emphasized as enabling human beings to increase compassion and freedom rather than diminish them. For the purposes of this essay, we trace the roots of our ethic of benemortasia to Jewish and Christian sources. This does not mean that such an ethic is confined to those traditions or to persons influenced by them any more than an ethic of euthanasia is confined to its Stoic origins or adherents.

The moral life of Jews and Christians alike is and has been guided by the Decalogue, or Ten Commandments. "Thou shalt not kill" is one of the clear constraints upon human decisions and actions expressed in the Decalogue. It is precisely the nature of this constraint that is at stake in decisions regarding euthanasia.

Modern biblical scholarship has discovered that the Decalogue, or Mosaic Covenant, is in the form of a treaty between a Suzerian and his people (Mendenhall, 1955). The point of such a treaty is to specify the relationship between a ruler and his people, and to set out the conditions necessary to form and sustain community with that ruler. One of the most significant purposes of such a treaty is to specify constraints that members of a community must observe if the community is to be viable at all. Fundamentally, the Decalogue articulates the indispensable prerequisites of the common life.

Viewed in this way the injunction not to kill is part of a total effort to prevent the destruction of the human community. It is an absolute prohibition in the sense that no society can be indifferent about the taking of human life. Any act, insofar as it is an act of taking a human life, is wrong, that is to say, taking a human life is a wrong-making characteristic of actions.

To say, however, that killing is prima facie wrong does not mean that an act of killing may never be justified (Ross, 1930). For example, a person's effort to prevent someone's death may lead to the death of the attacker. However, we can morally justify that act of intervention only because it is an act of saving a life, not because it is an act of taking a life. If it were simply an act of taking a life, it would be wrong.[1]

A further constraint upon human freedom within the Jewish and Christian traditions is articulated in a myth concerning the loss of paradise.

---

[1] One may be perplexed that societies with their roots in Jewish and Christian traditions have been able to justify capital punishment. If one believes that capital punishment will have a deterrent effect, i.e., will save lives, its justification is at least understandable. We have raised serious doubts in recent years as to its deterrent effect and hence now have good reason to question this practice.

The loss of Eden comes at the point where man and woman succumb to the temptation to know good and evil, and to know it in the perfect and ultimate sense in which a perfect and ultimate being would know it (Revised Standard Version of the Bible, 1952). To know who should live and who should die, one would have to know everything about people, including their ultimate destiny. Only God could have such knowledge. Trying to decide who shall live and who shall die is "playing god." It is tragic to "play god" because one does it with such limited and uncertain knowledge of what is good and evil.

This constraint upon freedom has a liberating effect in the practice of medicine. Nothing in Jewish and Christian tradition presumes that a physician has a clear mandate to impose his or her wishes and skills upon patients for the sake of prolonging the length of their dying where those patients are diagnosed as terminally ill and do not wish the interventions of the physician. Thus the freedom of the patient to accept his or her dying and to decide whether he or she is to have any particular kind of medical care is surely enhanced. A patient, who has every reason to believe that he or she is dying, would lose the last vestige of freedom were he or she denied the right to choose the circumstances under which the terminal illness would take its course. Presumably that patient is someone who has not chosen to die, but who does have some choices left as to how the last hours and days will be spent. Interventions, in the form of drugs, drainage tubes, or feeding by injection or whatever, may or may not be what the patient wishes or would find beneficial for these last hours or days. People who are dying have as much freedom as other living persons to accept or to refuse medical treatment when that treatment provides no cure for their ailment. There is nothing in the Jewish or Christian tradition that provides an exact blueprint as to what is the most compassionate thing to do for someone who is dying. Presumably the most compassionate act is to be a neighbor to such a person and to minister to such a person's needs. Depending upon the circumstances, this may or may not include intervention to prolong the process of dying.

Our ethic of benemortasia acknowledges the freedom of patients who are incurably ill to refuse interventions that prolong dying and the freedom of physicians to honor such wishes. However, these actions are not acts of suicide and assisting in suicide. In our ethic of benemortasia, suicide and assisting in suicide are unjustifiable acts of killing. Unlike the ethic of those who would legalize voluntary euthanasia, our ethic makes a moral distinction between acts that *permit* death and acts that *cause* death. As George P. Fletcher notes, one can make a sharp distinction, one that will stand up in law, between "permitting to die" and "causing death." Jewish and Christian tradition, particularly Roman Catholic thought, have maintained this clear distinction between the failure to use extraordinary measures (permitting to die) and direct intervention to bring about death (causing death).[2] A distinction is also drawn between a drug administered to cause death and a drug administered to ease pain which has the added effect of shortening life (see, for example, Smith, 1970).

Why are these distinctions important in instances where permitting to die or causing death both have the effect of shortening life? In both instances there is a failure to try to prolong the life of one who is dying. It is at this point that one must see why consequential reasoning is in itself too narrow, and why it is important also not to limit the discussion of benemortasia to the immediate relationship between a patient and his or her physician.

Where a person is dying of a terminal illness, it is fair to say that no one, including the dying person and his or her physician, has wittingly chosen this affliction and this manner or time of death. The choices that are left to a dying patient, an attendant physician, others who know the patient, and society concern how the last days of the dying person are to be spent.

From the point of view of the dying person, when could his or her decisions be called a deliberate act to end life, the act we usually designate as suicide? Only, it seems to me, when the dying person commits an act that has the immediate intent of ending life and has no other purpose. That act may be to use, or ask the physician to use, a chemical or an instrument that has no other immediate effect than to end the dying person's life. If, for the sake of relieving pain, a dying person chooses drugs administered in potent doses, the intent of this act is not to shorten life, even though it has that effect. It is a choice as to how to live while dying. Similarly, if a patient chooses to forego medical interventions that would have the effect of prolonging his or her life without in any way promising release from death, this also is a choice as to what is the most meaningful way to spend the remainder of life, however short that may be. The choice to use drugs to relieve pain and the choice not to use medical measures that cannot promise a cure for one's dying are no different in principle from the choices we make throughout our lives as to how much we will rest, how hard we will work, how little and how much medical intervention we will seek or tolerate, and the like. For society or physicians to map out life styles for individuals with respect to such decisions is surely beyond anything that we find in Stoic, Jewish, or Christian ethics. Such intervention in the liberty of individuals is far beyond what is required in any society whose rules are intended to constrain people against harming others.

But human freedom should not be extended to include the taking of

[2] See, for example, an excellent discussion by the Protestant Paul Ramsey, *The Patient as Person*, pp. 113–164, which contains many references also to Roman Catholic literature on the care for the dying. For the Jewish views, see the classic text by Immanuel Jakobovits, *Jewish Medical Ethics*. Whereas Jewish law forbids active euthanasia, Jakobovits makes it clear that "Jewish law sanctions and perhaps even demands the withdrawal of any factor—whether extraneous to the patient himself or not—which may artificially delay the demise of the final phase."

one's own life. Causing one's own death cannot generally be justified, even when one is dying. To see why this is so, we have to consider how causing one's death does violence to one's self and harms others.

The person who causes his or her own death repudiates the meaningfulness and worth of his or her own life. To decide to initiate an act that has as its primary purpose to end one's life is to decide that that life has no worth to anyone, especially to oneself. It is an act that ends all choices regarding what one's life and whatever is left of it is to symbolize.

Suicide is the ultimately effective way of shutting out all other people from one's life. Psychologists have observed how hostility for others can be expressed through taking one's own life. People who might want access to the dying one to make restitution, offer reparation, bestow last kindnesses, or clarify misunderstandings are cut off by such an act. Every kind of potentially and actually meaningful contact and relation among persons is irrevocably severed except by means of memories and whatever life beyond death may offer. Certainly for those who are left behind by death, there can remain many years of suffering occasioned by that death. The sequence of dying an inevitable death can be much better accepted than the decision on the part of a dying one that he or she has no worth to anyone. An act that presupposes that final declaration leaves tragic overtones for anyone who participated in even the smallest way in that person's dying.

But the problem is even greater. If in principle a person can take his or her own life whenever he or she no longer finds it meaningful, there is nothing in principle that prevents anyone from taking his or her life, no matter what the circumstances. For if the decision hinges on whether one regards his or her own life as meaningful, anyone can regard his or her own life as meaningless even under circumstances that would appear to be most fortunate and opportune for an abundant life.

What about those who would commit suicide or request euthanasia in order to cease being a "burden" on those who are providing care for them? If it is a choice to accept death by refusing non-curative care that prolongs dying, the freedom to embrace death or give one's life in this way is honored by our ethic of benemortasis. What is rejected is the freedom to cause death whether by suicide or by assisting in one. (Dyck, 1968, distinguishes between *giving* one's life and *taking* one's life.)

How a person dies has a definite meaning for those to whom that person is related. In the first year of bereavement, the rate of death among bereaved relatives of those who die in hospitals is twice that of bereaved relatives of those who die at home; sudden deaths away from hospital and home increase the death rate of the bereaved even more (Lasagna, 1970).

The courage to be, as expressed in Christian and Jewish thought, is more than the overcoming of the fear of death, although it includes that

Stoic dimension. It is the courage to accept one's own life as having worth no matter what life may bring, including the threat of death, because that life remains meaningful and is regarded as worthy by God, regardless of what that life may be like.

An ethic of benemortasia stresses what Tillich has called the "courage to be as a part"—namely, the courage to affirm not only oneself, but also one's participation as a self in a universal community of beings. The courage to be as a part recognizes that one is not merely one's own, that one's life is a gift bestowed and protected by the human community and by the ultimate forces that make up the cycle of birth and death. In the cycle of birth and death, there may be suffering, as there is joy, but suffering does not render a life meaningless or worthless. Suffering people need the support of others; suffering people should not be encouraged to commit suicide by their community, or that community ceases to be a community.

This consideration brings us to a further difficulty with voluntary euthanasia and its legalization. Not only does euthanasia involve suicide, but also, if legalized, it sanctions assistance in a suicide by physicians. Legislation like the Voluntary Euthanasia Act of 1969 makes it a duty of the medical profession to take someone else's life for him. Here the principle not to kill is even further eroded and violated by giving the physician the power and the encouragement to decide that someone else's life is no longer worth living. The whole notion that a physician can engage in euthanasia implies acceptance of the principle that another person's life is no longer meaningful enough to sustain, a principle that does not afford protection for the lives of any of the most defenseless, voiceless, or otherwise dependent members of a community. Everyone in a community is potentially a victim of such a principle, particularly among members of racial minorities, the very young, and the very old.

Those who would argue that these consequences of a policy of voluntary euthanasia cannot be predicted fail to see two things: that we have already had an opportunity to observe what happens when the principle that sanctions euthanasia is accepted by a society; and that regardless of what the consequences may be of such acts, the acts themselves are wrong in principle.

With respect to the first point, Leo Alexander's (1949) very careful analysis of medical practices and attitudes of German physicians before and during the reign of Nazism in Germany should serve as a definite warning against the consequences of making euthanasia a public policy. He notes that the outlook of German physicians that led to their cooperation in what became a policy of mass murders,

> started with the acceptance of that attitude, basic in the euthanasia movement, that there is such a thing as life not worthy to be lived. This attitude in its early stages concerned itself merely with the severely and chronically sick. Gradually the sphere of those to be included in this category was enlarged

to include the socially unproductive, the racially unwanted, and finally all non-Germans. But it is important to realize that the infinitely small wedged-in lever from which this entire trend of mind received its impetus was the attitude toward the nonrehabilitable sick.

Those who reject out of hand any comparison of what happened in Nazi Germany with what we can expect here in the United States should consider current examples of medical practice in this nation. The treatment of mongoloids is a case in point. Now that the notion is gaining acceptance that a fetus diagnosed in the womb as mongoloid can, at the discretion of a couple or the pregnant woman, be justifiably aborted, instances of infanticide in hospitals are being reported. At Johns Hopkins Hospital, for example, an allegedly mongoloid infant whose parents would not permit an operation that is generally successful in securing normal physical health and development, was ordered to have "nothing by mouth," condemning that infant to a death that took 15 days. By any of our existing laws, this was a case of murder, justified on the ground that this particular life was somehow not worth saving. (If one argues that the infant was killed because the parents did not want it, we have in this kind of case an even more radical erosion of our restraints upon killing.)

Someone may argue that the mongoloid was permitted to die, not killed. But this is faulty reasoning. In the case of an infant whose future life and happiness could be reasonably assured through surgery, we are not dealing with someone who is dying and with intervention that has no curative effect. The fact that some physicians refer to this as a case of permitting to die is an ominous portent of the dangers inherent in accepting the principle that a physician or another party can decide for a patient that his or her life is not worth living. Equally ominous is the assumption that this principle, once accepted, can easily be limited to cases of patients for whom no curative intervention is known to exist.

With all the risks that attend changing the physician's role from one who sustains life to one who induces death, one may well ask why physicians should be called upon to assist a suicide?

M. R. Barrington, an advocate of suicide and of voluntary euthanasia, is aware of the difficulty of making this request of physicians and of the necessity for justifying legalization of such requests. She suggests that the role of the physician in assisting suicide is essential, "especially as human frailty requires that it should be open to a patient to ask the doctor to choose a time for the giving of euthanasia that is not known to the patient" (Barrington, 1971). This appeal to "human frailty" is very telling. The hesitation to commit suicide and the ambivalence of the dying about their worth should give one pause before one signs a declaration that empowers a physician to decide that at some point one can no longer be trusted as competent to judge whether or not one wants to die. Physicians are also frail humans, and mistaken diagnoses, research interests, and sometimes errors of judgment that stem from a desire for organs, are part of the practice of medicine.[3]

Comatose patients pose special problems for an ethic of benemortasia as they do for the advocates of voluntary euthanasia. Where patients are judged to be irreversibly comatose and where sustained efforts have been made to restore such persons to consciousness, no clear case can be made for permitting to die, even though it seems merciful to do so. It seems that the best we can do is to develop some rough social and medical consensus about a reasonable length of time for keeping "alive" a person's organ systems after "brain death" has been decided (Ramsey, 1970). Because of the pressures to do research and to transplant organs, it may also be necessary to employ special patient advocates who are not physicians and nurses. These patient advocates, trained in medical ethics, would function as ombudsmen.

In summary, even if the practice of euthanasia were to be confined to those who voluntarily request an end to their lives, no physician could in good conscience participate in such an act. To decide directly to cause the death of a patient is to abandon a cardinal principle of medical practice—namely, to do no harm to one's patient. The relief of suffering, which is surely a time-honored role for the physician, does not extend to an act that presupposes that the life of a patient who is suffering is not worthy to be lived. As we have argued, not even the patient who is dying can justifiably and unilaterally universalize the principle by which a dying life would be declared to be worthless.

Some readers may remain unconvinced that euthanasia is morally wrong as a general policy. Perhaps what still divides us is what distinguishes a Stoic from a Jewish and Christian way of life. The Stoic heritage declares that my life and my selfhood are my own to dispose of as I see fit and when I see fit. The Jewish and Christian heritage declares that my life and my selfhood are not my own, and are not mine to dispose of as I see fit.

In the words of H. Richard Neibuhr,

> I live but do not have the power to live. And further, I may die at any moment but I am powerless to die. It was not in my power, nor in my parents' power, to elect my *self* into existence. Though they willed a child or consented to it they did not will *me*—this I, thus and so. And so also I now, though I *will* to be no more, cannot elect myself out of existence, if the inscrutable power by which I am, elects otherwise. Though I wish to be mortal, if the power that threw me into being in this mortal destructible body elects me into being again there is nothing I can do about that. I can destroy the life of my body. Can I destroy myself? This remains the haunting question of the literature of suicide and of all the lonely debates of men to whom existence is a burden. Whether they shall wake up again, either here in this life or there in some other mode of being, is beyond their control.

[3] See Yale Kamisar, "Euthanasia Legislation: Some Non-Religious Objections" for copious documentation of medical error and other aspects of medical practice that would make euthanasia legislation hazardous.

> We can choose among many alternatives; but the power to choose self-existence
> or self-extinction is not ours. Men can practice birth-control, not self-creation;
> they can commit *bio*cide; whether they can commit suicide, self-destruction,
> remains a question.

Although one has the power to commit biocide, this does not give one
the right to do so. Niebuhr views our lives as shaped by our responses
to others and their responses to us. All of us are in responsible relations
to others. The claim that an act of suicide (biocide) would harm no one
else is unrealistic. To try to make that a reality would require an incredibly
lonely existence cut off from all ties of friendship, cooperation, and mutual
dependence. And in so doing, we would repudiate the value and benefits
of altruism.

The other points at which the proponents of euthanasia and the advocates of benemortasia part company concern the perception of the context in which all moral decisions are made. Here again the division has
religious overtones. Those who decide for euthanasia seem to accept an
ethic which ultimately privatizes and subjectivizes the injunction not to
kill. Those who oppose euthanasia see the decision not to kill as one that
is in harmony with what is good for everyone, and indeed is an expression
of what is required of everyone if goodness is to be pervasive and powerful
on earth. Once again, H. Richard Niebuhr has eloquently expressed this
latter position:

> All my specific and relative evaluations expressed in my interpretations and
> responses are shaped, guided, and formed by the understanding of good and
> evil I have *upon the whole*. In distrust of the radical action by which I
> am, by which my society is, by which this world is, I must find my center
> of valuation in myself, or in my nation, or in my church, or in my science,
> or in humanity, or in life. Good and evil in this view mean what is good
> for me and bad for me; or good and evil for my nation, or good and evil
> for one of these finite causes, such as mankind, or life or reason. But should
> it happen that confidence is given to me in the power by which all things
> are and by which I am; should I learn in the depths of my existence to
> praise the creative source, . . . all my relative evaluations will be subjected
> to the continuing and great correction. They will be made to fit into a total
> process producing good—not what is good for me (though my confidence
> accepts that as included), nor what is good for man (though that is also
> included), nor what is good for the development of life (though that also
> belongs in the picture), but what is good for being, for universal being, or
> for God, center and source of all existence.

Our ethic of benemortasia has argued for the following beliefs and
values:

1) that an individual person's life is not solely at the disposal of that person; every human life is part of the human community that bestows and
   protects the lives of its members; the possibility of community itself
   depends upon constraints against taking life;
2) that the dignity that attaches to personhood by reason of the freedom
   to make moral choices includes the freedom of dying people to refuse

noncurative, life-prolonging interventions when one is dying, but does not extend to taking one's life or causing death for someone who is dying;

3) that every life has some worth; there is no such thing as a life not worth living;

4) that the supreme value is goodness itself to which the dying and those who care for the dying are responsible. Religiously expressed the supreme value is God. Less than perfectly good beings, human beings, require constraints upon their decisions regarding those who are dying. No human being or human community can presume to know who deserves to live or to die.

At the same time, we have implied throughout that religion and the Jewish and Christian expressions of it are not obstacles to modern medicine and a better life; rather they help foster humanity's ceaseless quest to preserve and enhance human life on this earth.

REFERENCES

Alexander, L. 1949. Medical science under dictatorship. *New Engl. J. Med.* **241**:39–47. For a thorough study of the "edge of the wedge" argument as it applies to legalizing voluntary euthanasia, see Sissela Bok, "Voluntary Euthanasia," unpublished Ph.D. thesis.

Barrington, M. R. Apologia for suicide. *In* Downing, *op. cit.*

Downing, A. B., ed. 1971. Euthanasia and the Right to Death. New York, Humanities Press.

Dyck, A. J. Religious Views and U.S. Population Policy (prepared for the Commission on Population Growth and the American Future and available at the Institute of Society, Ethics and the Life Sciences, Hastings-On-Hudson, N.Y.). See also Population policies and ethical acceptability. *In* Rapid Population Growth: Consequences and Policy Implications. Roger Revelle et al., eds. Baltimore, Johns Hopkins Press, 1971. See also 1972. Perplexities for the would-be-liberal in abortion, *J. Rep. Med.* **8**(6):351–4.

Dyck, A. J. 1965. Questions for the global conscience. *Psych. Today.* **2**(4):38–42.

Editorial. 1970. A new ethic for medicine and society. *Cal. Med.* **113**:67–68.

Fletcher, G. P. Prolonging life: some legal considerations. *In* Downing, *op. cit.*

Fletcher, J. The patient's right to die. *In* Downing, *op. cit.*

Genesis, Chapter 3, The Holy Bible. 1952. Revised Standard Version. New York, Thomas Nelson and Sons.

Jakobovits, I. 1967. Jewish Medical Ethics. New York, Bloch Publishing Co.

Kamisar, Y. Euthanasia legislation: some non-religious objections. *In* Downing, *op. cit.*

Lasagna, L. 1970. The prognosis of death. *In* The Dying Patient. O. G. Brim et al., eds. New York, Russell Sage Foundation. Pages 80–81.

Mendenhall, G. E. 1955. Law and Covenant in Israel and the Ancient Near
    East. Pittsburgh, Biblical Colloquium.
Morison, R. S. 1971. Chairman's introduction. *In* Early Diagnosis of Human
    Genetic Defects. M. Harris, ed. H. E. W. Publication No. (NIH) 72-25.
    Page 9.
Niebuhr, H. R. 1963. The Responsible Self. New York, Harper & Row.
Ramsey, P. 1970. The Patient as a Person. New Haven, Yale University
    Press.
Ross, W. D. 1930. The Right and the Good. Clarendon, Oxford University
    Press. (See pp. 19–21 for an explanation and a list of *prima facie* duties.)
Smith, H. L. 1970. Ethics and the New Medicine. New York, Abingdon
    Press.
Tillich, P. 1952. The Courage To Be. New Haven, Yale University Press.

CHAPTER 9

ETHICS AND EUTHANASIA

JOSEPH FLETCHER

It is harder morally to justify letting somebody die a slow and ugly death, dehumanized, than it is to justify helping him to escape from such misery. This is the case at least in any code of ethics which is humanistic or personalistic, i.e., in any code of ethics which has a value system that puts humanness and personal integrity above biological life and function. It makes no difference whether such an ethics system is grounded in a theistic or a naturalistic philosophy. We may believe that God wills human happiness or that man's happiness is, as Protagoras thought, a self-validating standard of the good and the right. But what counts *ethically* is whether human needs come first—not whether the ultimate sanction is transcendental or secular.

What follows is a moral defense of euthanasia. Primarily I mean active or positive euthanasia, which helps the patient to die; not merely the passive or negative form of euthanasia which "lets the patient go" by simply withholding life-preserving treatments. The plain fact is that negative euthanasia is already a fait accompli in modern medicine. Every day in a hundred hospitals across the land decisions are made clinically that the line has been crossed from prolonging genuinely human life to only prolonging subhuman dying, and when that judgment is made respirators are turned off, life-perpetuating intravenous infusions stopped, proposed surgery canceled, and drugs countermanded. So-called "Code 90" stickers are put on many record-jackets, indicating "Give no intensive care or resuscitation." Arguing pro and con about negative euthanasia is therefore merely flogging a dead horse. Ethically, the issue whether we may "let the patient go" is as dead as Queen Anne.

Straight across the board of religious traditions there is substantial agreement that we are not morally obliged to preserve life in *all* terminal cases. (The religious-ethical defense of negative euthanasia is far more generally accepted by ministers and priests than medical people recognize or as yet even accept.) Humanist morality shows the same nonabsolutistic attitude about preserving life. Indeed, not only Protestant, Catholic, and Jewish teaching take this stance; but it is also true of Buddhist, Hindu, and Moslem ethics. In short, the claim that we ought always to do everything we can to preserve any patient's life as long as possible is now discredited. The last serious advocate of this unconditional pro-vitalist doctrine was David Karnofsky—the great tumor research scientist of the Sloan-Kettering Institute in New York. The issue about *negative* euthanasia is settled ethically.

Given modern medicine's capabilities always to do what is technically possible to prolong life would be morally indefensible on any ground other than a vitalistic outlook; that is, the opinion that biological survival is the first-order value and that all other considerations, such as personality, dignity, well-being, and self-possession, necessarily take second place. Vestigial last-ditch pro-vitalists still mumble threateningly about "what the Nazis did," but in fact the Nazis never engaged in euthanasia or mercy killing; what they did was merciless killing, either genocidal or for ruthless experimental purposes.

THE ETHICAL AND THE PRE-ETHICAL

One way of putting this is to say that the traditional ethics based on the sanctity of life—which was the classical doctrine of medical idealism in its prescientific phases—must give way to a code of ethics of the *quality* of life. This comes about for humane reasons. It is a result of modern medicine's successes, not failures. New occasions teach new duties, time makes ancient good uncouth, as Whittier said.

There are many pre-ethical or "metaethical" issues that are often overlooked in ethical discussions. People of equally good reasoning powers and a high respect for the rules of inference will still puzzle and even infuriate each other. This is because they fail to see that their moral judgments proceed from significantly different values, ideals, and starting points. If God's will (perhaps "specially revealed" in the Bible or "generally revealed" in his Creation) is against any responsible human initiative in the dying process, or if sheer life is believed to be, as such, more desirable than anything else, then those who hold these axioms will not find much merit in any case we might make for either kind of euthanasia—positive or negative. If, on the other hand, the highest good is personal integrity and human well-being, then euthanasia in either form could or might be the right thing to do, depending on the situation. This latter kind of ethics is the key to what will be said in this chapter.

Let's say it again, clearly, for the sake of truly serious ethical discourse. Many of us look upon living and dying as we do upon health and medical care, as person-centered. This is not a solely or basically biological understanding of what it means to be "alive" and to be "dead." It asserts that a so-called "vegetable," the brain-damaged victim of an auto accident or a microcephalic newborn or a case of massive neurologic deficit and lost cerebral capacity, who nevertheless goes on breathing and whose mid-brain or brain stem continues to support spontaneous organ functions, is in such a situation no longer a human being, no longer a person, no longer really alive. It is *personal* function that counts, not biological function. Humanness is understood as primarily rational, not physiological. This "doctrine of man" puts the *homo* and *ratio* before the *vita*. It holds that being human is more "valuable" than being alive.

All of this is said just to make it clear from the outset that biomedical progress is forcing us, whether we welcome it or not, to make fundamental *conceptual* changes as well as scientific and medical changes. Not only are the conditions of life and death changing, because of our greater control and in consequence our greater decision-making responsibility; our *definitions* of life and death also have to change to keep pace with the new realities.

These changes are signaled in a famous surgeon's remark recently: "When the brain is gone there is no point in keeping anything else going." What he meant was that with an end of cerebration, i.e., the function of the cerebral cortex, the *person* is gone (dead) no matter how many other spontaneous or artificially supported functions persist in the heart, lungs, and vascular system.[1] Such noncerebral processes might as well be turned off, whether they are natural or artificial.

This conclusion is of great philosophical and religious interest because it reaffirms the ancient Christian-European belief that the core of humanness, of the *humanum,* lies in the *ratio*—man's rational faculty. It is not the loss of brain function in general but of cerebral function (the synthesizing "mind") in particular that establishes that death has ensued.

Using the old conventional conceptual apparatus, we naturally thought about both life and death as events, not as processes, which, of course, they are. We supposed that these events or episodes depended on the accidents of "nature" or on some kind of special providence. It is therefore no surprise to hear people grumbling that a lot of the decision making that has to be carried out in modern medical care is "playing God." And given that way of thinking the only possible answer to the charge is to accept it: "Yes, we *are* playing God." But the real question is: Which or whose God are we playing?

The old God who was believed to have a monopoly control of birth and death, allowing for no human responsibility in either initiating or terminating a life, was a primitive "God of the gaps"—a mysterious and awesome deity who filled in the gaps of our knowledge and of the control

[1] The "brain death" definition of the Harvard Medical School's *ad hoc* committee is far too imprecise, effecting no real difference from the traditional clinical definition. The recent Kansas statute (Ann. Supp., 77-262, 1971) which is based upon it changes nothing since it requires absence of *brain* function, whereas what is definitive is cerebration, not just any or all brain functions regardless of whether they are contributory to personal quality.

which our knowledge gives us. "He" was, so to speak, an hypothecation of human ignorance and helplessness.

In their growing up spiritually, men are now turning to a God who is the creative principle behind things, who is behind the test tube as much as the earthquake and volcano. This God can be believed in, but the old God's sacralistic inhibitions on human freedom and research can no longer be submitted to.

We must rid ourselves of that obsolete theodicy according to which God is not only the cause but also the builder of nature and its works, and not only the builder but even the manager. On this archaic basis it would be God himself who is the efficient as well as the final cause of earthquake and fire, of life and death, and by logical inference any "interference with nature" (which is exactly what medicine is) is "playing God." That God, seriously speaking, is dead.

ELECTIVE DEATH

Most of our major moral problems are posed by scientific discoveries and by the subsequent technical know-how we gain, in the control of life and health and death. Ethical questions jump out at us from every laboratory and clinic. May we exercise these controls at all, we wonder—and if so, then when, where, how? Every advance in medical capabilities is an increase in our moral responsibility, a widening of the range of our decision-making obligations.

Genetics, molecular biology, fetology, and obstetrics have developed to a point where we now have effective control over the start of human life's continuum. And therefore from now on it would be irresponsible to leave baby-making to mere chance and impulse, as we once *had* to do. Modern men are trying to face up in a mature way to our emerging needs of quality control—medically, ecologically, legally, socially.

What has taken place in birth control is equally imperative in death control. The whole armory of resuscitation and prolongation of life forces us to be responsible decision makers about death as much as about birth; there must be quality control in the terminating of life as in its initiating. It is ridiculous to give ethical approval to the positive ending of subhuman life in utero, as we do in therapeutic abortions for reasons of mercy and compassion, but refuse to approve of positively ending a subhuman life in extremis. If we are morally obliged to put an end to a pregnancy when an amniocentesis reveals a terribly defective fetus, we are equally obliged to put an end to a patient's hopeless misery when a brain scan reveals that a patient with cancer has advanced brain metastases.

Furthermore, as I shall shortly explain, it is morally evasive and disingenuous to suppose that we can condemn or disapprove positive acts of care and compassion but in spite of that approve negative strategies to achieve exactly the same purpose. This contradiction has equal force whether the euthanasia comes at the fetal point on life's spectrum or at some terminal point post-natally.

Only man is aware of death. Animals know pain, and fear it, but not death. Furthermore, in humans the ability to meet death and even to regard it sometimes as a friend is a sign of manliness. But in the new patterns of medicine and health care patients tend to die in a moribund or comatose state, so that death comes without the patient's knowledge. The Elizabethan litany's petition, ". . . from sudden death, good Lord, deliver us," has become irrelevant much if not most of the time.

It is because of this "incompetent" condition of so many of the dying that we cannot discuss the ethical issues of elective death only in the narrow terms of voluntary, patient-chosen euthanasia. A careful typology of elective death will distinguish at least *four* forms—ways of dying which are not merely willy-nilly matters of blind chance but of choice, purpose, and responsible freedom (historical ethics and moral theology are obviously major sources of suggestion for these distinctions):

(1) Euthanasia, or a "good death," can be *voluntary and direct,* i.e., chosen and carried out by the patient. The most familiar way is the overdose left near at hand for the patient. It is a matter of simple request and of personal liberty. If it can be held in the abortion debate that compulsory pregnancy is unjust and that women should be free to control their own bodies when other's lives (fetuses) are at stake, do not the same moral claims apply to control of the lives and bodies of people too? In any particular case we might properly raise the question of the patient's competence, but to hold that euthanasia in this category is justifiable entails a rejection of the simplistic canard that all suicide victims are mentally disordered.

Voluntary euthanasia is, of course, a form of suicide. Presumably a related issue arises around the conventional notion of consent in medical ethics. The codes (American Medical Association, Helsinki, World Medical Association, Nuremberg) all contend that valid consent to any surgery or treatment requires a reasonable prospect of benefit to the patient. What, then, is benefit? Could death in some situations be a benefit? My own answer is in the affirmative.

(2) Euthanasia can be *voluntary but indirect.* The choice might be made either in situ or long in advance of a terminal illness, e.g., by exacting a promise that if and when the "bare bodkin" or potion cannot be self-administered somebody will do it for the patient. In this case the patient gives to others—physicians, lawyers, family, friends—the discretion to end it all as and when the situation requires, if the patient becomes comatose or too dysfunctioned to make the decision pro forma. There is already a form called the Living Will, sent upon request to thousands by the Euthanasia Educational Fund (although its language appears to limit it to

merely negative methods). This perfectly reasonable "insurance" device is being explored by more and more people, as medical prolongation of life tends to make them more afraid of senescence than of death.

Since both the common law tradition and statute law are caught practically unequipped to deal with this medical-legal lag, the problem is being examined worriedly and behind the scenes by lawyers and legislators. They have little or no case law to work with. As things stand now the medieval outlook of the law treats self-administered euthanasia as suicide and when effected by a helping hand as murder.

(3) Euthanasia may be *direct but involuntary*. This is the form in which a simple "mercy killing" is done on a patient's behalf without his present or past request. Instances would be when an idiot is given a fatal dose or the death of a child in the worst stages of Tay-Sachs disease is speeded up, or when a man trapped inextricably in a blazing fire is shot to end his suffering, or a shutdown is ordered on a patient deep in a mindless condition, irreversibly, perhaps due to an injury or an infection or some biological breakdown. It is in this form, as directly involuntary, that the problem has reached the courts in legal charges and indictments.

To my knowledge Uruguay is the only country that allows it. Article 37 of the *Codiga Penal* specifically states that although it is a "crime" the courts are authorized to forego any penalty. In time the world will follow suit. Laws in Colombia and in the Soviet Union (Article 50 of the Code of Criminal Procedure) are similar to Uruguay's, but in their codes freedom from punishment is exceptional rather than normative. In Italy, Germany, and Switzerland the law provides for a reduction of penalties when it is done upon the patient's request.

The conflict and tension between the stubborn prohibitionism on the one hand and a humane compassion on the other may be seen in the legal history of the issue in the United States. Eleven cases of "mercy killing" have actually reached the courts: one was on a charge of voluntary manslaughter, with a conviction and penalty of three to six years in prison and a $500 fine; one was for first-degree murder, resulting in a conviction, which was promptly reduced to a penalty of six years in jail with immediate parole. All of the other nine cases were twisted into "temporary insanity" or no-proof judgments—in short, no convictions.

(4) Finally, euthanasia might be *both indirect and involuntary*. This is the "letting the patient go" tactic which is taking place every day in our hospitals. Nothing is done for the patient positively to release him from his tragic condition (other than "trying to make him comfortable"), and what is done negatively is decided *for* him rather than in response to his request.

As we all know, even this passive policy of compassion is a grudging one, done perforce. Even so, it remains at least theoretically vulnerable to malpractice suits under the lagging law—brought, possibly, by angry or venal members of the family or suit-happy lawyers. A sign of the times was the bill to give negative euthanasia a legal basis in Florida, introduced by a physician member of the legislature.

But *ethically* regarded, this indirect-involuntary form of euthanasia is manifestly superficial, morally timid, and evasive of the real issue. I repeat: it is harder morally to justify letting somebody die a slow and ugly death, dehumanized, than it is to justify *helping* him to avoid it.

MEANS AND ENDS

What, then, is the real issue? In a few words, it is whether we can morally justify taking it into our own hands to hasten death for ourselves (suicide) or for others (mercy killing) out of reasons of compassion. The answer to this in my view is clearly Yes, on both sides of it. Indeed, *to justify either one, suicide or mercy killing, is to justify the other.*

The heart of the matter analytically is the question of whether the end justifies the means. If the end sought is the patient's death as a release from pointless misery and dehumanization, then the requisite or appropriate means is justified. Immanuel Kant said that if we will the end we will the means. The old maxim of some moral theologians was *finis sanctificat media*. The point is that no act is anything but random and *meaningless* unless it is purposefully related to some end or object. To be moral an act must be seeking an end.

However, to hold that the end justifies the means does not entail the absurd notion that *any* means can be justified by *any* end. The priority of the end is paired with the principle of "proportionate good"; any disvalue in the means must be outweighed by the value gained in the end. In systems analysis, with its pragmatic approach, the language would be: the benefit must repay the cost or the trade-off is not justified. It comes down to this, that in some situations a morally good end can justify a relatively "bad" means, on the principle of proportionate good.

The really searching question of conscience is, therefore, whether we are right in believing that *the well-being of persons* is the highest good. If so, then it follows that either suicide or mercy killing could be the right thing to do in some exigent and tragic circumstances. This could be the case, for instance, when an incorrigible "human vegetable," whether spontaneously functioning or artificially supported, is progressively degraded while constantly eating up private or public financial resources in violation of the distributive justice owed to others. In such cases the patient is actually already departed and only his body is left, and the needs of others have a stronger claim upon us morally. The fair allocation of scarce resources is as profound an ethical obligation as any we can imagine in a civilized society, and it arises very practically at the clinical level when triage officers make their decisions at the expense of some patients' needs in favor of others.

Another way of putting this is to say that the crucial question is not whether the end justifies the means (what else could?) but *what justifies the end?* And this chapter's answer is, plainly and confidently, that human happiness and well-being is the highest good or *summum bonum,* and that therefore any ends or purposes which that standard or ideal validates are just, right, good. This is what humanistic medicine is all about; it is what the concepts of loving concern and social justice are built upon.

This position comes down to the belief that our moral acts, including suicide and mercy killing, are right or wrong depending on the consequences aimed at (we sometimes fail, of course, through ignorance or poor reasoning), and that the consequences are good or evil according to whether and how much they serve humane values. In the language of ethics this is called a "consequential" method of moral judgment.

I believe that this code of ethics is both implicit and explicit in the morality of medical care and biomedical research. Its reasoning is inductive, not deductive, and it proceeds empirically from the data of each actual case or problem, choosing the course that offers an optimum or maximum of desirable consequences. Medicine is not a-prioristic or *prejudiced* in its ethos and modalities, and therefore to proscribe either suicide or mercy killing is so blatantly nonconsequential that it calls for critical scrutiny. It fails to make sense. It is unclinical and doctrinaire.

The problem exists because there is another kind of ethics, radically different from consequential ethics. This other kind of ethics holds that our actions are right or wrong according to whether they follow universal rules of conduct and absolute norms: that we ought or ought not to do certain things no matter how good or bad the consequences might be foreseeably. Such rules are usually prohibitions or taboos, expressed as thou-shalt-nots. Whereas this chapter's ethics is teleological or end-oriented, the opposite approach is "deontological" (from the Greek *deonteis,* meaning duty); i.e., it is duty-ethics, not goal-ethics. Its advocates sometimes sneer at any determination of obligation in terms of consequences, calling it "a mere morality of goals."

In duty-ethics what is right is whatever act obeys or adheres to the rules, even though the foreseeable result will be inhumane. That is, its highest good is not human happiness and well-being but obedience to a rule—or what we might call a prejudiced or predetermined decision based not on the clinical variables but on some transcending generality.

For example, the fifth of the Ten Commandments, which prohibits killing, is a no-no rule for nonconsequentialists when it comes to killing in the service of humane values like mercy and compassion, and yet at the same time they ignore their "moral law" when it comes to self-defense. The egocentricity and solipsism in this moral posture, which is a very common one, never ceases to bemuse consequentialists. You may end your neighbor's life for your own sake but you may not do it for his sake! And you may end your own life for your neighbor's sake, as in an act of sacrificial heroism, but you may not end your life for your own sake. This is a veritable mare's nest of nonsense!

The plain hard logic of it is that the end or purpose of both negative and positive euthanasia is exactly the same: to contrive or bring about the patient's death. Acts of deliberate omission are morally not different from acts of commission. But in the Anglo-American *law*, it is a crime to push a blind man off the cliff. It is not, however, a crime to deliberately not lift a finger to prevent his walking over the edge. This is an unpleasant feature of legal reasoning which is alien to ethics and to a sensitive conscience. Ashamed of it, even the courts fall back on such legal fictions as "insanity" in euthanasia cases, and this has the predictable effect of undermining our respect for the law.

There is something obviously evasive when we rule motive out in charging people with the crime of mercy killing, but then bring it back in again for purposes of determining punishment! It is also a menacing delimitation of the concepts of culpability, responsibility, and negligence. No *ethically* disciplined decision maker could so blandly separate right and wrong from motives, foresight, and consequences. (Be it noted, however, that motive is taken into account in German and Swiss law, and that several European countries provide for recognition of "homicide when requested" as a special category.)

It is naïve and superficial to suppose that because we don't "do anything positively" to hasten a patient's death we have thereby avoided complicity in his death. Not doing anything is doing something; it is a decision to act every bit as much as deciding for any other deed. If I decide not to eat or drink any more, knowing what the consequence will be, I have committed suicide as surely as if I had used a gas oven. If physicians decide not to open an imperforate anus in a severely 21-trisomy newborn, they have committed mercy killing as surely as if they had used a poison pellet!

Let the reader at this point now ask himself if he is a consequentialist or an a priori decision maker; and again, let him ask himself if he is a humanist, religious or secular, or alternatively has something he holds to be better or more obliging than the well-being of the patient. (Thoughtless religious people will sometimes point out that we are required to love God as well as our neighbors, but can the two loves ever come into conflict? Actually, is there any way to love God other than through the neighbor? Only mystics imagine that they can love God directly and discretely.)

Occasionally I hear a physician say that he could not resort to positive euthanasia. That may be so. What anybody would do in such tragic situations is a problem in psychology, however, not in ethics. We are not asking what we would do but what we should do. Any of us who has an intimate knowledge of what happens in terminal illnesses can tell stories of rational people—both physicians and family—who were quite clear ethically about the rightness of an overdose or of "turning off the machine," and yet found themselves too inhibited to give the word or do the deed. That is a phenomenon of primary interest to psychology, but of only incidental interest to ethics.

Careful study of the best texts of the Hippocratic Oath shows that it says nothing at all about preserving life, as such. It says that "so far as power and discernment shall be mine, I will carry out regimen for the benefit of the sick and will keep them from harm and wrong." The case for euthanasia depends upon how we understand "benefit of the sick" and "harm" and "wrong." If we regard dehumanized and merely biological life as sometimes real harm and the opposite of benefit, to refuse to welcome or even introduce death would be quite wrong morally.

In most states in this country people can and do carry cards, legally established (by Anatomical Gift Acts), which explain the carrier's wish that when he dies his organs and tissue should be used for transplant when needed by the living. The day will come when people will also be able to carry a card, notarized and legally executed, which explains that they do not want to be kept alive beyond the *humanum* point, and authorizing the ending of their biological processes by any of the methods of euthanasia which seems appropriate. Suicide may or may not be the ultimate problem of philosophy, as Albert Camus thought it is, but in any case it is the ultimate problem of medical ethics.

CHAPTER 10

ETHICAL AND MORAL PROBLEMS IN THE USE OF ARTIFICIAL AND TRANSPLANTED ORGANS

J. RUSSELL ELKINTON

One of the dramatic achievements of medicine during the past two decades has been the development of the use of artificial and transplanted organs. This development has required the surmounting of many difficult technical problems in the fields of medicine, surgery, immunology, and biomedical engineering. The difficult problems, however, have not been limited to these fields; as these techniques have been developed and applied, it has become apparent that the procedures pose grave issues of a moral and ethical nature. What these issues are, how they have been met to date, and what they may be in the future, are the subjects of this chapter.

Many different organs have been transplanted with more or less success, and a number of different organs and parts of the human body have been replaced with artificial substitutes. For the purposes of this chapter, however, the discussion will be limited to the transplantation of the kidney and the complementary use of mechanical substitutes (dialyzers) for that organ, and to the transplantation of certain other major organs, chiefly the heart and the liver. It is these drastic procedures that have compelled attention to what is right and what is wrong for the various persons involved: the patient or recipient, the organ donor (living or dying), the other members of the families, the professional team, and, indeed, society at large.

Attempts by the medical profession and by other groups in society to deal with these ethical problems have evolved rapidly during the past few years. Less than a decade ago only a few of the physicians and surgeons undertaking renal transplantation and dialysis (Scribner; Merrill, 1964; Hamburger et al., 1964; Woodruff; Moore, 1965), and a number of medical editors (Page, 1963; Elkinton, 1964), began to write on the subject. Over the next few years the medical profession started to examine the subject more extensively (Wolstenholme and O'Connor; Starzl; Reemtsma; Hamburger and Crosnier; Schreiner and Maher; Page, 1969; Moore, 1972). Then, as the experimental programs expanded and increasing degrees of success came with improvement in technical procedures, other professional groups became involved. The lawyers were turned to for help with the legal problems concerned with consent for the removal of organs from healthy and dying donors (Sadler et al.; Dukeminier). The psychiatrists and psychologists were brought in to assist with the complex emotional situations that rapidly surfaced in donors, recipients, and their families (Castelnuovo-Tedesco; Shea et al.; Abram). The theologians entered the arena with points of view ranging from that of catholic natural law to that of situation ethics (Fletcher; Ramsey; Thielicke). More recently, the sociologists have begun to analyze this whole process and to point out that it is a paradigm of the broader ethical issues arising in the rapid expansion of our present day technological society (Fox). And finally, that forgotten man, the layman, has begun to express both his enthusiasm and his doubts about the whole development (Schmeck, Rosenfeld).

Given this brief background, let us turn to the specific ethical issues as they concern each category of person involved.

THE PATIENT-RECIPIENT

The man or woman whose continued existence is jeopardized by the relentless progression of disease and failure of an organ has every right to seek, and consent to, any therapeutic procedure that may prolong life and alleviate distress. The crucial question is: what are the chances of success or rehabilitation as compared to the physical, mental, and financial risks or stresses involved in the procedure. To develop appropriate expectations for making this decision, the patient and those responsible for him must lean heavily on their medical advisors. But the patient, if competent, must make the primary decision himself.

Prediction of success is easiest where experience with the procedure has been greatest—as in the use of dialyzers and transplantation of the kidney in patients with progressive renal failure. In 1964, such a patient receiving a renal allograft had about a 5 percent chance of surviving 1 year; now his chances appear to lie between 50 and 75 percent, or even greater. This tremendous increase in survival rate is due, in the main, to great improvements in techniques of immunosuppression and to a very much wider experience on the part of the transplanting teams. A similar increase in survival rate has been achieved for those patients who have been maintained solely by hemodialysis. Thus, such a patient knows that he has a reasonable chance of life as opposed to death for at least a few years. The quality of that life in terms of rehabilitation is more difficult to predict, but few patients hesitate to try for survival.

In the case of the transplantation of single organs such as the heart or the liver, medical experience has been much more limited and the survival rate has been very low. Here, the patient who consents to such an operation is really offering himself as an experimental subject, more for the benefit of others in the future than for himself. The transplanting team has the ethical obligation to be sure that his consent is completely voluntary and fully informed, and that the proper scientific standards are maintained in the study, as spelled out in the second part of the Declaration of Helsinki (World Medical Association).

In a word, the patient who undertakes to make use of an artificial or transplanted organ must understand clearly what it is that he is consenting to, that is, what risks he is subjecting himself to in his attempt to survive. In these circumstances there is no moral reason why he should not make the attempt.

THE LIVING DONOR

The healthy person who agrees to give one of his two kidneys to another person submits to certain short-term surgical and long-term medical risks. Is it right that he should do so? The surgical risks are small and are estimated be in the range of 0.1 to 0.2 percent mortality (Hamburger and Crosnier). The donor is usually a parent or sibling of the recipient and runs such a risk, however small, for altruistic reasons. The first moral requirement therefore is that the prospective donor understand the risks involved and be under no external or abnormal psychological pressures to make the donation. Physicians tend to be suspicious of apparent altruistic actions (perhaps because of their experiences with so many mentally disturbed patients); laymen appear to be less skeptical (Fellner and Schwartz). Doctrine in most religions supports genuine altruistic actions on the part of one person toward another. A kidney freely given for appropriate motives, therefore, is an admirable and ethical act.

The prospective donor should understand that there are other hazards besides the medical and surgical risks. The emotional and psychological relationship between donor and recipient may become difficult. If the allograft does poorly or fails, the donor may feel guilty or angry at what in hindsight seems to have been an unnecessary sacrifice or risk on his part. If the allograft does well, the donor and even the recipient may feel undue proprietary rights in the life of the other. Such possible psychologic hazards are not a moral objection to the donation of a kidney so long as the donor and his physician are on the alert to minimize them.

THE POTENTIAL CADAVERIC (DYING) DONOR

Transplantation of an organ from a dead body avoids most of the ethical difficulties just outlined; in their place there are others. Until techniques are perfected for preservation of the vitality of organs for long periods after the death of the donor, the principal ethical problem is to ensure that the dying potential donor receives every care that is due him as a human being in his own right. Thus, he needs to be under the care of a medical team that is independent of the team caring for the recipient. Furthermore, because of the need to preserve the circulation in the allograft until the last possible moment, the determination of the moment of death, and indeed the definition of death, becomes crucial. The traditional medical and legal definitions of death depend on the presence or absence of the circulation and the beat of the heart. Circulation and respiration of moribund patients sometimes are maintained artificially for considerable periods of time by mechanical means. If such a patient has no chance to recover, is it ethical to remove an organ for transplantation before turning off the supporting apparatus? Some physicians now hold the opinion that irreversible failure of the brain is what really determines the death of a patient as a human being, and great efforts are being made to establish reliable diagnostic criteria for such "brain death." But other physicians (Toole), as well as laymen and jurists, are dubious of abandoning the traditional definition of death; legal rulings on the matter are slow in being made and, to date, are not very encouraging. Nevertheless, it seems to this writer that the essence of human personality lies in the conscious and unconscious mind with its accumulated conditionings and memories and that the physical substrate of this mind is the brain. Hence, if the irreversible failure of function of the brain can be established with certainty, such failure means that the patient as a human person has died. In such a view, mechanical support of the circulation until an organ is removed would be morally justifiable. But the criteria for establishing such a diagnosis are still uncertain, and ethical judgments in such situations are correspondingly difficult. In any case, it is clear that the welfare of the dying patient must not be jeopardized.

FAMILIES OF RECIPIENTS AND DONORS

Relatives of patients whose lives can only be prolonged by the use of artificial or transplanted organs are subject to many psychological and emotional stresses that may lead to ethical problems. Expectations of results from the procedures should not be raised unduly for the relatives any more than for the patient. Nor should excessive intra-family pressures on certain members to give one of their kidneys to the sick member be permitted or encouraged; resentment, fear, and guilt are usually the consequences. The same may be said about putting pressure on relatives of a dying patient for permission to remove one of his organs at the moment of death; emotional agitation and apprehension may be added to the grief already stemming from the occasion. The medical advisors bear the first responsibility for preventing these wrong and undesirable consequences, but the press and lay science writers also need to educate the public on the issues. Uniform anatomical gift acts should be supported for enactment into law, and the public should be encouraged to designate in times of health organs for removal at the time of death.

THE MEDICAL TEAM: PHYSICIANS AND SURGEONS

The original initiative for the development of the use of artificial and transplanted organs came from the natural desire of doctors to prevent death in, and restore to a useful life, those of their patients with certain organs undergoing irreversible damage. To prolong life and to prevent suffering is the accepted role of the physician. Nevertheless, physicians in charge of patients so circumstanced are faced with ethical and moral problems.

Choice of patients is one of the first moral hurdles for the medical team. Where facilities for chronic hemodialysis or transplantation, or both, are limited, only some of the patients who might benefit can be treated; the rest must be left to the inexorable course of their disease. Someone has to choose who shall be given a chance to live and, as a consequence, who must be left to die. In the lay press this has been labeled "playing God" and, labeled or not, the situation is distressing to those who must make the decision. The Seattle group that pioneered the hemodialysis program for chronic uremics initially enlisted the help of an anonymous committee made up of different members of the community to choose which patients should be saved. Inevitably, such a procedure results in assigning relative worths to different lives—an act that is ethically and religiously repugnant to most people. Other dialyzing and transplanting centers have attempted to avoid this consequence by taking patients on a "first come, first served" basis. But it is very hard for the medical team to avoid at least subconscious evaluations of the relative desirability of the life to be saved: the young vs. the old, the talented vs. the untalented, the family breadwinner vs. the ne'er-do-well. The only way to get completely off the horns of this dilemma is to make the therapies available to all who need them—a resolution that has its own set of difficulties (this is discussed further below). Meanwhile the members of the medical profession who are endeavoring to carry out these programs to save at least some of their patients must act according to the best lights of their own consciences and of enlightened public opinion.

These therapeutic programs are limited in part because medical time and skills are limited; physicians and surgeons have to choose how to expend their professional efforts. When is it right to put time, effort, and hospital and laboratory facilities into saving the lives of a relatively few patients requiring these elaborate procedures as against many others who need definite, but less dramatic, medical assistance? Again, each doctor has to make his own choice as to how he will use his own professional skill, but the effect of the sum total of such individual choices is a justifiable concern of the whole community, of society at large.

There are other ethical and moral problems for the medical personnel engaged in these programs. Have they adequately informed the patient-recipients, the donors, and their families of the nature and the chances of success of the anticipated procedures? Have they endeavored to minimize the physical, psychological, and financial hazards involved? Have they tried to maintain a helpful psychological relationship with their patients, avoiding antagonism and undue dependence? All doctors have such problems with many different kinds of patients, but these problems tend to be especially acute in carrying out the hemodialysis-transplantation programs. And has the medical team acted for the sake of the patients they are treating and for gain in scientific knowledge to benefit future patients, rather than for their own prestige and publicity? This last ethical question is not pertinent to most of the professional teams working in this field. But the dramatic nature of these procedures—and especially the events associated with the first cardiac transplantations—has underscored the necessity for the profession to be very careful in this respect.

The medical profession has certainly tried to exercise caution. Various codes and guidelines have been promulgated to this end by various professional societies and organizations; these include the Board on Medicine of the National Academy of Sciences, The Council for International Organizations of Medical Sciences, American College of Cardiology, American Heart Association, American Medical Association, and the National Heart Institute (for references, see Elkinton, 1970). More recently the Committee on Morals and Ethics of the Transplantation Society has issued a statement (Merrill, 1971) that deals with specific ethical issues involved in the care of patients and donors. The Society says that renal allografts are now therapeutic procedures in the hands of a trained team and that transplantation of other organs, except the brain, is acceptable as an experimental procedure; that in the choice of recipients risks must be weighed against benefits; that the health of the living donor is primary; that cadaveric sources of organs are morally desirable; that death of a person occurs in the brain rather than in the heart; that the death of a prospective cadaveric donor must be certified by two physicians not in the transplant team. Xenografts (transplantation of organs from species other than man) are acceptable experimentally; the sale of human organs is indefensible. With regard to publicity, the public has a right to be informed, but the privacy of donors and recipients must be respected, and no news release should be made before an innovation has been formally presented to a group of medical peers. Quite clearly, the medical profession is concerned and anxious about the ethical problems arising from this field of professional activity.

SOCIETY

Beyond the issues facing the various individuals involved, the use of artificial and transplanted organs poses fundamental ethical and moral problems to society at large. These include the conflict between the patient's right to privacy and society's right to know what is being done and learned in this complex field, the determination of priorities for the use of limited resources to meet competing medical and social needs, and the development of wise attitudes in society toward its biological future and the role of death in human life.

The perennial conflict between the rights of the individual and the rights of society is here exemplified by the need of the patient and his family to undergo these therapeutic procedures in privacy as opposed to the need of the public to be informed about these dramatic and important medical advances. Resolution of this conflict in each instance depends upon the conscientious efforts of members of the medical profession and members of the public press to understand each other's obligations. Medical personnel have to shield their patients from undue publicity and see to it that the primary reporting of the medical results is presented in the proper professional and scientific forum. Reporters and science writers should inform the public about the character and directions of important advances in medical science and practice. To make basic judgments about the proper goals for these medical advances and the extent to which to support them, society must be adequately informed and educated.

One of the difficulties in developing any new and complex procedure in our technologic society is the initial high cost and limitations in various resources. The development of the use of artificial and transplanted organs is no exception. Any doctor who has participated in such a program knows the tremendous drain on time, energy, skill, hospital and laboratory facilities, and funds. Theoretically, when a human life is saved or prolonged, the cost should not be counted. Yet to what extent are other patients penalized by such a diversion of resources? There is nothing new about this problem; society has always had to make such choices. When tuberculosis was one of the chief scourges of the population, extensive resources were spent on sanitariums and public health measures to control it; preventive action and the development of effective antibiotics eventually reduced the demand on facilities and efforts. In the case of chronic hemodialysis, home dialysis programs, cheaper dialyzers, and wider use of paramedical personnel are beginning to reduce the cost in time, effort, and money. A successful renal transplantation has the same effect, and presumably advances in technique will reduce the cost of that procedure. But society must be alert in order to foster research in areas that will prevent the very diseases that ultimately lead to necessity for these elaborate and expensive treatments in the end-stages of the disease.

Competition also is keen in the allocation of society's total resources between medical needs and other social needs. Health care must compete in the public arena with education, housing, transportation, welfare and antipoverty programs, aid to the elderly, and—apparently—the maintenance of a massive military machine. These choices are ethical in nature, for in making them society decides what is the greater good and the lesser good for its various members. Thus, the ethical issues arising from the development of artificial organs and organ transplantation mirror the increasing difficulties of present-day society in judging priorities and controlling limited medical and social resources with maximum consideration for human values and the quality of human life.

Judgments about the quality of the life depend ultimately on the philosophical and religious beliefs of those who are making the judgments. In deciding on the desirable use of artificial and transplanted organs in the future, society will have to decide what is good in terms of human values for the biological future of the race. To what extent and under what circumstances is it good to patch bodies and to prolong life in the face of fatal disease? This question requires examination of men's attitudes toward death. Whether a man believes in God and a future life, or whether he is a humanist, agnostic, or atheist, he should be able to see that death is a natural part of the process of life and plays an essential role in its evolution. As such, the timely death of each individual should be accepted as a good, and not feared as an evil. It is, of course, the untimely death of individuals who have not completed their normal spans of life that is the concern of the medical programs under discussion. Such concern is reasonable and good for both the individual and for society when acted upon with due regard for the quality of human life.

THE FUTURE

Many of the ethical problems in the use of artificial and transplanted organs of the present day have now been outlined; what will these problems be in the future? These are some of the probabilities as they appear to me.

For the patient with chronic renal failure, the medical prospects probably will continue to improve as technical progress is made in simpler, cheaper, and safer methods of dialysis, in tissue typing, in immunosuppression, and in in vitro preservation of organs after removal. When living donors are used, improvements in methods for determining histocompatibility will increase the chances for success. Where such preferable allografts cannot be obtained, greater use will be made of kidneys from cadavers. The availability of such cadaveric organs will increase as uniform anatomical gift acts are enacted into law and as the public is educated to use them. Legal precedents for changing the definition of death are unlikely in the near future, but improved technique for the preservation and transport of organs should go far to counterbalance this difficulty. The major problem of death from infection probably will always be present as the immune responses of the recipient are artificially suppressed to prevent rejection of the allograft. But techniques of immunosuppression will continue to be improved to the end that the risk of failure in either direction will be decreased. Technical progress, therefore, will do much to diminish or obviate the physical, psychological, financial, and ethical difficulties facing this type of patient.

For the patient with failure of an unpaired organ, such as the heart or the liver, the future is much more uncertain. Technical difficulties are great and donors are limited; the ethical difficulties attending this category of organ transplantation are correspondingly large. Efforts will surely be expanded on artificial substitutes for such organs and on measures to prevent disease of the organs in the first place.

The medical profession and society will have to make many choices. Dialysis and transplantation programs will have to be balanced against other medical and social programs, and the balancing will of necessity take place in the social and political arena. As man must condition and modify a wide range of his technological activities to improve rather than to harm the quality of his life, so he will have to weigh the assets and liabilities of these programs in terms of human values. If he can do this to the enhancement of the human spirit and the whole man, these particular medical developments will stand as good and worthwhile achievements for the society from which he has sprung.

REFERENCES

Abram, H. S. 1968. The psychiatrist, the treatment of chronic renal failure, and the prolongation of life: I. *Amer. J. Psychiat.* **124**:1351–1358.

Castelnuovo-Tedesco, P., ed. 1971. Psychiatric Aspects of Organ Transplantation. New York, Grune & Stratton, Inc.

Dukeminier, J., Jr. 1970. Supplying organs for transplantation. *Mich. Law Rev.* **68**:811–866.

Elkinton, J. R. 1964. Moral problems in the use of borrowed organs, artificial and transplanted. *Ann. Intern. Med.* **60**:309–313.

Elkinton, J. R. 1970. The literature of ethical problems in medicine—Part 3. *Ann. Intern. Med.* **73**:863–870.

Fellner, C. H., and S. H. Schwartz. 1971. Altruism in disrepute. Medical versus public attitudes toward the living organ donor. *New Engl. J. Med.* **284:**582–585.

Fletcher, J. 1968. Our shameful waste of human tissue: an ethical problem for the living and the dead. *In* Updating Life and Death: Essays in Ethics and Medicine. D. R. Cutler, ed. Boston, Beacon Press. Pages 1–29.

Fox, R. C. 1970. A sociological perspective on organ transplantation and hemodialysis. *In* New Dimensions in Legal and Ethical Concepts for Human Research. I. Ladimer, ed. *Ann. N.Y. Acad. Sci.* **169:**406–428.

Hamburger, J., and J. Crosnier. 1968. Moral and ethical problems in transplantation. *In* Human Transplantation. F. T. Rapport and J. Dausset, eds. New York and London. Grune & Stratton, Inc. Pages 37–44.

Hamburger, J., J. Crosnier, and J. Dormont. 1964. Problèmes moraux posés par les méthodes de suppléance et de transplantation d'organes. *Rev. Franc. Etud. Clin. Biol.* **9:**587–591.

Merrill, J. P. 1964. Clinical experience is tempered by genuine human concern. *J.A.M.A.* **189:**626–627.

Merrill, J. P. 1971. Statement of the Committee on Morals and Ethics of the Transplantation Society. *Ann. Intern. Med.* **75:**631–633.

Moore, F. D. 1965 (April 5). Ethics in the new medicine—tissue transplants. *The Nation.*

Moore, F. D. 1972. Transplant: the Give and Take of Tissue Transplantation. Simon and Schuster, New York.

Page, I. H. 1963 (October 14). Prolongation of life in affluent society. *Mod. Med.* 89–91.

Page, I. H. 1969. The ethics of heart transplantation. *J.A.M.A.* **207:**109–113.

Ramsey, P. 1970. The Patient as Person: Explorations in Medical Ethics. New Haven and London, Yale University Press.

Reemtsma, K. 1968. Ethical problems with artificial and transplanted organs: an approach by experiential ethics. *In* Ethical Issues in Medicine. E. F. Torrey, ed. Boston, Little, Brown, and Company. Pages 249–263.

Rosenfeld, A. 1969. The Second Genesis: The Coming Control of Life. New Jersey, Prentice-Hall, Inc.

Sadler, A. M., et al. 1970. Transplantation and the law: progress toward uniformity. *New Engl. J. Med.* **282:**717–723.

Schmeck, H. M., Jr. 1965. The Semi-Artificial Man: A Dawning Revolution in Medicine. New York, Walker and Co.

Schreiner, G. E., and J. F. Maher. 1965. Hemodialysis for chronic renal failure. III. Medical, moral and ethical, and socio-economic problems. *Ann. Intern. Med.* **62:**551–557.

Scribner, B. H. 1964. Presidential address: ethical problems of using artificial organs to maintain human life. *Trans. Amer. Soc. Artif. Intern. Organs.* **10:**209–212.

Shea, E. J., D. F. Bogdan, R. B. Freeman, and G. E. Schreiner. 1965. Hemodialysis for chronic renal failure. IV. Psychological Considerations. *Ann. Intern. Med.* **62:**558–563.

Starzl, T. E. 1967. Ethical problems in organ transplantation: a clinician's point of view. *In* The Changing Mores of Biomedical Research: A Colloquium on Ethical Dilemmas for Medical Advances. J. R. Elkinton, ed. *Ann. Intern. Med.* **67** (Suppl. 7):32–36.

Thielicke, H. 1970. The doctor as judge of who shall live and who shall die. *In* Who Shall Live? Medicine Technology Ethics. K. Vaux, ed. Philadelphia, Fortress Press. Pages 146–194.

Toole, J. F. 1971. The neurologist and the concept of brain death. *Perspect. Biol. Med.* **14:**599–607.

Wolstenholme, G. E. W., and M. O'Connor, eds. 1966. Ethics in Medical Progress: with Special Reference to Transplantation. Ciba Foundation Symposium. London, J. & A. Churchill, Ltd.

Woodruff, M. F. A. 1964. Ethical problems in organ transplantation. *Brit. Med. J.* **1:**1457–1460.

World Medical Association 1964. Declaration of Helsinki: recommendations guiding doctors in clinical research. *World Med. J.* **11:**281.

CHAPTER 11

MANAGEMENT OF THE SICK WITH KINDNESS, COMPASSION, WISDOM, AND EFFICIENCY

ROBERT H. WILLIAMS

The status of health is extremely important in decisions about who should live and die, as well as when and how we die. The physician plays an important role in these decisions. He is almost always present at birth and death and is consulted frequently about physical and emotional problems in life. Particularly during these times of extensive family, community, national, and international turmoil, with the attendant insecurity, anxiety, frustration, and other changes that influence health and happiness, the physician is especially needed to supply guidance and to ease discomforts. This chapter deals with some of the factors that contribute to optimal medical care and satisfaction for both patients and physicians.

MEDICINE AS A CAREER

There are many attractions that prompt a young person to respond to the call of medicine as a career; certainly these include the social, economic, and scholastic status that physicians enjoy. To me and many others, however, the most important attraction has been the possibility of transforming a person who is in physical agony to one who is well and happy. The following letter from a patient conveys the type of satisfaction that can be experienced.

> I am expressing to you how my heart is brimming over with gratitude and deepest appreciation for your giving me back 'the gift of life.' It is almost impossible for me to realize that my disease has been eliminated; it is miraculous that this has been accomplished in such a short time. It has been a rough and rugged road at times, but with your standing by it has made it so much easier. I knew some day that I would be a well person and could walk again. The laurels of victory go to you and the other doctors who have given to my case a highly specialized knowledge.

This letter was from a patient who had suffered for at least 22 years. During that time, she had become extremely weak and bedridden and had extensive skin, muscle, bone, and other changes, including mental changes that necessitated hospitalization for more than a year. Although she had seen many doctors, her condition had not been diagnosed. She experienced dramatic recovery after removal of her adrenal glands, which had produced Cushing's disease.

For centuries, physicians have basked in the limelight of a noble heritage. This profession has enjoyed great admiration, respect, appreciation, and sometimes glorification; even recent polls tend to substantiate this. Through the centuries medicine has stood out as an art, but as a real science it has gained its status chiefly in the last few decades. However, it has been claimed that with this change there has been a decrease in the art of medicine. The art of medicine consists of a skillful application of the science of medicine in the hopes of improving the overall welfare and happiness of the patient, his family, and others. Indeed, too many physicians have been fascinated by the progress in science and have rested confident that a given drug would soon cure the patient's disease. They have failed to recognize that most diseases are associated with varying degrees of emotional upheaval and that the patient may be in great distress even though the drug administered is working magically upon a specific disease.

During my lifetime I have had the pleasure of witnessing the greatest progress that has ever been made in medicine. The first clinical diagnosis of coronary thrombosis was made in 1912; the first clinical diagnosis of appendicitis was made only 27 years earlier. A large number of diseases that were once rampant are now cured rapidly, and some have largely been prevented, e.g., typhoid, malaria, poliomyelitis, and smallpox. The cause and treatment of numerous genetic disorders have been discovered. Advances in other areas of science have helped medicine: the elucidation of many aspects of nuclear physics and the development of atomic energy; knowledge of the actions and synthesis of nucleic acids and proteins; the coding, transcription, and translation of genetic information; recognition of the structural and functional aspects of cell components; new discoveries in many areas of immunology and virology.

Despite great scientific progress, there is much criticism of the medical profession by the public, while the medical profession in turn is disturbed by the philosophies and actions of some of the laity. Hippocrates remains pre-eminent among outstanding physicians of the past, and his code has been greatly publicized and much of it followed—some of it too little and some too much. Hippocrates, Osler, and some of the other great men of medicine who have enunciated important guidelines probably would alter many of them in accordance with present-day problems. The great Fuller Albright, when presenting some of his policies, often emphasized that he might change them at any time, depending upon subsequent observations. This is a thesis that should be applied to religious policies, laws, and other guidelines.

Progress in medicine benefits from many types of approach. Indeed, formalized training in science is not always required for a person to make great contributions. For example, many leading physicians believe that Senator Lister Hill, through his wise legislative leadership in health measures, has done more for the health of the United States than any other one man. Physicians can make great contributions by working as teachers or investigators in basic science or clinical science departments, or as practitioners of medicine, or as administrators in medicine. It has been said that William H. Welch, a renowned pathologist, contributed more to the Johns Hopkins Medical School than any one man, chiefly through his administrative skills. Differing qualities are needed for success in these different spheres of medicine. The person who chooses to practice medicine should be very interested in humanity and in the health and welfare of people and should be prepared to attend to both the art and science of medicine. His personality can greatly affect his progress.

SETTINGS FOR OPTIMAL PRACTICE

There is an enormous amount to learn about the actions and reactions of the human body in different circumstances. Consequently, preparation of the physician must be of high quality and extensive quantity. Since there is far more knowledge required than any one individual can master (Fig. 1), each trainee should decide early which sphere of medicine he wants to enter and prepare for it in the best manner. We need physicians well trained in one of a large variety of special areas, and others with excellent training in many different spheres of medicine. The latter type of doctor is called a generalist or family physician. The need for the generalist has become quite apparent to both physicians and nonphysicians. The members of an organization composed of the heads of the departments of medicine of each medical school (the Association of Professors of Medicine) voted unanimously to cooperate in considering plans for this type of specialist. Various medical schools have already established a department of family medicine. The generalist must be aware of the distinct limitations in his depth of knowledge in a large number of fields and must seek consultation often. Sometimes he receives suggestions about diagnosis and treatment from several specialists at the same time, but he is the coordinator. Often he conducts the recommended diagnostic and therapeutic procedures, although the more intricate ones are dealt with directly by a specialist. The goal is to offer the best possible patient care, irrespective of who may be needed to render service. The generalist should be trained predominantly in internal medicine, pediatrics, psychiatry, and emergency care.

HIGH-PRESSURE INFUSIONS

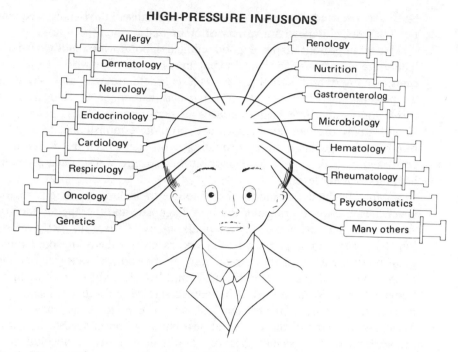

Fig. 1. No physician, no matter how brilliant, can master a major proportion of medicine, even with greatest determination (from *J. Amer. Med. Assoc.* 1958. **167**:192.

Premedical education should give most trainees a solid background in the major principles of biology, genetics, physiology, chemistry, psychology, philosophy, sociology, and economics. Trainees would also gain from a moderate amount of traveling, general reading, observations of patterns of life, and other activities that give some idea of many types of careers and living patterns. Once out of medical school, the physician should not curtail his graduate training, since this is when he gets most specifically trained for his career.

His proper training acquired, the physician must establish the most appropriate office, laboratory, and hospital arrangements, as well as consultation facilities for optimal practice. An increasing number of physicians are avoiding or leaving solo general practice either for specialization or for group practice. Many physicians in practice by themselves become distressed because of overwork and because they are unable to solve their patients' problems satisfactorily. A group practice may consist of a well-integrated clinic or of an aggregation of physicians in an office building, carefully selected to include a wide diversity of medical specialties. In either instance the objective is cooperation and coordination that will permit appropriate attention to patients 24 hours a day, seven days a week.

Such groups need generalists as well as specialists. Physicians frequently need to work closely with a variety of other well-trained specialists.

It is important to have good clinical laboratories readily available. There are numerous laboratories, but many do inferior work. In a recent questionnaire that I submitted to 165 graduate trainees and physicians, 91 percent voted in favor of requiring certification of all clinical laboratories and establishing high standards of performance. These goals would abolish many existing laboratories and promote establishment of a greater number of large laboratories providing a broader spectrum of service of consistently high quality. Such laboratories require well-trained specialists at a professional level.

Most hospitals should be big enough to include numerous medical specialties and a wide range of the best diagnostic and therapeutic facilities. At present there are too many hospitals, many of them distinctly inferior. Small hospitals in a populous area are rarely justified. In some remote geographic areas, a small hospital may be of some advantage, but most of the major and complex problems should be referred to a well-equipped, larger hospital. With improved helicopter service and other transportation measures, good hospital and medical service can be readily available to essentially all parts of the United States. Nursing homes need to be considerably improved, especially because of the high costs of hospitalization. Many nursing homes should be visualized as hospitals for the chronically ill, but they should have excellent service by physician assistants, nurses, physical therapists, dietitians, as well as well-trained physicians, sociologists, and psychologists. It is becoming increasingly popular to have a dormitory-type of medical facility built close to hospitals and clinics, so that out-of-town patients can be placed in the nearby unit at a reasonable price; 78 percent of those questioned in the survey mentioned above favored this plan. This facility must include personnel trained to carefully supervise the collection of specimens and many diagnostic and therapeutic procedures.

Various segments of the government can help significantly in establishing optimal patterns of patient care. The accomplishments of the National Institutes of Health demonstrate how effective the government can be when proper counsel and wise leadership from others are used. The federal government is rapidly becoming intensively involved in all phases of health and, indeed, must become much more so. There must be far greater government support for health education at both the undergraduate and the graduate levels as well as for continued education for graduates. Special inducements must be provided to promote appropriate health care based on geography, specialty, and patterns of practice. Much more study and action are needed to supply enough of the appropriate types of hospitals where they are needed and to facilitate transportation between hospitals and remote areas. Our methods for disposing of the dead must be improved; this includes cutting costs markedly. An increase in cremation and placement of the ashes in homes or small vaults would be beneficial.

As discussed in Chapter 7, one of the greatest problems, especially for the future, is the need for policies to reduce the birth rate and the number of people with agonizing problems. Also, laws must be instituted to reduce the rapidly increasing number of malpractice suits and to improve the manner in which they are dealt with; exorbitant awards should be curtailed. Legislation is required that will protect patients appropriately yet avoid the many gross injustices that occur today.

These various goals will best be attained by collaboration and cooperation between many groups: government, medical societies, medical schools, insurance companies, and others. The National Institute of Medicine can play a key role in integrating many activities, acquiring information, and stimulating action.

THE PHYSICIAN'S MANAGEMENT OF THE PATIENT

The best patient care requires a good relationship between the physician, the patient, and the family; each has certain obligations. Some of the complaints that physicians most commonly voice about their patients are: (1) too many patients are psychoneurotic; (2) some try to use social, economic, or political status to gain special privileges; (3) they telephone too frequently and speak for too long; (4) they are impatient regarding diagnosis and treatment and they fail to show appreciation; (5) they frequently fail to follow instructions; (6) they complain excessively about fees; (7) they shop for physicians; and (8) many of them have objectionable personality patterns. Many of these problems arise through insufficient communication and understanding on the part of the patient, the physician, or both.

We often see medical students with essentially the same grade point average attain very different levels of success in their careers. The physician's success in dealing with his patients is very much affected by his general attitudes, the principles and policies by which he operates, and the type, timeliness, and extent of his actions. These characteristics are influenced by many factors, including the physician's own genetic pattern, his relationship with his family and others, his own experiences, and especially his own health. When a physician has emotional problems of his own or feels insecure or uncomfortable, his dealings with patients tend to be different from those of one who is happy and at ease. Dr. B., a prominent surgeon, once told me that a famous neurosurgeon was being severely critical of his assistants during an operation. Eventually Dr. B. became exasperated and started to withdraw from the operation early. The neurosurgeon went to him to express his apologies, explaining that he felt particularly uncomfortable and irritable because he had a bad case of hemorrhoids and one was giving him great discomfort at the time. Dr. B. told the neuro-surgeon that he had better get his hemorrhoids fixed, and soon, if he expected him to continue as his assistant.

Like others, I feel greatly rewarded when I can help people to feel better and to experience success in various ways. I delight in the challenge of trying to conquer a patient's problems. A vast amount of knowledge if required to deal with medical problems and there is no good substitute for this. However, in the end success depends not only on one's knowledge but also on how the knowledge is applied, so I will discuss some of the ways I feel help one to attain success. First, application of the golden rule has put a new light on many questions in my professional and home life. The physician should try to project himself into the patient's position and ask himself how he would want to be treated in such a situation. For example, several years ago one of our brilliant residents told me that he wanted to subject a patient to a thyroidectomy. Since we knew the proper diagnosis and treatment, I asked him why he wanted her to have an operation. He stated: "It would be very interesting to see her thyroid tissue under the microscope." However, when I asked him whether he would still recommend the operation if his wife were the patient, he smiled and said: "No." Application of the golden rule helps one to be objective and to remove prejudices and false rationalizations. However, we must also consider the patient's own philosophies and wishes, because they may differ from those of the physician.

Although it has often been stated that the physician should have *sympathy* for his patients, *empathy* is more appropriate. With empathy, one recognizes and perceives the feelings of his patient, whereas with sympathy, the physician's perception of the patient's problems may be so keen that he actually experiences some of the patient's discomforts. Unfortunately, such subjective reactions on the part of the physician may interfere with the wisest treatment. A physician can perceive the patient's symptoms without actually experiencing them. He must be able to keep his head even though the patient and others may be losing theirs in a distressing situation.

Many patients have not only physical discomfort but also much emotional upheaval. Hospitalization makes many feel lonely, discouraged, and depressed. Especially at these times, kind, tender, loving care, rendered with a genuine display of interest and determination to help can be very beneficial. This is a time when there should "abide faith, hope and love; these three, but the greatest is love" (I Corinthians 13:13). Indeed, the greatest thing in the world is love, so beautifully described by Drummond as composed of patience, kindness, generosity, humility, courtesy, unselfishness, good temper, guilessness, and sincerity. Many physicians do often react in this way, but tend not to display such traits when facing a patient with obnoxious behavior. However, this is an extremely important part of our challenge and can be faced directly much better when one considers that *all behavior depends upon the physical and/or chemical status of the brain.* In patients with abnormal behavior, we must search for physical or chemical abnormalities. Even when we don't find them, we must realize that they are present.

Major emotional and psychiatric problems often distress the patient, his family, and his physician. There is a widespread lack of understanding of causative factors and of how to deal with them appropriately. The cost of managing such problems is often enormous. Patients resist being told that they have a psychiatric disorder; moreover, because their management can be so perplexing, many physicians hate to be involved with them. Some emotional disturbance is present in a large proportion of major medical problems. Presumably no symptoms can be manifested to the patient except through mentation. For example, with deep anesthesia, all symptoms are abolished. The type and extent of reactions to different conditions with which patients are confronted depend very much upon previous conditioning. Thus, an individual who has been preconditioned to react to certain experiences with fear, anxiety, and agitation, tends to hyperreact to related stimuli. Such conditioning is associated with increased release of adrenalin and noradrenalin, which in the brain may increase nervousness, anxiety, fear, frustration, agitation, insomnia, and even panic. Excess adrenalin and noradrenalin also influence the cardiovascular and gastrointestinal systems and the liver, lung, pituitary, adrenal, thyroid, and all other organs. The anxiety can be beneficial if it alerts a person to possible danger and causes him to apply protective measures, or it can be a hindrance if it is too intense or lasts too long.

Suggestion plays a highly important role in symptoms. It is on this basis that faith healers, soothsayers, and other quacks thrive. Suggestion is the basis for response to hypnosis. For example, one of my patients was a girl, aged 21, who had become paralyzed in her right arm at 3 a.m. eight months before. Subsequently, no one had seen her move any part of her arm; its muscles had become atrophied. Pin-pricks and other means of producing pain caused no discomfort nor did extreme flexion of the wrist. Two minutes after hypnosis was started she moved all portions of her arm freely and experienced pain in her wrist, although she had had none during the four days since its hyperflexion. Suggestion is the basis for the fact that as many as 25 percent of subjects react to placebos (capsules of sugar which look like a specific drug being tested) with skin rashes, nausea, and vomiting; they fear that they may be getting a toxic drug.

Until recently, diagnosis and treatment in psychiatry have been based chiefly upon the physician's subjective reactions. Consequently, many activities of psychiatrists have fallen into the class of art rather than of science. With increasing research using objective evaluations, the specific basis for abnormal mentation is found more often (Chapter 2). All illness is associated with metabolic changes—some local, some general, and some involving the brain very significantly. Thus, in all instances of psychiatric disturbances, it is important to consider what metabolic changes may be producing the psychiatric pattern. Of course, certain types of psychological conditioning, as discussed above, can bring about many metabolic changes, but a number of the metabolic changes can be primary and cause psychiatric disturbances. In one instance (presented in greater detail in Chapter 2) a boy was considered to have schizophrenia and epilepsy and was treated for them for years. It was later found that his schizophrenia and epilepsy were caused by hypoparathyroidism, and his symptoms were abolished by correction of the associated low blood calcium levels. In another case the mother of a physician was treated for a psychiatric disorder for 20 years before it was suspected that her trouble was caused by low blood levels of glucose. With removal of an insulin-secreting tumor (which caused the low blood sugar level) her psychiatric disorder disappeared.

A patient may have a classic psychiatric syndrome plus underlying unrelated organic disease. For example, a woman who was the second wife of a minister was admitted to the hospital with what was considered to be classic hysteria. She was pounding on her chest and shouting that she was dying of a heart attack. The minister's first wife, who had been a highly popular person, had died of a heart attack, and failure of the second wife to be as popular provided a setting for hysteria. This psychiatric pattern was so prominent that little attention had been given to the possibility of heart trouble but her last heart beat was heard during examination.

The foregoing cases should emphasize the need to investigate many types of metabolic changes as possible causes of behavioral disorders, while also considering the effects of social, environmental, philosophical, psychological, familial, and other features. When we see a patient with one leg shorter and weaker than the other we are not surprised to see him walk with a limp, but the bases for mental "limps" usually are less obvious. Since primary or subsidiary metabolic changes are always present we must search for them as best we can. Meanwhile, we must continue to show kindness, considerateness, and compassion, although there are times when these can be overextended and keep the patient from progressing through his own determination and efforts. The patient must realize that we cannot always pinpoint the primary cause of his behavioral difficulty and must resort to certain psychotherapeutic and drug approaches in alleviating some of the problems involved.

ATTITUDES AND RESPONSIBILITIES OF PATIENTS

Patients often voice the following complaints about their physicians: (1) high costs; (2) not enough genuine interest; too impersonal; (3) inadequate personal respect; (4) examinations too hurried; (5) insufficient discussion about findings, diagnosis, treatment, and prognosis; (6) excessive waiting in office; (7) too much delay in appointments (some complain of too many appointments); (8) inaccessibility during nonoffice hours; (9) too little interest, consideration, and aid from office assistants; (10) too little or too much consultation; (11) implication or designation of troubles as psychiatric; (12) too old or too young; (13) too unknowledgeable; and (14) "I just don't like him." Many of these problems are related to the physician's failure to orient the patient and key members of his family and to win their friendship, respect, and full cooperation. When the patient understands the significance and possible benefits of certain diagnostic and therapeutic procedures, he is less bothered by the time, cost, and effort involved. He also tends to become more relaxed and cooperative, more loyal to and respectful of his physician.

Patients often expect and demand a tremendous amount from a physician; knowledge, appearance, personal charm, genuine interest, determination to give his most, ready availability, and many other such things. However, patients should exhibit many of the same characteristics to obtain the best care. Intense illness often brings out the real character of the patient, for better or for worse. Some patients radiate pleasant personality traits when all is going relatively well, but exhibit unattractive characteristics when the going gets tough. At the other extreme are some who appear more admirable when their troubles are intensified.

The patient should select a regular physician in whom he has sufficient confidence and then give him full cooperation, loyalty, and respect. I find that I am stimulated to do my very best when a patient tells me: "Dr. Williams, I have utmost faith in you and will do at all times whatever you recommend." This makes me feel my full responsibility keenly. Since physicians and patients can differ greatly in philosophies and approaches, when a patient and the physician do not seem to be able to operate on the same wavelength, despite earnest efforts, it is wise to change physicians.

Some patients want to have their own physician available at nights and on weekends and holidays, but since this is impractical, it is advantageous for him to be a member of a well-organized group clinic. In this way, the patient's full record is available to competent physician colleagues who can contact the regular physician for emergency assistance.

Each physician must have enough time for further education, rest, recreation, and family association. However, many patients think that the physician should take time for these things only when they do not need attention. Many patients fail to realize that other patients may have a greater need for their physician at a particular time. Some patients with extra wealth, social status, or political power use such status for demanding special privileges. Now we are rapidly reaching a situation where essentially everybody is a pay-patient, through one means or another, and where we must not discriminate because of wealth, social status, sex, race, or other factors, except the nature and extent of illness. Each patient must be given excellent care, but some of the luxuries in physical surroundings need to be restricted, since the costs are exorbitant.

The key members of the patient's family should be given basic information about the diagnosis, treatment, and course of the patient's disease. This will help them to care for the patient. Not providing enough information may cause the family to be misled by certain statements the patient makes and to take actions that could hamper his recovery.

A recent national survey is of interest in view of the fact that so many patients complain about physician's "high fees." The survey revealed that the average physician earns $12 an hour when regular, overtime, night and weekend services are considered. By comparison, plumbers, bricklayers, pipe-fitters, carpenters, and roofers average $9 to $9.50 an hour. Overhead is about 50 percent in each group and has been deducted. Of course, the physician's formal training is far more expensive and extensive than that of the other workers mentioned. For example, most of the physicians in Seattle have had 10 to 14 years of formal training after finishing high school. Moreover, many physicians spend considerable time dealing with patients by telephone and do not charge for these services. Some physicians must pay more than $12,000 a year for malpractice insurance. Actually, the increasing frequency of malpractice suits has caused more and more expenditure because so many unnecessary tests and other procedures are conducted to prevent malpractice suits. The public at large is paying for this situation.

Some of the laboratory tests prove to be of no value in certain patients; on the other hand, if the physician orders tests sequentially only as they are indicated, the patient's stay in the hospital will be spread over several days, and costs will be that much higher. Hospital charges have skyrocketed because of increasing salaries for hospital personnel and increasing costs of supplies, but some conditions not properly managed in the acute stages may result in chronic disturbances, which may then cause even higher costs and much discomfort.

Some physicians, especially general practitioners, say that they do not have time to perform more than a cursory examination on many of their patients, because they see more than 40 people a day. However, more thorough attention may make it unnecessary for some patients to return so often. While certain patients complain of their physician's haste, others dislike lengthy examinations, preferring chiefly palliative therapy, such as medicine to alleviate symptoms of a cold or of a gastrointestinal upset.

History-taking can be relatively brief but thorough if it is performed in a highly skilled manner. The physician must demonstrate a keen ability to know what aspects to pursue, as well as how to pursue them and to what extent. This is comparable to a bird dog running rapidly over a field, yet knowing when to slow down to proceed meticulously in pointing the birds.

Occasionally a patient complains because the contents of his record are kept secret from him. However, this is a wise measure because there often are brief statements that the patient would get out of context or would not understand and that might cause him unnecessary distress. Also, there may be remarks that are subsequently helpful to his or another physician, such as "exaggerates complaints," "poor historian," "poor memory." More orientation is desirable for females, especially young ones, when it is necessary to discuss sexual activities and to examine the breasts, clitoris and other sexual organs.

More consultation, collaboration, and coordination among physicians are of distinct advantage to patients. Some persons complain about being seen by more than one physician, partly because of the additional charges, the time involved, and their unfamiliarity with another physician. Others, who feel that their physician may not have diagnosed and treated their condition properly, want examinations by other physicians. Additional consultation may provide distinct improvement, but when it does not, the patient is assured that every effort has been made.

Most patients cooperate well when it comes to participating in teaching and research activities, but a few insist that they want to be examined by only their own physician and not by any trainees. They fail to recognize the advantages of additional care from very good interns and residents. Patients must realize that we cannot produce good physicians without giving them training experience with patients. To some extent research is involved in the management of essentially every patient no matter who is the physician. Since patients vary in the way that they respond to drugs, we must observe individual responses and make appropriate adjustments in the type of medicine and the dosage.

The general pattern of research has improved greatly in the last few decades. This includes the major goals, experimental designs, methods, accumulation and analysis of data, and publications. Although a vast amount of research is performed upon animals and upon certain specimens from man, there is no good substitute for some of the clinical investigations. Since such research can be highly valuable to all of us, it is important that we all be used as subjects to an appropriate extent.

The policies protecting individuals involved in clinical research have in recent years swung from one extreme to the other (see Fig. 2, Chapter 1). Until a few years ago, some research was performed without the patients' knowledge or consent, even though the patients were not expected to benefit from the research. This applied especially to certain projects that used cancer patients because death was impending anyhow. Some of the experiences were sufficiently abusive to lead to the institution of regulations demanding that with any form of clinical research the patient must be well informed and must have given his written consent. The principle involved is good, but it has been so extended in some instances that it has caused much unnecessary trouble for investigators and patients alike. Indeed, the nuisance has been sufficient that some very good research projects have been dropped. Certain administrators insist that the potential research subject should have presented to him a detailed description of *all* of the possible complications that could accompany a given research project. This means that a person who is subjected to even a mild operation would need to be told that he could: (a) bleed to death, (b) die from a blood clot, (c) develop a wound infection which could cause death, and (d) die from anesthesia. Relatively few lay persons would be willing to consent to even the simplest operation if it were presented in this manner. Such a situation occurred when 66 subjects, of whom 64 were female hospital or medical school employees, were asked if they would be willing to take two tablets of acetylhydroxybenzoate when they next had a headache. There was an inverse relationship between the number of volunteers and the length of the description of possible hazards. When told that the drug was actually aspirin, 20 of 21 who had refused to take it under the other name said that they would continue to take aspirin. Sound judgment and the golden rule are the best guides.

Although there has been marked improvement in drugs marketed, there is still room for much progress. Approximately 500 drugs are introduced each year. Some of these are essentially the same drug assigned a different trade name; only generic names should be official. Drugs have been used to tremendous advantage, but many of them can cause death. This applies even to such commonly used compounds as aspirin, cold tablets, and birth control pills. More than is commonly realized, ill-effects can occur when certain compounds are taken daily for many months or years. For example, a prominent business man who was in great pain with a bone disorder, became nervous and was placed on reserpine therapy. After a few months he developed depression which increased over several years. He lost his job, most of his money, and his home. He was contemplating suicide, but a few weeks after another physician stopped the reserpine, all was well again and he got a position. Prolonged usage of reserpine produces depression.

Many compounds are used to relieve symptoms but do not correct the fundamental disorder, and consequently the patient's condition may be worsened. For example, a patient who consults a physician because of headache, nervousness, insomnia, abdominal cramps, and diarrhea, may end up with one compound to relieve the headache, a second for the abdominal cramps, a third for the diarrhea, and a fourth for the insomnia. When these therapies are discontinued, the symptoms may become intensified. In reality all of them may have been produced by a family conflict that could be resolved.

DEATH

When we deal with death—its prevention, promotion, and management—we must call on both the art and the science of medicine. New policies and laws are needed concerning the role of physicians and others in (a) prolonging life, and (b) pointlessly delaying death. We must condition the public to recognize the following points: (a) Everyone must die; our genetic and metabolic patterns assure death; (b) sometimes it is best for the individual, his family, and society not to prolong life; death may be a welcome relief; (c) the last few minutes or hours of life often are not associated with much suffering; (d) during all phases of impending death there is much that the physician, the family, the patient, and others can do to reduce physical discomforts and to decrease feelings of loneliness, anxiety, fear, and other psychologic discomforts.

Death is said to be the permanent end of *all* life. However, we usually pronounce death a few minutes after gross body movements, breathing, and heartbeat have ceased. Yet we know that some of the cells can be removed after this time and, when cultured, will continue to multiply and to proceed with certain functions for weeks thereafter. Hela cells grow luxuriantly in many laboratories although the donor (Helen Lane) died many years ago. Criteria have been formulated for pronouncing death in patients with irreversible coma, although the heart continues to beat forcefully and most of the cells of the body are fully alive. When mentation is gone permanently, there is no good reason to maintain life in the other portions of the body, because the main purpose of the body and of life has been lost.

Death, of course, can occur within a few minutes, without any previous warning, or it can develop over a period of several years. It can occur in many different ways. However, I will describe here what seems to be one of the common patterns, considered in four stages: (1) impending death, which lasts for weeks, months, or years, (2) imminent death, which lasts for days, (3) cardiorespiratory failure, which lasts for hours, and (4) the Hereafter, which lasts infinitely.

The stage of *impending death* begins when maintenance of life seems relatively hopeless. Even with this status some patients may feel relatively good and continue working. Members of the family should be given (a) the diagnosis, if it has not been given earlier, (b) the proposed plan of therapy—largely to relieve symptoms, and (c) orientation with respect to the most probable course. Certain psychological, financial, and other adjustments for death should be made. Often it is difficult to predict the various phases accurately, but the physician's best thinking with the information at hand is usually of benefit.

Some patients experience prolonged and intense physical suffering as well as emotional trauma during the first stage. Until recently, with death impending many physicians have deliberately withheld much information that would aid the patient in visualizing his current and future status. We physicians have tended to follow our predecessors in presenting an unduly optimistic picture, as well as in attempting to prolong life as long as possible in all patients—making use of all facilities, artificial and otherwise, even when delaying death increases the agonies of the patient, his family, and society. When the prognosis is hopeless and especially when there also is much suffering, discussions should be held with the patient and certain members of the family to decide how much effort should be devoted to prolonging life as opposed to merely making the patient as comfortable as possible. If the patient and the physician think the latter has priority, they should proceed accordingly. When the patient is incompetent, this decision could be made by his next of kin and his physician. In the earlier-mentioned questionnaire for medical school faculty and trainees, only 4 percent voted to do everything conceivable for prolonging life in each patient.

In some decisions regarding euthanasia, in addition to the approval by the patient and his physician, opinions should be sought from members of a special committee that is competent to deal wisely with such measures.

The *imminent stage* is when death seems relatively certain and is expected reasonably soon. The patient needs to be prepared and comforted in this stage with regard to the actual dying process, and assurance must be given concerning the physician's ability to alleviate suffering. During this period and preceding it preparations for death are made by the patient, his family, and others.

The *third stage, cardiorespiratory failure,* is the one that most individuals associate with the greatest fears, anxieties, and horrible sensations. During this stage the patient eventually becomes unconscious. Moreover, drugs are usually used to alleviate discomfort and to dull the consciousness. I have witnessed hundreds of deaths in individuals who were under good medical care, and I believe that this stage is probably associated with the least discomfort of any of the three stages. Indeed, I myself have experienced this stage, and the discomfort I felt was probably equivalent to that felt by many others as they passed through this stage. Over a period of two days, due to heart stoppage, I was resuscitated 97 times; I lost consciousness with 35 of these episodes and had convulsions with many of them. On a number of occasions my heart stopped beating for more than 10 seconds, but between these spells, I was fully conscious. My death was considered almost inevitable. Although I had not been sick until three days before these episodes began, for several years I had conditioned myself to the concept that dying per se need not be associated with significant discomfort. Despite my being essentially dead numerous times, I would estimate that many individuals with psychoneurosis have suffered far more, although their "physical status is excellent."

Another example of the value of conditioning for death concerns my mother. By the age of 78 she had had heart failure for several years, and she expressed to me great fear of the final stages of dying. I described what would most probably be many of the characteristics and recounted some of the methods that we could use to prevent significant suffering. She accepted the orientation with full faith and confidence, and the subsequent year of her life was very happy. Two hours before death, she said that she knew the time had come, but that she was reasonably comfortable and well prepared for the end.

The *Hereafter* remains a mystery; it is discussed in Chapter 13. There are many who maintain that the Hereafter consists chiefly of persisting memories, good or bad, with regard to the deceased. The status of the victim's spirit and its entrance into hell or heaven remains mysterious. The existence of heaven or hell is doubted by many.

REFERENCES

Drummond, H. The greatest thing in the world. Reproduced by Harper & Row, N.Y. (initial publication 1890±)

Epstein, L. C. and L. Lasagna. 1969. Obtaining informed consent. *Arch. Int. Med.* **123:**682.

Williams, R. H. 1958. Future training in medicine and medical specialties. *J. Amer. Med. Assn.* **167:**192.

CHAPTER 12

LIFE AND DEATH: LESSONS FROM THE DYING

Elisabeth Kübler-Ross

INTRODUCTION

People are like stained glass windows; they sparkle and shine when the sun is out, but when the darkness sets in, their true beauty is revealed only if there is a light from within.   Unknown Author

I must have looked at my kitchen calendar a hundred times and read this saying often, without really grasping its meaning. It was not until years later that I became aware of the symbolical meaning of the statement, when I started to work with dying patients and followed them from the day of admission to the hospital until the time of their death.

There was Eva, who was in her last year of college, planning for a summer marriage and hoping that she would be "an exception to the rule"—that her acute leukemia could be conquered. She died six weeks after my first meeting with her. And there was little seven-year-old Susan, wiser and "older" than many adults, who was anticipating her death and looking forward to meeting her little sister and Jesus in heaven. She was better prepared for her death than were most of the staff, the members of the helping profession!

In our studies (Kübler-Ross, 1969), we followed over 500 patients who were faced with the knowledge of their limited life span and were struggling to find some sense and meaning in it. Originally, the idea was to learn from them—to ask them to be our teachers. And by sharing with us their needs, hopes, and fears, they would ultimately enable the professional and paraprofessional personnel to assist them better in this final crisis. We sat with them during days and nights, mainly listening to what they were able to impart and teach us. The results of these studies have helped many to accept death, and to face not only others in their dying but also to accept their own finiteness.

We may one day be grateful for the lessons we learned from these terminally ill patients, when it is our turn to face a crisis, whether final or not. This chapter is an attempt to share some of these lessons, which may be learned by those of us who are not critically ill. Perhaps we can thus benefit from the experience of those who have gone before us.

THE MEANING OF DEATH IN THE HISTORY OF MAN'S LIFE

While studying terminal patients, a series of questions arise that cry for an answer. Who are the patients who die "easily" and who are those who struggle in anguish and agony? Is the quality of life a measure of the ultimate quality of death? Do religious people die more peacefully than those who have lived without any religious faith? How can children often die with so much more equanimity and speak about their impending death when adults struggle to deny the reality of their impending demise? Is this pathological fear of death a result of our death-denying society? a problem of the Western culture? of modern man? or simply of the Judeo-Christian culture? And perhaps the question encompassing all the others is simply: How shall man live in order to be prepared for his own death without fear and anxiety?

Seeking the answers to these questions, one can look back through the history of man. In studying the philosophy of life and death we may examine art, music, poetry, or literature—all of which may shed some light on why man struggles with his own finiteness.

Probably the first poem in recorded history, the Babylonian *Gilgamesh,* is one of the most stirring poems in the literature of the world. King Gilgamesh visits Enkidu, his friend who represents mortal man. Enkidu is in the realm of death and involved in an almost superhuman struggle with death. King Gilgamesh is not successful in leading his friend back to the light, for "when the Gods created man they also created death for mankind." The king learns that the fate of men in the "beyond" is determined by the type of death they die![1]

If we follow the literature through history, we see how man tried to cope with the awareness of his finiteness. "Man is but a reed—and the weakest in nature; but then he is a reed that thinks," wrote Blaise Pascal. "It does not take the universe to crush him: a breath of air or a drop of water will kill him. Even if the material universe should overwhelm him, man would be more noble than that which destroys him; because he knows that he dies, while the universe knows nothing of the advantage which it obtains over him."

A similar philosophy of death is shared by the more contemporary American philosopher George Santayana, when he writes that, "Every knowledge raises man, in a sense, above mortality, by making him a sharer in the vision of eternal truth."

[1] This literature review is an excerpt from *The Meaning of Death,* to be published by Elisabeth Kübler-Ross and the late René Fueloep-Miller.

The price that man has to pay for his unique knowledge is the pain of anticipatory fear of death and the painful certainty that death is inevitable. Just as Gilgamesh lamented over the frightening aspect of his friend's death and his own death in 3000 B.C., patients and their families struggle today from denial to ultimate acceptance of death.

The Old Testament deals with death in Genesis and later on in the lamentations of Job. The fact that God's own chosen people were also subjected to the fear of death is borne out by the Psalms of David, in which death appears as a punishment of the wrathful Jehovah. Solomon makes death the measuring stone of all things when he cries: "All is vanity and straining after the wind." The prophets Isaiah and Jeremiah perceive death's inevitability and bemoan it or long for it. While the Old Testament only touches on death, the New Testament is based upon death entirely. It is the death of Christ that finds its glorification in the New Testament, and the salvation of mankind was brought about not really by Christ's life but by His death.

Some 1,500 years before Christ, the Hindu Vedic literature, in the third book of Rigveda, pronounced the dead holy. And the Vedic *Upanishads,* dating ca. 1000 B.C., contain the mystical teaching on all the riddles of life and death. Schopenhauer (and my own father!) said that this teaching has been the consolation of his life and would be his consolation in death!

Gauthama Buddha's poem *The Past of Truth* contains eternal words of wisdom on death. And the Hindu poem *The Self Is Not Born, Neither Does It Die,* from the Bhagavad Gītā (second century B.C.), is in its peculiar fashion one of the most inspiring Indian death poems. In the Indian view, the reading of this chapter from the death epic *Mahābhārata* during the funeral ceremony brought the soul of the newly dead inexhaustible happiness in the next world.

In the Chinese literature, it is above all the *Lot of Man* and *Proverbs* of Confucius that deserve mention. Later, the great Li-T'ai-Po wrote *Drinking Song on the Misery of this Earth.*

The main work of ancient Egyptian literature is the so-called *Book of the Dead* (ca. 1570–1100 B.C.), which contains detailed instructions for and descriptions of the life of the soul after its departure. The "Hall of Two-fold Justice," in which the dead man speaks with the God of Death and the judge, forms the chief scene. The "Book of Things in the Depth" and "The Book of Fools" describe the ghosts of the kingdom of death. An old pyramid text written about 3000 B.C. considers death with utmost serenity. The last verse of it reads: "Death is before me today as man longs to see his house when he has spent years in captivity." It is only toward the end of the Middle Kingdom that skepticism appears in the Egyptian concept of death. We find its literary expression in the "Talk Between One Tired of Life and a Soul."

In the pagan death poems of the old Germanic North, we find the glorification of the heroic death. They concede a happy afterlife only to the hero who dies on the battlefield.

It was certainly in Greek culture that man attained the most harmonious outlook on life and death. In Greece, death took the shape of a beautiful young man, resembling Eros. The Greeks compared Death with his brother Sleep, and they called their burial grounds "cemeteries," which means "sleeping rooms." Their tombs were fashioned in such a way that when Shelley saw them for the first time, he compared them enthusiastically with bridal rooms of immortal spirits. And yet, the Greek culture, which apparently seemed reconciled with the idea of death, was not spared the bitter horror of death. What else could it have been but the fear of death that made Homer put the following gloomy words in the mouth of departed Achilles: "Nay, speak not comfortingly to me of death. Oh great Odysseus, far rather would I live on earth the hireling of another, with a landless man who is himself destitute, than bear away over all the dead that be departed!"

Euripides, the great Greek tragedian, conveyed in moving scenes the dread of death in his times. In his *Iphigenia in Aulis,* we see the heroine pained by the thought of death, imploring her father to spare her life, which is to be sacrificed. "To die, how horrible," she exclaims; "the worst life is much better still than death." And in his *Hippolytus*, we hear:

> And so we are sick for life and cling
> on earth to this nameless and shining thin.
> For other life is a fountain sealed
> And the deeps below us are unrevealed
> And we drift on legends forever.

Socrates, perhaps the wisest man of all time, reiterates frequently that his contemporaries were troubled by the fear of death.

The most striking remark about the fear of death in Greece came, however, thousands of years later. It was written by the German poet and philosopher Herder, who tried to destroy the myth that the Greeks were free from the fear of death. Herder explained that Thanatos, the Greek God of Death, was feared and hated to such an extent that they not only hated to utter his name, but also considered the first letter of his name an evil omen.

The widespread fear of death in ancient Rome was similar to our own fear of death in modern America. This is well illustrated in the custom of talking about a deceased man as someone "who had lived" and not "someone who is dead." The Roman poets did not stress the irrevocability of death but elaborated on the shortness of life and advised man to enjoy it to the utmost. This is the message of Horace in his "Ode to Maecenas": "The joys I have possessed, in spite of fate, are mine. Nor Heaven itself upon the past has power, but what has been, has been, and I have had my hour."

The most powerful document of death literature is to be found in the third book of Lucretius' *On the Nature of Things:*

> What has this bugbear Death to frighten man,
> If souls can die, as well as bodies can?
> For as before our birth we felt no pain . . .
> so when our mortal frame shall be disjoin'd,
> the lifeless lump uncoupled from the mind,
> from sense of grief and pain we shall be free;
> we shall not feel, because we shall not be.

If we look at death in the Orient, we are not surprised that Saadi, the Persian poet, in his deeply moving description of his own agony and grief at the burial of his child, sounds no different than any parent we have ever accompanied to the funeral of his child in our time. Even the wise Omar Khayyam in his *Rubaiyat* wonders why we really know so little about the stranger death:

> Strange, is it not? that of the myriad who
> before us pass'd the door of Darkness through,
> not one returns to tell us of the Road,
> which to discover we must travel too.

During the Christian era, the fear of death was increased by the anxiety about the spiritual welfare after death. This apprehension reached its height during the Middle Ages, when the idea of Hell and eternal perdition, which threatened the sinner after death, became so prevalent that whole centuries were shaken with the fear of death. The terror of death is perhaps best seen in the paintings of this time, which picture death as a devil, killer, or revengeful destroyer, using a sword, scythe, spade, arrow, rope, or net during its incessant attempts to trap man.

The poetry of the Middle Ages is obsessed with the thought of death. Dante, the author of the *Divine Comedy,* is possessed by a deeply mystical feeling for death, as he progresses through the three spirit kingdoms of the beyond. For him, death is only a transition and an entrance to something divine and new. Petrarch also returns in his death poem for "Laura" to the brighter conception of antiquity.

Shakespeare's *Julius Caesar* shows the same kind of acceptance when he writes:

> Cowards die many times before their death;
> The Valiant never taste of death but once.
> Of all the wonders that I yet have heard,
> It seems to me most strange that men should fear;
> Seeing that death, a necessary end
> Will come when it will come.

In the seventeenth century we have the great *Horatian Ode Upon Cromwell's Return from Ireland* by Andrew Marvell. And with Thomas

Gray's *Elegy Written in a Country Churchyard,* the English poetry of death of the eighteenth century reaches its zenith.

In German poetry, the folk song *There Goes a Reaper, Named Death* initiated the writing of many powerful poems devoted to the subject of death. Paul Gerhardt's *O Sacred Head Now Wounded* has been set to music and has become a familiar church song. Klopstock glorified death. Goethe was able to rise above the fear of death in *Wanderer's Night Song.* His philosophy can be summarized in three words: "Die and become." Novalis said: "Death is life; life is only understood in death." We can look at Kleist, who terminated his own life, or at the writings of others such as Hebbel, Hugo von Hofmansthal, Rilke, or Hesse—each one of whom tried to see a positive side of death from many different angles.

The most outstanding German modern work, in which death plays a leading part, is Thomas Mann's *The Magic Mountain.* Mann calls death the "genius principle" and states that there are two roads to life. One of these is the usual and direct one, the other the hard and unusual one, which leads through death and is the road of genius.

In American literature, different attitudes toward death can be seen in Edgar Allan Poe's frightening poem *The Raven* or in the tender love poem *Annabel Lee.* Walt Whitman sings a hymn to death in his *I Heard the Universal Mother* and his poems in memory of President Lincoln. Emily Dickinson's little poem *Quiet Dust* is impressive in its simplicity. Charlotte Brontë also wrote in an eloquent manner, mourning the death of her sister. Thornton Wilder and Thomas Wolfe, the two noted authors, also dealt with the meaning of death. In his play *Our Town,* Wilder looks at the whole of life of a small town from the perspective of death. In *The Bridge of San Luis Rey,* he expresses the tender and consoling thought: "There is a land of the living and a land of the dead and the bridge is love; the only survival, the only meaning." Wilder's statement is no different from the Jewish concept that we shall continue to live as long as we are not forgotten and as long as we have loved and have been loved.

THE QUALITY OF LIFE AND THE ACCEPTANCE OF DEATH

It is irrelevant whether our concept of an afterlife includes a heaven with a golden gate, reincarnation, or a land of the dead. What is relevant is how we have lived, how we have loved, and how much trust and faith we have had in our lifetime.

Patients who are genuinely religious, no matter what denomination they belong to, go through an initial shock and temporary denial when they face their own impending death. They quickly pass, however, through the anger, bargaining, and depression, to reach a final acceptance without bitterness and anguish. People who are "a little bit religious" often feel guilt and remorse before death. They grieve not only their impending death, but also the irreversible loss of opportunity for love, faith, and true living.

If one can be aware and enjoy and live for today, he will be able to face death when it comes. This is perhaps best expressed in a letter from one of my dying patients:

> . . . I have a wonderful husband, whom I can talk with freely, and a couple of sisters; but other than that, the subject of my illness is taboo. People shy away from any mention of it . . . . We had a wonderful Christmas, and I am thankful that after almost two years since the diagnosis, I feel as good as I do. The overwhelming weakness is the worst, and trying to keep up with five boys (2½ to 8 years old) wears me down real fast. But you get a little less particular about dust in the corners, and you enjoy the boys as they are *right now* and you don't wonder about their futures. The Lord will take care of that. There are so many things I would like to say to them, so I am writing alot of thoughts down on paper. Someday their dad can read it to them, when they are old enough to comprehend the thoughts I want to leave with them.
>
> We live in such a fast-paced world, very few people really and truly enjoy their everyday living; they are always planning for tomorrow and next year! My husband and I have gone through so much, but we have lived life fuller and enjoyed it more than some people do in a whole lifetime. . . . Nobody but the Lord knows what is going to happen, so I am going to enjoy life *right now*.

A mother of a child with leukemia expressed the same feelings in a poem she gave to me entitled "Future Shock" (Kübler-Ross, in preparation):

> I cram it all in as much as I can,
> For today is tomorrow for our little man.
> Make memories now and hold them fast,
> For the future is but a thing of the past.
> The feeling of panic is slow to leave;
> I've spent so much time getting ready to grieve.
> Why is he going? Does nothing last?
> The future should not be a thing of the past.
> Some songs are short and some are long—
> Four years of perfection, but still—a short song.
> But *today* he does sing, and he's lively and loud,
> And the future has become the present, the now.

David Cole Gordon stated in his book *Overcoming the Fear of Death* that man does not fear death itself but that he associates death with the fears of time, decay, the unknown, irreversibility, the loss of pleasure and thought, and the loss of the self. Gordon helps us realize that we have allowed the clock to tyrannize us and to control our lives. He further elaborates on a theory of unification, which views man's basic motivation as the attainment of spontaneous peak experiences in which man is unified with himself, others, and the world, and in which his thought processes are momentarily stilled. Death for him is not associated with destruction but is seen as the ultimate unification experience, something we are all longing for.

He describes modern man in his pursuit of happiness, joining with business partners to make money, his search for security and control. But he also wisely shows how soon such interpersonal relationships turn from love to hate—basically, how vulnerable they are when they are not based on love, which culminates in this unification experience. Gratifying sexual experiences and enjoying hobbies and creative work, sports, or dancing may produce this unification experience. The best example is perhaps the one of the mountain climber who lives for the moment, who concentrates on the next step and the next handhold. He thinks fewer and fewer random thoughts. In mountain climbing, he, nature, in form of the mountain, and his other companions become more and more closely unified. Of sleep, Gordon says, "Sleep at least represents a cessation of totally conscious thought and a merging into a world that is less egotistically affirmed and more universal. . . . As we know from the personal experience we have all had, before we fall asleep our thoughts become fewer and fewer until they finally cease altogether. Just before losing consciousness we would not think even if we wanted to. So falling asleep is also a unification process that involves the gradual reduction of thought until there is no thought, and finally unification ensues."

Of death, he says: "Death does not represent destruction, evil, meaningless oblivion, or the dark forces of man. It is the quintessence of what man has always desired most and what has been the chief motivational factor in his life; the search for, and repetition of, the spontaneous unification experience he has encountered sporadically and at random during the course of his life and existence. It is the final, ultimate, and external experience of unity."

If we believe this theory and try to verify these concepts in the clinical setting, we begin to see why certain patients die with much more peace and equanimity.

Let us take the example of Miss T., a single, black woman who was in her early thirties when she was found unacceptable for a kidney dialysis program. This meant basically that she had to die in a society that had the means to keep her alive. It was our task to give her the bad news and our hope that we would be able to "be with her" during this final great crisis. Her physician, nurses, chaplain, and her social worker were all upset, and the patient ultimately consoled *us* with her statement: "Don't be so upset about it. I know I am going to die very soon, but it will be like being transplanted from this garden into God's garden."

A few evenings later, shortly before she died, Miss T. requested my presence. All was quiet in the hospital when I sat by her side, silently holding her hand. Neither of us thought about things and people outside the stark walls. I wondered what helped this young woman to accept her fate so peacefully. She apparently had a single problem on her mind that she needed to share with me. She kept repeating, "I am bad, I am bad," and together we sought to learn why she felt this way. We enumerated a number of things that could be regarded as bad in our society, and nothing seemed "right." I finally gave up and blurted out, "God only knows why you should feel bad!"

Her face lit up. "This is my answer. I have called God for help so many times these last few days and I hear Him say in the back of my mind, 'Why are you calling me *now*? Why did you not call me before when things were all right? What do you say to that Dr. Ross?"

I asked her what would happen if a boy would fall when playing outside and hurt his knee while mother was in the house. Without hesitation, she responded that the mother would go outside and console and help her child. I then continued the questioning and asked what would happen after the boy was all right and returned to play. She said, "The mother would go back into the house." And I asked, "The boy would have no use for her then?" After her, "No," I questioned further: "Does the mother resent this terribly?" Surprised, she said, "No, a mother would not resent that!" Looking at her, I said, "Strange; a mother would not resent it, and Father should?"

A bright smile came over her face. At that moment there was the greatest feeling of peace and acceptance in both of us. It was almost as if all thoughts ceased to be. There were no more doubts and no more questions, and no more fears. Unification experiences like this, especially with dying patients, not only make it possible for the terminally ill to die in peace, but also help us to accept our own finiteness with equanimity and without dread. This woman had experienced great love in her life and an equally solid faith in God, both of which helped her face this final crisis. I have a feeling that when I die, I will be thinking of these moments when I was at peace with myself, with another human being, and with this world.

If we believe that the quality of life is ultimately what counts in the face of death, then we see why bitter, resentful, money-hungry, and greedy people have more difficulties in accepting death. For, quality of life does not mean material riches. It refers entirely to the moments in our lives when we were at peace with ourselves and the world we lived in. It also refers to the truly meaningful relationships that we have had, the moments that we will reflect upon when we are lonely, old, or full of cancer. In those last few weeks and days, my dying patients did not reflect on how many fur coats they possessed or how many fancy handbags they showed off. Material things gradually lose their values as man reflects on the deeper meaning of life and death.

My final example is perhaps best documented by a black cleaning woman I met in the hospital where I held my seminars with dying patients. It was during the time when an almost insurmountable wave of hostility and resistance on part of the staff seemed to make these interviews with dying patients impossible. In my search for answers, I became very observant of the environment in which I had to function. During my daily rounds I noticed that this cleaning woman left some sort of imprint on my troubled patients. They did not talk about her, but I noticed that they appeared more comfortable each time she had been in their room.

One day I asked her what she did with my patients, and she became very defensive. She was concerned that I suspected her of "getting involved" with patients, while her job was simply to clean the floors! Weeks later, we finally had a cup of coffee together, and she opened up. She shared in simple language her life in the ghetto, her upbringing in poverty and hunger, hours of sitting with her dying child in the waiting room of a county hospital. The child died in her lap. There was no bitterness in her voice—simply statements of the summary of her life. But then she added, "Death is not a stranger to me any more, he is an old acquaintance. I am not afraid of him anymore. Sometimes I walk into the room of one of your dying patients and they look so scared. I cannot help but go over to them and touch them and say, "don't be scared, it is not so terrible."

This woman taught me that it is not what we say or do that is so important, but how we feel inside about it. Her suffering had truly enriched her life, and through her simple acceptance and love, she had helped others to come to peace with death.

Is it then not understandable that, in our materialistic and competitive world, we have little time to reflect on the deeper meaning of life? Is it not understandable why we have become the most death-denying society of all time? How can people who go from war to war, who develop atom bombs, who have little or no use for their old and their dying patients, be at peace with their own finiteness?

If we could stop our pursuit of more and more material things, if we could reflect for a while on what really counts, if we had the courage to think and reflect about life *and* death, we would raise our children differently. We would not allow 80 percent of the population in the United States to die in institutions. We would not allow our children to be excluded from visiting sick and dying patients in hospitals. We would make death and dying part of life again. We would then be able to raise a generation that would say with peace, "I have lived and therefore I will be able to die."

REFERENCES

Kübler-Ross, E. 1969. On Death and Dying. New York, Macmillan.
The literature review is an excerpt from *The Meaning of Death* to be published by Elisabeth Kübler-Ross and the late René Fueloep-Miller.
"Future Shock" poem is part of a book in preparation, *Children and Death,* by Elisabeth Kübler-Ross, to be published by Macmillan.
Gordon, D.C. 1970. Overcoming the Fear of Death. New York, Macmillan.

CHAPTER 13

THE HERE AND THE HEREAFTER: REFLECTIONS ON TRAGEDY AND COMEDY IN HUMAN EXISTENCE

JAMES LYNWOOD WALKER

In *Civilization and Its Discontents,* one of his germinal works, Sigmund Freud's basic thesis regarding civilization is that it issues from the struggle in human existence between Eros and Thanatos, love (life) and death. He claimed that it is the agonies of this struggle which nursemaids attempt to alleviate with their lullabies of Heaven. Regardless of our disagreements with detailed elaborations of this thesis by Freud and his followers, we cannot deny the basic truth in his assertions. Death is a central fact of human existence. It is the conclusion of aging, which we call, in the early years, growth and, in later years, deterioration. Aging, and therefore death, are implicit in birth.

Every culture has conceptions of life, death, and life after death. Man is human, the existentialists say, because he can be aware of himself as a separate, unique individual; he can transcend himself, that is, stand outside himself, as it were, and observe himself as he acts and is acted upon; and he can imagine, giving him the capacity to recall the past and to anticipate the future. Indeed, each man is capable of *projecting* himself into the future, in order to imagine his death and to wonder about life, if any, beyond death.

Conceptions of life after death are statements, also, about life before death. These conceptions provide direction to one's aspirations, delineate the nature and style of one's interaction with his environment, and determine the emotional tone of one's philosophy of life. Life-after-death theories represent attempts to elucidate the meaning of human existence against the background of its ultimate end. In a popular blues ballad, the lover's rationale for enhancing and sustaining an ecstatic moment is expressed simply in these words: "Tomorrow may never come, for all we know."

In various idioms, each man, regardless of his commitment or indifference to codified or institutionalized religious expressions, conceptualizes the relationship between the here and the hereafter and lives by the basic principles and implications of that conceptualization. A recent poster quotes Shakespeare as follows: "Life is a tragedy to those that think and a comedy to those that feel." Tragedy and comedy are themes through which we can illuminate our understanding of the relationship between the here and hereafter.

The final fact of human existence is death, a fact which each man either overemphasizes or ignores at his own peril. Throughout life, man vibrates between pride of uniqueness and fear of mortality. On the one hand, he feels exhilarated by his potentialities as a unique being. On the other hand, he feels frustrated by the ultimacy of death. Between the polar extremes of birth and death, the drama of the wandering spirit is enacted through the two basic dimensions of tragedy and comedy, both of which can be varied and embellished endlessly. Death can be seen as both the irrevocable tragedy and the ultimate comedy of human existence, for awareness of death implies that the fulfillment or completion of each act or event signals death's approach and that one must seize the time as if each moment were his last. Man's perennial challenge is to be aware of death and of the preciousness of each moment of life, without becoming either somber or flippant about life.

In the drama of the self, basic life attitudes are limited to the emphasis of the tragic or comic perspectives, or to a fusion of the two into a tragicomic orientation. Some persons focus on tragedy to the relative exclusion of comedy. To them, life is filled with travail and woe. Often, elaboration of the tragic perspective leads to consideration of psychosis, suicide, and murder as life's most salient alternatives. The tragic figure may begin to feel that life is utterly hopeless and meaningless, with little or no chance for change and renewal. Or, in some cases, he feels that improvement in his condition is contingent upon his ability to make others suffer and perhaps die. The result is a basic sadomasochistic style of life. Other persons emphasize comedy to the relative exclusion of tragedy. If the comic perspective is overelaborated, one's responses to life can become circumscribed by fatalism, passivity, and vanity. He can begin to feel that all furious action to make life meaningful and worthwhile is silly and futile.

Overemphasis of either tragedy or comedy can lead to a sense of hopelessness and despair, and only the *apparent* responses to that hopelessness and despair distinguish the tragic from the comic figure. The tragic figure tends to respond to his condition with an explosive self- or other-destructive act, whereas the comic figure tends to respond to his condition with a feigned courage, expressed through a happy-go-lucky faith that things will work out somehow, or with a mask of foolishness that guards him against being taken seriously. Still others recognize both tragedy and comedy as necessary, although separately insufficient, ingredients for the creative, wholesome self. Life, when viewed as the tragicomic drama of each self in its strivings for completion and wholeness, can be appreciated as an enterprise to be taken seriously, although not so seriously that one is overwhelmed by the pathos and sorrow, the absurdity and folly, which define the ambiguity and contingency of human existence. Those who are able to achieve and maintain the tragicomic perspective—which holds the reality of both suffering and release in creative tension—are those most likely to cope with, rather than to avoid, the experience of dying and, therefore, of living.

In literature, the purpose of the tragedy is to appeal to serious thoughts and emotions, concerning especially the profound sufferings of man. The focus is generally on some tumultuous passion or weakness of the leading character that leads him to a catastrophic end. Usually, as the tragedy unfolds toward the denouement, the hero, often admirable in many ways, achieves insight into the meanings of his conflicts, and the tragic act signifies an achievement for the hero of some sense of unification of an inner self. Contrariwise, comedy highlights man's follies and absurdities and usually comes to a happy ending. There was, for example, a fairly long period in America when most movies ended on a happy note, with the implication that the heroes, with whom we were supposed to identify, "lived happily ever after." In retrospect, we can see that the happy-ending trend in movies reflected American's unwillingness to face the tragic dimension of life, as well as it reflected America's need for periodic release from the inescapable tragedies of daily life, no matter how allegedly inane the liberating agent. Moreover, one can denigrate comedy only if he remains unaware that comedy usually contains satirical, chiding, and mocking aspects which challenge the spectator to entertain fresh perspectives and to undertake new action. Although the ostensible purpose of comedy is to excite mirth, its deeper purpose is to excite, ultimately, the alertness of wit, serious reflection, and deep involvement which tragedy demands. Consequently, we are inaccurate when we merely oppose the ostensible light-heartedness of comedy to the deeper emotions of tragedy, rather than seeing tragedy and comedy as different ways of conceptualizing events and actions.

The difference between tragedy and comedy in the search for self is the difference between taking oneself too seriously and being able to acknowledge one's ridiculously human limitations which, when seen clearly and experienced fully, can be fairly easily transcended. In short, the difference between tragedy and comedy is the difference between man's age-old heritage of alienating pride and his ever-present potentiality for reconciling humility. Clearly, the tragic perspective is the prime source of the martyr complex and, consequently, of the waiting game in which one expects that some apocalyptic or eschatological event will deliver him from all his pains and ills. It is also the perspective that challenges us to take life seriously and to do battle with the forces of destruction which plague us.

Equally clearly, the comic perspective is the prime source of that self-destructive flippancy that allows us to be foolhardy and noncommital about life's deeper meaning. Yet, it is also the perspective which enables us to achieve the liberating awareness that we are free to determine how we will respond to our conditions and to participate in the continuing creation and recreation of our world, regardless of how determined or limited we are by physiological, psychological, and sociological reality and heritage. From the serious perspective, all of life can be viewed as unqualifiedly tragic, as a cruel joke perpetrated on man by a company of diabolical gods. From the light-hearted perspective, all of life can be viewed as hilariously, unspeakably comical, which gets funnier as we get more and more serious about it. The *whole truth* is in the middle: instead of being either totally tragic or totally comic, life is a tragicomic pilgrimage from cradle to grave in which each man strives to discover, over and over, a sense of self through which he creates his own meaning and through which meaning is perceived and revealed in interpersonal communion.

There are two songs which illustrate the necessary unification of tragedy and comedy in the self. The first is a song titled "Who Am I?," as interpreted by Nina Simone, a fascinating black musician, who has been variously described as High Priestess, mystic, preacher, and artist. (At the very least, she is a masterful interpreter of music, both instrumentally and vocally.) Following are the words of the song:

Who am I? Who am I?
Was it all planned in advance,
Or was I just born by chance
   in July?
My friends only think of fun;
They're such a curious lot.
Must I be the only one
Who thinks these mysterious thoughts?
Some day I'll die.
Will I ever live again
As a mountain-lion, or a rooster
   or a hen, or a robin or a wren,
   or a fly?
Oh, who am I?
Do you believe in reincarnation?
Do you believe in reincarnation?
Were you ever here before?
Have you ever had dreams that you knew
   were true some time before in your life:
Have you ever had that experience?
So, you must question all the truths that
   you know,
All the loves and the lives that you know, and say:
Who am I?
Will I ever live again

> As a mountain-lion, or a rooster
> 　or a hen, or a robin or a wren,
> 　or a fly?
> Oh, who am I?

On the surface, these lyrics represent merely the sad and terrified wailing of a youngster who is mystified by the origins, meanings, and promises of life. She evinces the tendency of the tragic ones to view their plights as utterly unique and outside the experience of others: "Must *I* be the only one who thinks these mysterious thoughts?" She entertains questions about freedom and determinism, life and death, death and resurrection, separateness and relatedness, and wonders if they are entertained by others. Yet, on the underface, these lyrics represent the striving of a mystified self to overcome alienation, to recover a sense of healing perspective which allows one to acknowledge that all truths, all love, all life must be questioned if the self is to be renewed and is to grow. It is also this healing perspective which saves one from unmitigated arrogance and despair, for "if I'm one of those lives that have been reincarnated again and again and again and again and again, [then] who am *I*?" Summarily, the lyrics give at least a hint of self-ridicule which affirms a rudimentary awareness that the youngster must not take this particular plight too seriously. There is also, in the artist's playful tinkering with and serious command of the piano, evidence of the wholesome mixture of tragedy and comedy which characterizes the unifying or unified self.

Another song which illuminates our topic is titled "Blues for the Weepers," as interpreted by Lou Rawls, Al Hibbler, and Della Reese, who are outstanding contemporary blues singers. The lyrics are:

> The gay lights of glamour are darkened by drama,
> 　for the blues that I sing is the theme,
> Of the sob-singing sisters and the torch-bearing
> 　misters,
> Who just come to listen and dream.
> The soft lights are glowing;
> The champagne is flowing;
> In each customer's eye there's a gleam.
> They are the weary and weepless,
> 　the sad-eyed and sleepless,
> Who just come to listen and dream.
> Now, the black of the night
> Brings the blues in the night.
> Somehow they both seem to belong.
> They're the sad-eyed and the gay ones,
> 　the real hip, hooray ones;
> They hang on to each and every word of my song.
> For I sing of their drama,
> 　their fast-fading glamour;
> And the blues that I sing is my theme
> 　for the sob-singing sisters and the torch-bearing
> 　misters,
> Who just come to listen and to dream.
> Blues for the weepers!

In the rendition of this song, the singer and the band present a light-hearted treatment of apparent tragedy, though the primary, pervasive seriousness of the artists is equally clear. While describing objects as truly as possible, the singer reminds us that true meanings of the objects are to be discerned only through the overtones and undertones of the total setting.

Picture a night-club scene: dark lights, gay decor, mod fashions, waiters and waitresses, a singer and band members dressed in flashy costumes. The band goes into soft blues changes and the vocalist begins: "The gay lights of glamour are darkened by drama, by the blues that I sing for my thing . . . ." As he sings, one can almost picture him strutting across the stage, assuming various postures and expressions—some serious, some mocking and sarcastic. Throughout, the singer astutely reproduces all the phenomena of deep pathos, while also hinting that he is simply entertaining. Yet, for those who are listening with the third ear, that is, with the total organism, and who are therefore participating in the singer's experience, there are insights and perspectives which can be used in the search for self and release from the blues. The singer continues: "For I sing of their glamour, their fast-fading glamour; and the blues that I sing is the thing . . . ." The band then gives a playfully syncopated rendition of the title, a trill of notes which seem to suggest: "Now we will playfully mock the sadness of the tragic ones. We will mock their sadness both in the sense of feigning sadness ourselves and by poking fun at them for wasting their precious energies on needless self-pity." Sure enough, just when we begin to think that the musicians could not render blues changes and phenomena so accurately if, indeed, they did not have the blues themselves, the band reminds us, through playful syncopations, that we must not mistake the entertainment for the real thing. At this point, the spotlight returns to the vocalist, who repeats, with the same obvious seriousness, mockery, and sarcasm:

> For I sing of their drama,
>   their fast-fading glamour;
> And the blues that I sing is my theme
>   for the sob-singing sisters and the torch-bearing
>   misters,
> Who just come to listen and to dream.

In this short drama of song, the entertainers achieve the difficult task of interpreting, powerfully and sympathetically, the phenomena of tragedy and pathos and simultaneously poking gentle fun at the self-pitiers. It is essentially this creative synthesis of tragedy and comedy that defines the wholesome self.

To learn how to conjoin the power of compassion and understanding with the soothing gentleness of sensitivity and perspective is the ever-present challenge to each curer of souls, be he priest or prophet, medical man or witch doctor, loved one or stranger. When I can identify with and participate in another's suffering fully enough to understand the dynamics and depths of his struggle, I am able to reflect to him the totality of his experience in all of its seriousness and ludicrousness. The ability to see and to accept the ludicrousness of one's suffering can lead to deep laughter which represents, simultaneously, astonishment over one's ridiculous self-pity and joy over the unspeakable feeling of release. However, this comic laughter does not obliterate the seriously tragic realities of life, and it is generally followed by tears of joy which melt into deep weeping, representing unfinished grief over the pains and sufferings which accumulate in the agonizing struggle for life against the forces of death.

I am continually astounded at how ill-prepared our culture is to accept either deep laughter or deep weeping. We tend to adjudge those who enjoy laughter as guilty either of flippancy or of sinful indulgence in sensuality. We often characterize such persons as thinking only of fun. Furthermore, we tend to adjudge those who dare to weep openly as guilty of weakness, especially if they are men, or of taking matters too seriously. In a culture in which unfinished business is the norm and in which we are encouraged to save the completing of unfinished business for the "life to come," one who perceives possibilities of creating or discovering heaven in his own time and space must work through the comic gaiety and the tragic reflection of his unfinished business here and now. Only thus can he reclaim the life-giving energies with which he can participate in the death of the old and the exhilarating birth of the new. Only thus can he realize that life is to be both suffered and enjoyed.

Nevertheless, we must realize that the tragedy-oriented search for self can be, and often is, a most effective way to avoid the self. It can serve as a rationalization of one's existence when one is afraid that there is no authentic raison d'être and that the self, on its own terms, is not worthy of time and space. Comedy, also, can be, and often is, a means of resisting and avoiding change and growth. Yet, when combined into a wholesome tragicomic perspective, seriousness and light-heartedness can become the means whereby we see, acknowledge, and accept truths about ourselves which we have hitherto rejected. For example, the Jews' self-conscious identity as a suffering people seems to be one prime source of their concept of themselves as God's chosen people. When carried too far, this serious concept resulted in a very narrow, nationalistic understanding of the Messiah as one who would fit all their expectations and magically deliver them from the position of weakness into a position of prominence and power. Yet, despite this narrow perspective—if not because of it—the Jews have produced not only some of the world's most astute thinkers, but also some of the world's most intuitive comedians, who do not hesitate to poke fun at their own people. Moreover, in the current struggle of blacks for identity and integrity, we also see the tension between tragedy and comedy. Some authors and spokesmen assert that blacks are singularly oppressed and blessed. While there is profound truth in this assertion, which must not be taken lightly, there is also profound danger of arrogance and pride which can issue in self-justification and acquiescence, rather than in confrontation and self-determination. On the other hand, James Baldwin's almost completely humorless, agonized writings which reflect, in part, his deeply personal pilgrimage, also illustrate how the self-consciously chosen and overemphasized dimension of tragedy becomes additional, even excess, baggage when added to the realities of evil and suffering which seem inherent in the human condition. Yet, in Baldwin, perhaps above all other contemporary visionaries, there remains a balance of perspective which frees him from the ultimate dangers of arrogance and makes possible in him the reconciliation between the opposing forces of joy and despair. Like the Jews, blacks have produced both cogent thinkers and sensitive comics, who fear neither serious nor light-hearted analysis of the contemporary state of man and society.

I do not fully understand the relative lack of profundity and gaiety in many, perhaps most, contemporary white Americans. Profoundly thinking and genuinely comic whites seem rare, perhaps because repression of vital aspects of both personal and group experience has been an integral feature of American history. It seems that American institutions have become so sterile that persons can neither suffer tragedy nor enjoy comedy within them. If this is true, then American institutions, peopled largely by whites, have become more than ample proof that people who cannot suffer, or who through various mental tricks are unaware of suffering, which they both inflict and experience, cannot live.

In the final analysis, the essence of the tragicomic tension in life is oscillation between arrogant pride and unself-conscious humility; between self-centeredness and self-transcendence; between self-pity and self-concern; between determinism and freedom; between permanence and impermanence; and between vitality in life and death in life. This tragicomic tension is a recurring phenomenon, appearing always in different guises or with different nuances. For example:

> A female student begins a group therapy session acknowledging that she detests being ridiculed and often refuses to risk contact with others because she is afraid they will ridicule her. She acknowledges also that she is sensitive to, indeed searches for, the minutest signals that others see her as ridiculous and that when she discovers such signals, she immediately terminates the encounter. The therapist ventures the suspicion that in this way she accumulates lists of persons whom she attempts to avoid for fear of being ridiculed. She smiles and begins to relate how she used to hide in hallways and on stairwells in apartment buildings to avoid encountering other tenants; how she used to peek out doorways before entering sidewalks to make sure that no one was coming whom she knew; and how she maintains little ways of avoiding situations in which she fears either being, or being thought of as, ridiculous. The therapist ventures further: "So you became utterly ridiculous in order to avoid being ridiculed." At which point the young lady's husband, the therapist,

and the young lady herself burst into laughter. No miraculous transformation has occurred necessarily, except that the young lady is now aware of how she makes herself ridiculous and no longer can blame her condition on others. We can now focus on how she adopted this as a style of relationship, what it reflects about her self-concept, and how she can move more freely into creative encounter.

Death is inevitable. The sharper our awareness of this fact, the more likely we are to seize our time and to make life livable through the assertion of our creative energies. No matter *how* we conceive of life after death, or whether we conceptualize such a thing, the meanings and consequences of our living are unfolding here and now. The tragedy is that denying death, we deny life also. The comedy is that actual death will come much too soon anyway.

Finally, it might be useful to comment more specifically on conceptions of life after death. Numerous conceptions of the hereafter are operative in American society. These conceptions range from the judgment that any conception of a hereafter is utter nonsense to profound belief in bodily resurrection of the dead. Between these extremes, there are various positions that can be summarized in general terms. First, some persons believe in the perpetuation of identity through what can be called "genetic immortality." Continued existence is achieved by passing genetic material to succeeding generations of offspring, ad infinitum. Second, some persons, while acknowledging the inevitable decay of the body, look toward life after death through the conversion of bodily substance into other forms of life—or at least into forms of nurture and sustenance for new life. Third, some persons believe in the passing of the soul at death into another body or other bodies. There are innumerable variations on each of these themes regarding life after death. In each case, the basis of speculation is some form of faith. We know that the body decays. We know also that the history, actuality, and imagination that characterizes a unique personal identity fade with the decay of the body. Even if one continues to live in the memory of others, he is remembered in terms of the peculiar perspectives of others, rather than in terms of his own self-concept of which he alone is fully aware. The entire issue of the hereafter, or life after death, is a matter of faith, to be adjudicated on none other than psychological or spiritual grounds, where the appropriate concern is the purpose served by one's faith as applied to particular spheres of life. My assumption is that a useful conception of the hereafter will, at every point, highlight the preciousness of the here and now. Implicit, of course, is the assumption that the mystery of "life now" is at least as fascinating as the mystery of life after death.

CHAPTER 14

TOO MANY AND TOO FEW LIMITATIONS FOR CHILDREN

MICHAEL B. ROTHENBERG

INTRODUCTION: THE NEED FOR HISTORICAL PERSPECTIVE

The conjunction in the middle of the title of this chapter seems to me to characterize the current status of this situation quite accurately. Too many *and* too few limitations plague our children and ourselves, and indeed, in the same family, both situations may be present simultaneously. As the pressure has increased on physicians, among others, to provide society with some solution to this dilemma, we have often tended to provide a prescription which draws heavily from what I call the "unholy trinity" of activity/authority/magic. Traditionally, our patients have expected us to go about solving their problems in a highly active manner, our actions carried out with maximum authority, and with both doctor and patient tacitly accepting the reassurance provided for both parties by the "magic" of medicine. It is my impression that we do our patients and ourselves a disservice when we attempt to respond in this manner to the highly complex issues which are represented by children's and parents' questions concerning too many and too few limitations. Paul Goodman (1964), whom many college students attempted to make into one of their folk heros, pointed out to those of our children who consider themselves in the vanguard of various "anti-Establishment" movements in recent years, that their greatest weakness, and thus the greatest danger to the success of their cause, is the fact that "they have no sense of history." We adults, as we attempt to respond to the question of limitations, also seem often to have little or no historical perspective.

Since the beginning of World War II, we have been living in a world of turmoil. Even the most superficial glance at this period reveals a pattern of continuous rebellion against authority, established value systems, and accepted behaviors. The basic pattern appears to be the same, whether expressed in the emergence of new nation-states from crumbled colonial empires, frequent changes of government in established nations themselves, prison riots, or campus riots. While it is true that the atomic age carries with it a special anxiety produced by man's technical ability to commit species suicide, a pendulum-like pattern of alternations of greater or lesser limitations on man's individual and collective behavior seems to date as far back as written history.

Noel Perrin (1972), in an article in *The New Yorker* magazine, comments that, "Millions before us have stayed loose, and swung, and rapped. Indeed, I suspect that what we perceive going on in the late twentieth century really amounts to little more than our unreforming the Reformation—which thus becomes an aberration in Western history, a brief period of up-tightness lasting less than 500 years. Look back even a few years before it began (. . . the Reformation in England) and you find people acting and talking very much as they do now. You find great verbal and sexual freedom; you find people who know each other's first names but not their last; you find controversy over hair length between fathers and sons; you find the pleasure principle; and you certainly find the violence that so marks the fabric of life in our own time." Mr. Perrin explains that his comments resulted from his having read a book published in London in 1530, in the last five years of Catholic England. The book was a French grammar, with an attached dictionary, written by the Reverend John Palsgrave, "Les Clarcissement de la Langue Francoyse." Father Palsgrave used the first person and sample sentences in defining the various words in the dictionary section of his book, and it is these sentences that give a vivid picture made up of six or seven thousand vignettes of pre-Reformation life. Mr. Perrin points out that the best thousand, which are practically all bits of dialogue, amount to one-line, sixteenth-century plays. The verb "burst," for example, is described via the author's imagining someone coming late to a meal and finding his favorite dish gone. "The devil burst him," a late medieval voice exclaims. "He hath eaten all the cream without me!" With "bare," we get a sample of sixteenth-century wit, which seems to have quite a lot in common with twentieth-century wit. "What, barest thou his arse," someone says sarcastically, "weenest thou he have an eye there to see with?" And so the dictionary continues, with equally vivid descriptions of behavior in the areas of sexual morality, drinking, gambling, marriage, divorce, hair styles, hygiene, violence, etc. Perrin concludes, "This was an entire age of flower people. Throughout the dictionary shines a sense of joy in the mere act of living, a sense of wonder and delight that for the four centuries of the Reformation was practically confined to children." Palsgrave's "I take the world as it cometh, and love God of all" could well have been the motto of that age.

AND TODAY

Today, as we look at the industrialized Western world in which the great majority of the readers of this book are living, we can understand immediately how difficult it is to arrive at simple explanations of or simple solutions to the question of too many or too few limitations for our children. Among lower socioeconomic groups, rebellion against "Establishment repression" produces trouble with parental limit-setting. Among the working class, increased anxiety due to the pressure of the rebellion of the lower class, especially disadvantaged inner-city ghetto dwellers, tends to lead to a reactive, firm (if not out-and-out harsh) limit-setting, in the image of the "hard-hat." Among the middle class, affluence supports yippies, hippies, and drop-outs who have "turned on" and "tuned out." Here we find a group for which introspection is a highly valued subcultural activity which has produced, for example, a high percentage of Jewish youth who are using drugs and dropping out in the face of the pressure of a centuries-old value system which clearly interdicts both these behaviors. Among the upper class, increased anxiety is also seen, as a result of the decreased tolerance by society at large of concentration of power among the few. Once again, anxiety causes confusion, and confused parents cannot set limits, at least not consistently.

For many, the current situation is poignantly summarized by Ruth-Jean Eisenbud (1971) in some comments about adolescents which are applicable to children of all ages. She writes, "Far and wide the old, revered lines of authority have been tested and broken. Abdication became revolution. Although leaders in education everywhere seek ways to heal the rift and to reach the isolated, angry student, thousands of young people from comfortable, educated homes are still skipping school and setting record truancy figures. The degree of truancy, the drift away from home and family, the restless search for magic—all speak of a void.

"Where and why is the new truant? He is engaged in exciting new music, in mixed media, and in coast-to-coast safari. He is also shivering, cold, under-nourished, lost, drifting, or huddling in the park. His loneliness, fear, his sense of failure, his crying need to belong render him terribly vulnerable to membership in the drug culture, in spite of the tragic price such membership costs. Clinging to his own like to a magnet, the distance grows between the young adolescent and needed adult help. Instead of the homesickness when away from mother suffered by immature adolescents in the 1950's, the new adolescent suffers depression when alone with adults and away from his dearly needed peers.

"Today, to establish relationship with him, he must be approached as a member of his group. He now fights for his exiled group as he once fought negatively for his individuation at home and at school. Now, more than ever, his identity includes the *others*. Still, we know an adolescent's search for closeness does not stop with closeness to his peers. All along he also demands identification and closeness with adults, in spite of flight, anger, and insult. In the very act of protest he cries out, 'listen to me,' 'talk to me.' Sometimes with love and sometimes with fear, sometimes openly and sometimes covertly, he pleads with the adults for mutuality. 'Feel for me,' 'share your feelings with me,' are the messages that come across the gap.

"Indeed, as educators, either we join youth or lose them. But we must not lose ourselves in the process, and with ourselves the culture we carry for them. Educators who respond with 'other directedness' and impulsive anguished empathy to youth's demands by providing a 'free school' are not necessarily providing a *school for freedom*. If structure, motivation, and content are not an integral part of the new plan, no matter how strong the adult's empathy and compassion, the student's right to an education has been irresponsibly negated. Beneath youth's rejecting words are other words: 'stick to your authentic self, so that I can find my true self in an encounter with you'; 'be cool, be real, be knowing, be committed, and be available to me.' "

SOME CASES IN POINT

I can still recall vividly a story told to me with considerable dismay by a sensitive, intelligent, and sophisticated middle-class mother concerning her 13-year-old son, shortly after the Beatle craze had taken a firm hold in New York City. Her son and his three best friends had formed a rock music group and were vigorously pursuing longer hair and tighter trousers. Finding herself in what seemed to be a nearly continuous battle with her son over haircuts and trousers, this mother resolved to find a more rational solution to the conflict. Having armed herself both with some quiet, if agonized, introspection and the reading of some sensible literature on normal growth and development in adolescence, she approached her son calmly one day and announced to him that, to put an end to the conflict which had been so upsetting to both of them, he henceforth would be permitted to decide for himself when it was time for him to have a haircut and how much hair should be cut off at each sitting, and he would be permitted to use his mother's credit card to shop for his own clothing. Having delivered her carefully rehearsed speech, the mother was shocked when her son's response was to look at her incredulously and then promptly burst into tears. "What's the matter?" cried the mother. "Isn't this what you've wanted all along?" "You don't understand," sobbed her son. "I'm not ready for that yet!"

A few years ago (Rothenberg and Rothenberg, 1970), I submitted a story and commentary about violence and children to a new, "radical" magazine about schools. In the manuscript I pointed to the need to help disadvantaged children find alternative, nonviolent patterns of response to their admittedly destructive environment. In rejecting my manuscript, the magazine's editor commented: "The problem is not to find 'alternative patterns of response to their environment,' but to change the environment.

In this case, I think violence, like Fanon says, is the only healthy response. I find the more subtle and coercive violence we use on natives everywhere to be far more frightening. I think the 'alternative responses' educators are thinking of to be just that kind of coercion."

In contrast, I offer excerpts from a letter written by the headmaster of a private, progressive school in New York to the children's parents:

"Some parents may wish to know more precisely what is expected of them. The following are the School's expectations:

"Boys may wear suits, or slacks with jackets or sweaters. Slacks must be clean and pressed. Dungarees are not permitted. Shoes, not sneakers, are to be worn. Hair must be trimmed neatly, it should not overhang the forehead, and in no place should come below the line of the eyebrows. It should not overhang the ears or the collar. It should be clean.

"Girls should wear dresses, or blouses and jumpers. Slacks, cover-alls, or dungarees are not permitted. Shoes, not sneakers, are to be worn. Girl's hair should be clean and neatly trimmed and combed. It should not cover the forehead, and it must not reach below the line of the eyebrows.

"In the upper middle school, boy's hair is to be shorter, and girl's skirts are to be longer: *the permissible length of a boy's hair is a matter for the school authorities to decide.* A girl's hemline is not to be higher than one inch above the knee.

"It is sometimes said that school should concern itself with the child's mind rather than with superficial matters of dress and grooming, and that creativity is more important than costume. But a child who thinks that creativity is indicated by oddity of dress is getting a poor start in life. I'm afraid I must repeat the Handbook's warning that children who ignore the School's standards may be told to stay home until they meet them."

Contrast this with the story I have quoted elsewhere (Rothenberg, 1969) surrounding the events in still another private progressive school in New York City. A mother reported the following story to me:

Her child, who was in a four-year-old nursery group, came home within the first couple of weeks of school complaining that a little boy named Jimmy seemed to be taking a hammer to the heads of all the other children. When the child repeatedly reported this, the mother became sufficiently concerned to feel the situation warranted a visit to the school. She visited the school; and there followed a great deal of group discussion among the parents, teacher, and coordinator of that section of the school. Finally, the mother noted that only one little boy was somehow immune to Jimmy's hammer—a very small, quiet, retiring little fellow. One day after school she took the little boy's mother by the arm and said to her, "Would you mind explaining why your little fellow has never been smacked by Jimmy? I absolutely don't understand; he's the most helpless little boy in the group!" The mother shook her head and replied, "One day I was observing the class and I got one look at that Jimmy smacking

kids on the head with a hammer, so I grabbed him when no one was looking and said, 'listen, if you ever lay a hand on my kid, I won't even tell
you what's going to happen to you!' "

Finally, some old and still pertinent words of wisdom seem appropriate in closing this section of this chapter (J. S. Plant, 1937):

"Every child is an actor in a play; each phrase or deed is understood
only as a part of his total role, and that role is meaningless except as a
part of the total drama.

"This role was pressed into his tiny hands long before he stepped
upon the stage. Months before he was born, parents, relatives and neighbors 'hoped it would be a boy' or 'hoped it would be a girl'—lacking the
courtesy to wait upon his arrival before deciding the part he must play.
Indeed, his role goes farther back to the dreams, the tragedies, the triumphs of the early years of his parents. Who of us has not mended the
disappointments of youth and adulthood with the promise that this child
'will live it differently'? The role he is to play is often cast down to the
last dotting of the 'i' or crossing of the 't.' Children as actors differ markedly in what they do with their roles. Many, in comfortable security, accept
and play the role as given to them. Many are tragically unsuited for the
part they are expected to play—of the wrong sex, too intelligent, too retarded, too individualistic, too dependent, too frail for the titanic struggle,
or too eagerly adventuresome for a part that calls for docility. Some children forever grope in confusion to find the meaning of their roles, whereas
others in ritualistic manner grow, go to school, work, marry, have children,
amass a fortune, die—without ever having had the slightest idea of what
it is all about."

In summary, we appear to be confronted with the problem of a highly
polarized response to the question of too many or too few limitations for
children. But with this brief overview of the problem, its historical perspective, and some vignettes illustrating the variations in which it manifests
itself, we are still left with the question, "What can be done about it?"

SOME RECOMMENDATIONS

I am very much with Ralph Crawshaw (1967) when he says, ". . . it
seems to me there are two kinds of men in the world, those who think
persons must be changed, and those who think persons can change. For
one type of man, power and control comes first. They tell other men (or
patients) how and what to do. For the other type of man, understanding
and patience are the watchwords. They give room and knowledge. I always
hope to be the latter man. . . ."

It would be presumptuous and pretentious in the extreme for me to
attempt to offer a solution to the terribly complex problem expressed in
the title of this chapter. Rather, I should like to share with the reader

some thoughts and recommendations which may suggest directions in which we may find the "room and knowledge" necessary for the development of solutions.

To a striking degree, "discipline" is the subject most frequently chosen when parent groups meet and request a guest speaker to talk to them about their children. While "sex" and "drugs" are the subjects about which speakers are most frequently asked to speak when adolescents are being discussed, the "hidden agenda" is invariably once again "discipline," focused on these two highly charged areas of adolescent functioning.

It seems to me that parents have to find out why they need to keep asking "experts" how to discipline their children before they can find out what *kind* of discipline to exert. In a world characterized by an ever-increasing pace of social mobility and changing value systems, all instantly communicated via world-wide mass media, many parents have more questions about who they are and what they stand for than at any other time in human history. I expect that it is this anxiety about their own value systems and this awareness of the constant, massive challenges to those value systems that have led so many parents to reach out, often desperately, for expert advice and opinion. If parents are not helped first to become aware of the sources of their own anxiety, they cannot move into a position from which they can rationally implement specific limit-setting techniques for their children—techniques which, to be effective, require an awareness of the causes and manifestations of the children's anxieties. My impression is that it is the younger generation's greater sexual freedom (and license), made possible by the newer contraceptive devices and liberalized abortion laws with their attendant near eradication of the fear of pregnancy, that creates the most acute anxiety of all in parents by striking so deeply at many of the roots of the Judeo-Christian ethic by which most adults were reared. I wonder if it isn't this anxiety, with its attendant anger, resentment, yes—and perhaps some envy—that distorts adults' perception of youth's behavior and leads to the a priori assumption that the kids are out to "get" us, thereby blowing the "generation gap" issue out of all proportion. It is noteworthy in this connection that while, as Shoben (1969) and others have pointed out, some 10 percent at most of all college students were actually involved in the campus crises across the nation, the great majority of adults, including most legislators, reacted, and indeed continue to react, as if they were dealing with some sort of mass uprising. Available documentation indicates that the great majority of our young people are "straight" kids who, in fact, should worry us more for their failure to question sufficiently the status quo than for their potential to wreck the Establishment. Witness the typical premedical student who, having interrupted a lecture with vigorous handwaving, asks his professor, who may be anxiously anticipating a vigorous challenge, "Is this going to be on the exam?"

If we *listen,* children of all ages will "tell" us quite clearly exactly how many limitations they need. Two prerequisites, it seems to me, are required for listening that will be more than just hearing and that will provide undistorted input to us. The first of these has to do with our facing up to our own anxieties and to the degree to which these anxieties may produce in us a level of expectation for our children which results in our expecting the worst of them; and by so doing, getting the worst from them. In connection with this, we must be aware that none of us is immune to acting out our own unconscious antisocial impulses and fantasies through our children. Adelaide Johnson's (1949) paper on the subject has become a classic. The second prerequisite is that the understanding derived from our listening be based on solid knowledge of *normal* child development. A highly readable, healthily eclectic, and informative book such as that of Stone and Church (1968) should be on every physician's shelf and in the home of as many parents as possible. The phenomenology of normal child development in the four major areas in which a child grows—physical, intellectual, emotional, and social—can and should be taught to our children as they grow. Indeed, I would seriously recommend a course in normal child development as a prerequisite for graduation from all of our high schools and colleges. Presenting this material in a practical fashion, without the use of psychological jargon, would be a worthwhile project for parents in PTA, church, and any other available groups.

I commented above that our children, if we listen, will "tell'" us what limitations they need. Drawing from one of many possible developmental schemata (Erikson, 1950), let me attempt to illustrate how knowledge of a child's developmental status with its concomitant typical anxieties will result in our being able to understand the child's needs for the support, reassurance, and limit-setting that will promote successful achievement of the milestone in question:

Age	Major Psychosocial Developmental Milestone	Major Type of Anxiety
0–6 mo.	Sense of Basic Trust	Stranger Anxiety
1–3 yr.	Sense of Autonomy	Separation Anxiety
4–6 yr.	Sense of Initiative	Mutilation Anxiety
7–12 yr.	Sense of Industry	Anxiety Regarding Loss of Control
Adolescence	Sense of Identity	Anxiety Regarding Loss of Independence

Within such a framework, the mother of a two-year-old can understand that the child's negativism is an inevitable, outward manifestation of the child's normal movement toward greater autonomy and not a manifestation of the mother's failure as a parent. At the same time, the mother's awareness of separation anxiety as a central issue at this age can help her to define limits for the child's autonomous functioning. The guidelines for these limits can be based on knowledge that *total* autonomy is not the child's goal, but that the developmental thrust is focused on a relative autonomy from mother, on whom the child has hitherto been so totally dependent and with whom the child has so totally identified. By the same token, an adolescent, whose overall level of maturity warrants it, might be given the opportunity, when he's out with a date and using the family car, to choose his own curfew hour; but with the understanding that if he is going to return home later than the time which he has previously announced he will call his parents and let them know. In this instance, the adolescent can independently choose the hour of his return home, while making it possible for his parents to discharge their responsibility by sharing his decision with them.

With a modicum of insight into our own motivations and anxieties, and a solid base of knowledge of child development, it seems to me that as parents we would then be in a position to apply *consistently* limits for our children which would be appropriate to the child's age and the family's ethnic, religious, and political value system. Armed with this self-knowledge and knowledge of child development, I think we would find it a good deal easier to let our children win some of the smaller battles with us, thereby making it easier for them to lose the critical larger battles which indeed they must lose if they are to continue to grow and develop in a healthy fashion. The youngster's winning of clothing and hair battles, for example, can help him more gracefully to lose battles over drugs and delinquency.

A special word about the issue of consistency seems in order here. If I were asked to choose the single potentially most destructive element in parent-child relationships, I would choose inconsistency. Being consistent is something easier said than done for most of us. Yet, the utilization of insight and developmental principles in interaction with a child on one occasion and the absence of this approach and therefore of reasonable limit-setting on the next, identical occasion can lead to a situation in which the child stops responding to either approach because of his confusion as to what is really expected of him. The child who is screamed at or even beaten every Friday night by a drunken father can develop a set of self-protective defense mechanisms to cope with the violent interaction he knows is about to occur. The same child confronted with a drunken, violent father one Friday night and an ingratiating father the next Friday night is thrown off balance, as it were, and in the resulting confusion becomes much more vulnerable in the face of destructive parental behaviors. I feel that this same vulnerability supervenes after much less dramatic but equally inconsistent parental behaviors around such issues as those we have discussed above in relation to the two-year-old and the adolescent.

Finally, at a time when insistent demands for freedom have become a daily occurrence, a comment about the difference between freedom and license seems to me to be required. A. S. Neill (1966), in the introduction to his book, "Freedom—Not License," says, "freedom—over-extended, turns into license. . . . I define license as interfering with another's freedom." In his book, "Summerhill: A Radical Approach to Child Rearing," Neill (1960) pointed out that, "It is this distinction between freedom and license that many parents cannot grasp. In the disciplined home, the children have *no* rights. In the spoiled home, they have *all* the rights. The proper home is one in which children and adults have *equal* rights." For example, in the disciplined home, the arrival of dinner guests who are known to the children may require the simultaneous disappearance of the children to their own rooms for the evening, or at least a similar disappearance after a perfunctory greeting of the guests. In the spoiled home, we might find the same guests totally monopolized by the children who may be rushing in and out of the room to show the guests their latest interests and achievements. In Neill's proper home, one would expect the children to share the guests with their parents for perhaps the first half hour or so of their visit, after which they would leave the adults to each other's company for the rest of the evening.

In concluding, I feel that I can do no better than to leave the reader with these words of James Baldwin (1964): "We have, as it seems to me, a very curious sense of reality—or rather, perhaps, I should say, a striking addiction to irreality. How is it possible, one cannot but ask, to raise a child without loving the child? How is it possible to love the child if one does not know who one is? How is it possible for the child to grow up if the child is not loved? Children can survive without money or security or safety, or things; but they are lost if they cannot find a loving example, for only this example can give them a touchstone for their lives. THUS FAR AND NO FURTHER; this is what the father must say to the child. If the child is not told where the limits are, he will spend the rest of his life trying to discover them. For the child who is not told where the limits are, knows, though he may not know that he knows it, that no one cares enough about him to prepare him for his journey."

REFERENCES

Avedon, R., and J. Baldwin. 1964. Nothing Personal. New York, Dell Publishing.

Crawshaw, R. 1967. Letter. *In* Medical Opinion and Review, **3**, 2.

Eisenbud, R. 1971. Structured for freedom. *In* Notes from Stevenson, No. 2. Lucille Rhodes, ed. Robert Lewis Stevenson School, 24 W. 74th Street, New York, N.Y. 10023.

Erikson, E. 1950. Childhood and Society. New York, W. W. Norton.

Goodman, P. 1964. The Community of Scholars. New York, Random House.

Johnson, A. M. 1949. Sanctions for superego lacunae of adolescents. *In* Search-lights on Delinquency. New York, International Universities Press.

Neill, A. S. 1960. Summerhill: A Radical Approach to Child Rearing. New York, Hart Publishing.

Neill, A. S. 1966. Freedom—Not License. New York, Hart Publishing.

Perrin, N. 1972. Before fun city. *In* The New Yorker, February 26.

Plant, J. S. 1937. Personality and the Cultural Pattern. New York, Common-wealth Fund.

Rothenberg, E. B., and M. B. Rothenberg. 1970. Violence: story and com-mentary. *In* The Educational Forum, November.

Rothenberg, M. B. 1969. Violence and children. *In* Mental Hygiene, **53,** 4.

Shoben, E. J. 1969. Demonstrations, confrontations, and academic business as usual. *In* Western Humanities Review, **23,** 1.

Stone, L. J., and J. Church. 1968. Childhood and Adolescence. 2nd ed. New York, Random House.

CHAPTER 15

CAREERS AND LIVING

ROBERT H. WILLIAMS

Although there are hundreds of work patterns, the vast proportion of the population is concerned chiefly with meeting immediate needs for survival—food, clothing, shelter, and health care. At the other end of the spectrum are some for whom these basic requirements are readily available and who are free to choose the patterns of work and living that offer the greatest opportunity for happiness, glory, luxuries, and other amenities. People in this category have the chance to select what seems to be the most appealing career, to become well prepared for it, and to pursue it in an excellent manner. The extent of choice and the chance for success are influenced both by external factors—geographic, environmental, social, political, and cultural—as well as by internal factors—the mental and physical abilities of the individual. Therefore, work patterns and accomplishments differ markedly. In this chapter, I present only a few considerations concerning the careers of individuals who are blessed with relatively good capacities and opportunities to use them. For convenience, I mention chiefly men, but the same principles apply to careers for women.

The type of career chosen, and the satisfaction and happiness it does or does not offer, markedly influence the individual's life, including how he lives and the extent of his desire to live. Furthermore, within the family the father's career usually influences the reactions and courses of the rest of the family. Today, there are more career patterns from which to choose than at any time in history. The type of career selected and the manner in which it is pursued are of far greater common concern than at any other time. In general, the most rewarding careers require prolonged and expensive training, often in a much more restricted area than formerly. Many phases of a career can produce unhappiness, anxiety, depression, frustration, ill-health, and sometimes even suicide. Therefore, I now present some important factors that should be considered in planning careers for qualified people.

REWARDS FOR SUCCESS

Usually, people who make intensive efforts for success in a career are inspired by the possibility of rewards of one sort or another. Of course, it is assumed that *progressive successes produce progressive increases in reward*. Devoting extra work, taking rapid advantage of special opportunities, and making some sacrifices tend to promote rapid progress toward greater rewards later. Early successes also lead to a greater choice of areas in which to progress. Undergraduate success → excellent graduate school training → preparation of professional skills in certain areas → good position → better position, etc. It also is assumed that these progressions lead to material gains such as good clothing, food, and housing. Some individuals work for success as a basis for providing a luxurious home, yacht, cars, and extensive subservience. Others are gratified more by public praise, prestige, and honors, such as awards, medals, and honorary degrees. Some of these men have had as their major goal to generate a praiseworthy image in the public eye, and after receiving exaltation recognize that they have fooled the public, but not themselves. Others with outstanding abilities and performances work chiefly to bring happiness for themselves and others. They seem to be more concerned with *being* great than with being *called* great, believing that their actions speak louder than their words. Some individuals end up richly rewarded from all viewpoints.

SELECTING GOALS*

Some General Considerations

The wise formulation of future goals requires much intensive study. Many ambitious young men push hard for an outstanding career but remind me of Roy Riegel, who made an 85-yard run in a Rose Bowl game—a brisk and beautiful run, but in the wrong direction. It is highly important for each person to locate his "goal posts."

If a person is to have proper perspective in choosing his goals, he must acquire a great deal of information about both the general and the specific aspects of various careers. It is good to get much advice but *the individual must attempt to match his own characteristics with those of the career patterns that he is contemplating*. Just as in a jig-saw puzzle only certain pieces fit together to form a beautiful picture, for many individuals a successful career requires that they carefully match their own attributes with the characteristics needed for the career. Often, characteristics that produce criticism in some settings are praiseworthy in others. For example, William Halsted, the famous surgeon at Johns Hopkins University, was known for his personal finickiness. He regularly sent his shirts from Baltimore to Paris for laundering, he bought his hats in London, and he burned a type of wood that produced the hottest flames. He was critical of table-

---

* Some of these concepts on selecting a career and attaining the goals emerged during my conferences with numerous trainees at the Harvard Medical School and the University of Washington Medical School.

cloths with creases pressed in. However, these same characteristics—his meticulousness, his precision, his determination for the best results regardless of the work involved—were the very qualities that produced his great contributions to surgery. One of these contributions was the invention and extensive use of a clamp for very exact control of bleeding. Similarly, George Minot, a Nobel laureate, once stopped his car on a busy street in Boston where, ignoring the horn-blowing and shouts of stalled motorists, he studied a butterfly that had come flying across a side lot. Yet without this persistent curiosity and determination he would never have established the value of liver in the treatment of pernicious anemia, for he had to overcome many obstacles: certain leading scientists insisted that his thesis was wrong, and his chief asked him to transfer his study from an excellent hospital to a poor one where research was difficult, but where he nevertheless achieved his goal.

Although some people seem to be able to perform well in only one area, perhaps because their interests and motivation lie in only one field, others can perform magnificently in many areas and show a wide range of interests. An individual must decide whether he should follow his multiple interests or restrict himself to one area, becoming an expert in it. With the great increase in population and with the opportunities for rapid communication and travel, it appears that in general it is better for most people to select a restricted field for specialization, rather than for a large number of people to cover many fields without much expertise in any. Nevertheless, generalists play an important role in promoting coordination, integration, and collaboration in numerous activities. They also are very much needed as administrators. In other words, they can become experts in breadth rather than in depth, although it is important that their interests and activities not be overextended to the point of "everythingitis."

In advising about career selection I generally make the following statement: *"A person must consider both the field in which he has the greatest interest and the one in which he believes his performance will be the best.* These two aspects tend to involve the same field, because an individual rejoices in his handiwork." This concept helps to avoid one of the greatest problems of careers, namely, wide deviation between a person's goals and in his capacity to attain them. We cannot expect a person's performance to exceed his capacity, but we hope that it will not be below his capabilities. Ideally, the performance:capacity ratio should be 1:1, giving an excellent "performance efficiency index."

When the career pattern selected, or assigned, requires capacities far below the existing level, the performance efficiency index may be very inferior because the person may become unmotivated, discouraged, and lackadaisical. His dissatisfaction may lead eventually to anxiety, frustration, agitation, and depression, causing major problems both in the family and with others.

When an individual's capacities are grossly deficient for attaining certain goals, both the "goal attainment index" (capacity:goal) and the "performance efficiency index" are low. Eventually the person may become insecure, overwhelmed, discouraged, anxious, depressed, agitated, frustrated, and insomnic. Occasionally the feelings of inferiority and worthlessness may even cause deep depression and suicide (see Fig. 3 in Chap. 1).

Selection of Specific Goals

Too often, failure to select the most appropriate career leads to marked unhappiness; therefore, one should attempt to compare one's own capacities, interests, and motivation with the requirements for a specific career in every possible way—through reading, travel, discussion, and exposure to the career whenever possible. Then a number of other factors must be considered in selecting a specific career, including its importance, immediate and long-range, and the feasibility of making significant progress. It is important to explore new phases, to attempt to project their future values, and to estimate the opportunity for leadership in such areas (Fig. 1). Studying the past trends in certain careers can help one project

LEVELS OF PROGRESSIVENESS DISPLAYED BY DIFFERENT PHYSICIANS

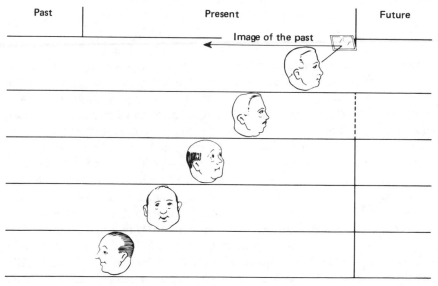

Fig. 1. Levels of progressiveness. Top character represents smallest proportion of individuals, who, after carefully studying past developments, extrapolate probable course of future events; second character gets less clear picture of future because of insufficient study of past; third character has desire but not ability to visualize the future; fourth subject represents largest proportion—those who are not sufficiently interested in past or future; bottom subject dwells in patterns of past and not only fails to contribute to progress but also often actively opposes it.

the future and avoid the pitfalls of the past. Unfortunately, too many, encouraged by their parents, follow the pathways of the past unthinkingly. Opportunities to work closely with individuals with outstanding careers have often proved advantageous because of the inspiration, philosophy, and knowledge transmitted; greatness breeds greatness. However, one reason the young often seem to make more major original contributions is that they are inquisitive, tend to avoid dogmas, and have not learned that a given procedure "has been tested and will not work." Many Nobel laureates initiated their major research before they were 30. Often certain phenomena that seem important have not previously received much attention. While I have emphasized the luster of the new, much remains uncovered in both old areas and new.

ATTAINING GOALS

It is important to receive training that is excellent in both quality and quantity. The optimal relationship between breadth and depth of training must be considered; either can be extended to the detriment of the other. In addition to learning facts, the trainee should attempt to understand their evolution and significance. This helps him to design new patterns for progress.

Ambitious goals usually mean competition. This need not be destructive but can be beneficial, particularly if viewed in a somewhat friendly way, as a game in sports. With alertness to opportunities, it is possible to gain a few extra yards of advantage periodically, thereby accelerating final attainment of one goal. However, at times it is wise to sacrifice a few yards for much greater yardage later. Conversely, negligence or poor judgment as to the relative value of certain measures for career advancement can cause one to fall far behind. Recoveries can sometimes be made, but it is like swimming against a swift current. I liken the situation to a series of concentric circles (Fig. 2); if a person in the inner circle slips to the periphery, much effort is required to regain the former preferred position. Establishing priorities based on the significance of different phases of the work is wise; such planning should often consider the role of personality. *It is important to include hard work in long-range planning but to keep it at a pace that is optimal for the individual and that permits maintenance of good health and happiness.* Work habits vary, so each individual must discover his best pattern. The situation can be likened to running a mile race. Each miler must learn how fast to attempt to run each of the four laps. If he runs earlier parts of the race too fast, he may become exhausted during the final lap and lose. On the other hand, if he runs the earlier laps too slowly he may be too far behind to win even though he has saved his energy for an outstanding final lap.

Even persons who have selected goals commensurate with their abili-

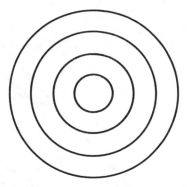

Fig. 2. With excellent ability and hard work in preparing for a career one can gain entrance into the enviable center circle. However, by judgment errors or lapses in work one can rapidly slip to outer circles. Many individuals cannot regain the center despite hard work.

ties may encounter major problems because of improper work habits. Prolonged excessive work may lead to severe chronic fatigue, nervousness, insomnia, inefficiency, anxiety, depression, and sometimes even suicide (Fig. 3). If such symptoms appear, it is desirable to face the problems squarely by taking a rest, getting reorganized, and adopting sounder work habits. One's attitude toward one's work also makes a considerable difference. *It can be helpful to view one's work as something of a game and as one that is reasonably simple, even though it may have to be played vigorously.*

Some people work best alone, whereas others work better as part of a team. Good teamwork sometimes accomplishes more than the same number of people working individually, just as a good mile relay team is faster than the fastest miler in the world.

Top career people must have excellent early training and must continue extensive education throughout life; they should make repeated adjustments for optimal progress. Unless they continue their education, they may suddenly find themselves hopelessly behind. Moreover, all of the real leaders, irrespective of the field, must continue to engage in research, because the research of today is the practice of tomorrow. Research is important both for evaluating the present and for planning the future.

OBLIGATIONS AND RESPONSIBILITIES

We must always remember that people are not born equal and do not subsequently have equal opportunities. A person with superior capacities should have a superior performance, yet this gives him an average "performance efficiency index" (Fig. 3). Top career persons should supply leadership in a larger number of ways. These people tend to be the ones

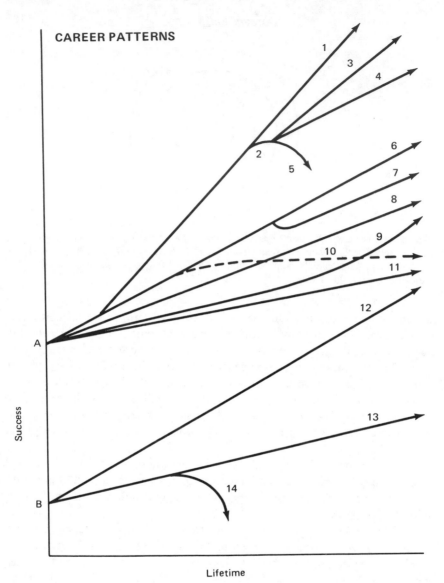

Fig. 3. The courses of some careers are depicted. The following factors are the main ones involved:

A. *Superior abilities:* (1) Maximal performances, maximal work; (2) overwork, health failure; (3) rest, work adjustment, total recovery; (4) acute recovery but chronic neurosis; (5) anxiety, severe depression, suicide; (6) performance:capacity ratio normal; (7) inadequate attention at critical periods; (8) not enough work; (9) inadequate training, but tremendous effort; (10) superior early, with continuation of hard work, but not of education; (11) poor goal selection; person incapable or uninterested.

B. *Moderate abilities:* (12) performance:capacity ratio normal (same as in 6); (13) parental, teacher, and traditional pressures cause selection of goals far above abilities, causing frustration, despair; (14) goals more overwhelming than in 13, causing marked fear, anxiety, agitation, depression, and suicide.

Of course, there are many more patterns possible for both A and B.

who were born with superior attributes. Many are aided extensively by members of their families, by special groups, and by the public. In return, each top career person is obligated to benefit those who aided his success and also to help many less fortunate people. As discussed in more detail in Chapter 11, there are considerations that are helpful to all of us in assisting others. Among them are the following: (a) mental behavior depends upon the physical and chemical status of the brain, (b) there are marked differences in these components among people owing to many factors, (c) because of differing capacities we must expect and encourage different types and amounts of performances, (d) by realistically applying the Golden Rule and the concept that the greatest thing in the world is love, we are better conditioned to help others, and (e) we must attempt to bring out the best in each person. My earlier discussion of career selection did not consider the value of various careers for society, but this is highly important. The need for progress is far greater in some areas than in others. Therefore, careers in psychology, philosophy, sociology, ecology, eugenics, genetics, criminology, marriage counselling, propagation and termination of life, and in many other areas that are important to the welfare of mankind should be considered carefully. Although the performance efficiency index may be lower thereby, the value of accomplishment may be much greater, as may be the gratification.

Of course, aid to others can and should be rendered in a vast number of ways. Great contributions can be made both by teaching and by training others to teach. Skilled administration is highly important, too, especially in planning and promoting patterns for progress. Unfortunately, administration is visualized too often as painful when it can be made pleasurable—like an enjoyably challenging game. Administration can be an art, a science, and a means of enormous progress.

THE ROLE OF LEADERS

The leaders in various fields can play an important role in advancing the benefits of career choices to both individuals and society. These leaders should (a) provide more and better information concerning career specialties, types and availability of training, and rewards; (b) plan for better selection, training, distribution, and reward of specialists in accordance with the needs for such specialists; (c) provide the most appropriate working conditions; (d) arrange for more and better coordination and collaboration in activities of specialists. Much work is needed to help trainees match their capabilities with career opportunities. *Far too little attention is given to establishing gradations in career standards; we follow excessively single standards.* Because people differ markedly in capacities and performances, we must have different standards, and should adjust aid and encouragement accordingly. In golf the matter is handled by establishing handicaps. Too often we give a single award for the best man in a given field. Indeed, we repeatedly reward the best people, even though their performance efficiency index is no better than that of numerous others with lesser abilities. Most recipients of such rewards would not seem to need encouragement as much as do many others who are less able, although rewards probably stimulate individuals at every level. Although we should encourage competition, it should not be so marked that it causes jealousies, selfishness, harmful secrecy, suboptimal performance, inadequate collaboration, and too little aid for others.

SUMMARY AND CONCLUSIONS

A person's career can bring enormous happiness or great unhappiness. Careful planning, associated with excellent orientation, is necessary to select the most appropriate goals and attempt to attain them. It is important to attempt to match the individual's goals with his desires and abilities. Since many people contribute to a successful career, the career person is obliged to demonstrate both gratitude and aid to others. Leaders in various segments of society can systematically contribute toward career patterns that will significantly benefit individual careers as well as society in general.

CHAPTER 16

ADVANTAGES AND DISADVANTAGES OF TECHNOLOGICAL ACHIEVEMENTS

ROBERT F. RUSHMER

The triumphs of technology have provided material wealth beyond the fondest dreams of kings and nobles of the last century. Having achieved this pinnacle of technological success, a large and growing proportion of our people insist that these amazing accomplishments are not what they wanted after all. The younger generation, for whom these riches were intended to be priceless heritage, increasingly disclaim the goals of the past 100 years and insist that the cost has been too great. Intelligent, educated, and well-endowed youth have been turning to communes, drugs, and violence to escape a world threatened by man's inability to control the products of his own creation. The complications of technological achievements have high priority among the targets of current protests. Widespread antagonism toward technology seems misdirected, because the fault lies more in human utilization of technology than in fruits of industrial innovation. The human animal has failed to attain the full potential of his technology or to forecast and control its complications. Individual intelligence, incentive, and innovation have created modern marvels; our greatest deficiency is a lack of group intelligence or judgment in identifying and assessing human needs, developing mechanisms for attaining or supporting essential requirements, and applying effective constraints to avoid excesses. Supersuccess and overabundance are the prime characteristics of our current crises. Unless industrialized nations are prepared to cast aside current creature comforts and regress to the simple life of the past, new techniques and technologies must be the prime hope for improving the total environment for future generations. Compounded complications of these new approaches can be avoided by improved understanding of human desires and requirements.

THE AMBIVALENCE OF HUMAN ASPIRATIONS

Man is a complex animal with many paradoxical and apparently incompatible drives and responses. He demands law and order but appears spellbound by spontaneous violence in mass communications and the contrived violence of sports. Mankind is intensely competitive with members of his own tribe but becomes highly cooperative with them when confronted by threats from outside. He is immune to the mass destruction on the highways but mobilizes enormous resources to rescue a man trapped in a mine or a child in a well. Desmond Morris identified in man the ambivalence of the "naked ape," combining the arboreal playfulness of vegetarian monkeys with the curiosity of the wide-ranging carnivorous apes living in highly organized troops. Resolving such conflicting wishes and aspirations seems impossible, but some kind of balanced compromise is essential. Abraham Maslow (in Wilson) has postulated that all mankind shares certain fundamental needs which can be arranged in a hierarchy of five levels as follows:

(1) *Physiological needs:* Humans require food, clothing, shelter, and rest as the most elemental requirements for survival.
(2) *Safety or security needs:* Having attained essential physiological requirements for the present, humans seek to protect and assure them for the future.
(3) *Social needs:* Most humans seek to establish stable relationships with others inside and outside the family groups. Identification and sharing with members of social, economic, political, and recreational groups appear to be fundamental drives.
(4) *Ego needs:* Each individual requires some degree of self-esteem, self-confidence, and self-satisfaction with added incentives from approval and respect by his peers.
(5) *Self-fulfillment needs:* Growth, development, and realization of potential are the last and highest of individual requirements which become manifest when all or most of the other requirements have been attained.

The priorities of these five needs become clear with the realization that food and shelter dominate all other considerations by individuals in want of them. A starving man is less concerned with future prospects or intellectual ideals. Future security becomes a prime goal when current essentials have been attained. Social interactions and sharing merge as a means or result of striving for security. Ego needs and self-fulfillment requirements are powerful psychological drives in an organized environment. The advantages and disadvantages of technologies can best be judged in terms of their success or failure in supporting these fundamental human aspirations.

AGRICULTURE

Vast areas of the world are occupied by agricultural societies so underdeveloped that most of the people (i.e., 90 percent) are struggling to produce sufficient food for the local population, leaving few to govern, to teach, or to develop resources and produce other essentials. The agricultural revolution has attained such efficiency that less than 10 percent of the people in the United States can produce more than ample food for its total population, with surpluses for export to other countries.

Technology has provided greatly increased yields. Food preservation techniques greatly expand the quantity, durability, and the spatial distribution of foodstuffs. A visit to any supermarket reveals a convergence of edible products from all parts of the globe available any season of the year—an astonishing logistic accomplishment. The value of agricultural technology is not limited to its economic contribution, for it also provides adequate and varied nutrition to the entire population which improves physical and intellectual development. Children living in poverty are known to display lower scores on tests of intellectual function and a lower educational achievement. These results may reflect malnutrition coupled with social and biological disadvantages of their environment. Enormous productivity has made it possible to meet fully the physiological needs of the entire United States' population with adequate supplies of food and the security of plenty throughout each year present and future, even with continued population growth. Modern social relationships in an industrialized society are inconceivable without efficient food production.

Massive agricultural machinery greatly expands productivity by each farm laborer, which in turn frees large numbers of the labor force to work in factories, services, research and development, and other pursuits of economic, educational, and cultural benefit to the entire country.

The benefits of agricultural mechanization are so visible and tangible that one rarely considers complications or disadvantages of the trend. Mass production of food requires large acreage through consolidation of small farms and opening of new vast areas to large-scale farming. Greater productivity has reduced farm labor requirements, initiating a major migration to urban areas in search of employment opportunities. Deterioration of the cities is attributable in part to the mass exodus from the farms. Substandard housing and poverty are generally viewed as a characteristic of central cities, but rural areas contain approximately 60 percent of substandard housing and nearly half of the nation's poor.

Thus, pressures for urban migration persist, but arrival at city limits provides few answers to unskilled labor. The ego requirements of farm labor have been undermined by deterioration of job satisfaction, strict government regulations, price controls, and subsidies. Despite major advances in telecommunications, rural populations feel divorced from the excitement and activity of urban life where the "action" appears to be glowing over the horizon. The future of farm communities is uncertain, and the opportunities for self-fulfillment are correspondingly in doubt.

One hundred years ago it was not predicted that such complications could result from techniques capable of providing an abundance of health-sustaining foods produced by greatly reduced physical exertion by fewer farm laborers. The defects which have emerged were not the result of inadequate or ineffective technology—quite the contrary. The complications result from "excessive" success, over-abundance, and an inability to forecast and deal with the rapid social changes which modern man can attain (Toffler). The farming community must share responsibility for environmental deterioration from many factors, including deforestation, lowered water level, depletion of topsoil, and excessive utilization of chemical fertilizers, weed killers, and insect control materials. The threats to future life and health are real and widely recognized. Excesses of production, dangerous byproducts, and resource depletion are characteristic of virtually all aspects of modern societies. A most important future requirement is the development of plans and incentives which will reverse the trend of migration back to rural areas and small towns to relieve intolerable congestion and problems of metropolitan areas. Technological developments in the areas of rapid transportation, air conditioning, and mass communication of arts, sciences, and current events could be oriented to provide all the essential amenities of metropolitan life in small towns even in relatively remote areas.

MASS PRODUCTION AND AUTOMATION

The agricultural revolution freed a major segment of the total labor force to engage in research, development, industrial production, packaging, advertising, distribution, and maintenance of an ever-growing abundance of goods and services. Technology has not only satisfied the material needs and wants of the masses to an unprecedented degree, it has provided luxuries and frills which have in turn become regarded as necessities. Automobiles, television, automatic dishwashers, stoves, powered lawnmowers, and other mechanized appliances have become transformed into essential requirements in the minds of major segments of the population. When the available markets become saturated with durable goods, we find "planned obsolescence" being openly practiced so that replacement must occur more frequently. We seem to be moving inexorably along pathways predicted with remarkable accuracy by thoughtful men such as Aldous Huxley in *Brave New World*.

The physiological requirements of most people in industrialized societies have been fully attained. Good nutrition, housing, clothing, healthy environment, and control of many diseases have produced generations with increasing size, strength, and life expectancy. The abundance of food and products is coupled with an increasing degree of individual security through social, economic, and political evolution. Governmental protection against unfulfilled individual needs is greater now than ever before and is still increasing. The major attainments in assuring both physiological needs and security have been accompanied by deterioration of major factors among social needs, ego needs, and self-fulfillment. Primitive man may have been cold, hungry, and insecure, but at least he was not bored. The rewards of self-satisfaction, success, and status were not denied him. Modern workers in mass production industries perform repetitive operations, or work with parts or fragments of the manufactured item. The pride of craftsmanship and the satisfaction of a job well done have been denied many modern workers by mass production techniques and automation.

Clearly, technology attained astonishing success in providing for the physiological needs of man and in ensuring security for his future physiological needs with leisure time to enjoy his affluence. Modern technology has achieved all these ends and in addition has proved able to "control nature" to an extensive and even brutal degree. The widespread reaction against technology is primarily a response to excessive success in attaining these ends without adequate restraint or control. The citizens of industrialized societies are manifestly discontented, and their futures are clearly threatened in the presence of a most munificent fulfillment of human needs and aspirations. The principal deficiency is the failure of social structures to manage and channel mankind's astonishing creative ability, so that he can attain real and proper objectives while avoiding the complications which threaten his future.

We are currently witnessing the mobilization of resources to eliminate major causes of environmental pollution. Many industrial plants are spending enormous sums to reduce air and water pollution. There is no doubt that these efforts can prove successful to a major degree. It is characteristic that the attack on this problem necessarily involves virtually all components of modern society, including farming, industry, transportation, communication, health service, and recreation. The technology which was responsible for deterioration of our environment is fully capable of restoring it if the dedication and the effort are adequate.

SHELTERS

Beyond the distant mists of time, primitive man smoothed the ground to ease his tired frame for sleep under a tree or in a natural cave (Fig. 1). After untold eons, shelters were fabricated from the materials at hand: sticks, skins, mud, ice, grasses. The size, shape, and characteristics were dictated by the environmental conditions and the materials used. The resulting shelters were remarkably effective, and the intrusion of modern

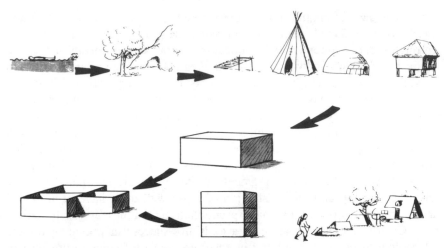

Fig. 1. The development of shelters began with leveling of ground under a tree or in a cave and progressed through habitats made of materials readily at hand to suit the environment. Enclosed rectangular spaces are particularly suited to close packing horizontally and vertically. The current trend is back to nature.

technology may be a backward step. For example, many Alaskan Eskimos are suffering cold and discomfort in rectangular dwellings made of wood and tar paper after abandoning the snug, traditional igloo to emulate "civilized" approaches.

The rectangular shape and dimensions of modern dwellings are most convenient for packing many rooms in close proximity both horizontally and vertically (Fig. 1). The need for packing increasing numbers of people in close proximity is the direct result of the agricultural and industrial revolution. The amazing affluence of goods, services, and leisure is producing a "return to nature" through hiking, camping, bicycling, and recreational housing away from the cities. As the work-week is reduced from six days to five days and soon possibly to four days, a growing portion of the population can realistically aspire to spending nearly half of any week in temporary or more permanent shelters remote from metropolitan areas.

Meanwhile, homes have become progressively more comfortable, convenient, and versatile by widespread installation of furnishings and appliances. Heating, cooling, food storage, cooking, cleaning, and other labor-saving devices have failed to provide the contentment and tranquility that was expected. The greatly increased leisure available to the homemaker has failed to provide the enrichment and expanded horizons that were surely intended. Instead, a vigorous "women's liberation" movement has emerged. A widening generation gap between the younger generation and their parents has resulted at least in part from the fact that children are no longer necessary to the running of the household. On the isolated farms of the last century, children could justifiably feel needed and wanted, but they have no essential role in urban settings. The concept of "chores" has been largely abandoned or clearly distorted by contrived jobs. Children in cities feel unneeded and unwanted, seeking satisfaction in escape but more often trying to attain some kind of identification with an unknown, threatening future. Paradoxically, the more tightly packed the people become, the more isolated they are from their neighbors, until occupants of adjoining apartments may not even speak to each other. Increasing interdependence of man on his fellow man has unexpectedly caused him to look inward, seeking seclusion in a crowd. These untoward effects are not the necessary result of technology but rather the result of man's adaptation to its accomplishments.

SETTLEMENTS

Industrialization requires geographical concentration of manpower and other necessary ingredients including materials, transportation, and communication utilities. The development of human settlements began with the conversion of the hunter to the farmer in prehistoric times. As shelters became grouped, the distance from home to fields was generally less than five miles (approximately 1 hour at walking rates). As cities were formed, most had a radius of about 10 minutes walking time or about 1 kilometer.

During the past century, most settlements have remained small but some have grown progressively, often in a radial pattern or more recently in grid patterns (Fig. 2). With improved transportation, the limits of travel in 10 minutes or 1 hour have greatly expanded along lines of communication (Doxiadis). Currently, whole areas or regions are becoming major metropolises or megalopolises through the confluence of adjacent cities into highly complex organizational units (Fig. 2). In general, metropolitan areas and megalopolises have grown rapidly and uncontrollably through simultaneous developments by individual entrepreneurs, groups, and governmental agencies with totally inadequate planning or integration. The individual components of cities, the utilities, transportation systems, logistics, and distribution are quite miraculous individually, but they are generally unsatisfactory as a total complex.

Virtually every step of the process has revealed unexpected complications. For example, in eighteenth century cities, individual wells were replaced by water piped to central distributing points. A direct result of this was a series of devastating epidemics of cholera that destroyed large numbers of citizens in major cities until methods of purifying water were introduced in the early 1900's. Water purification is clearly a desirable goal, but it created unpredicted complications in the form of poliomyelitis epidemics. When all infants are exposed to poliomyelitis during the first few months of life, which would occur naturally when the water is unpurified,

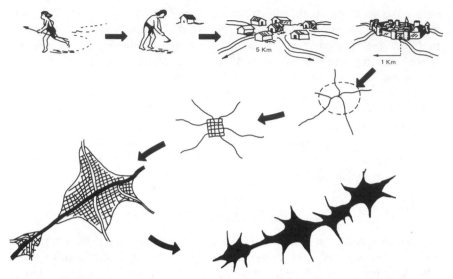

Fig. 2. The earliest hunter and food gatherer ranged widely but development of agriculture restricted the average daily travel to about 5 km from village to farm (about 1 hour walking), and 1 km within most cities up until the industrial revolution occurred. Now, cities have grown uncontrollably and metropolises are expanding and converging into megalopolises, principally along the lines of communications.

demonstrable paralysis rarely develops. However, if infection with the virus is delayed until childhood or adult life, when natural immunity has disappeared, paralytic poliomyelitis becomes much more common. This threat to life and health has been countered recently by the development of an effective vaccine providing widespread immunity for those fortunate enough to receive this preventive care.

The persistent deficiency of long-range planning is all too obvious in cities where water systems, sewers and streets, power, and other essentials are installed separately with sequential disruption of all of them each time one is modified or extended. The typical American approach to technology has been to forge ahead in some direction with little or no planning, and with unjustified confidence that we will solve the complications as they arise. We now confront the fact that virtually all aspects of the cities' survival are becoming saturated and threaten major breakdown. For example, major power failures are now capable of paralyzing large areas or regions. Telephone communication is provided by one of the most efficient private enterprises in the country, yet saturation threatens breakdown in the largest cities. Disposal mechanisms are barely keeping up with the accumulation of solid wastes. New technologies are not required to remedy most if not all civic ills. We need to use what is now known in accordance with carefully conceived regional plans. The central portions of cities are deteriorating, partly because they are no longer truly essential in a modern industrial society. Functions of big cities can now be fulfilled in smaller communities or suburbs at sites removed from the congestion and clamor of metropolitan centers. Even decentralization of mass-production industries can be achieved if their prime logistical requirements can be met by trucks instead of railroads or ships.

We require neither new technology nor individual imagination but only a far greater amount of group intelligence in the approaches to the problems we share. It seems entirely possible that the increasing complexity of modern society can be successfully controlled by more effective management through improved or realigned forms of government. Individual citizens may be called upon to relinquish certain individual rights and privileges for the good of the community, and our aim should be to attain the most beneficial form of group management or control with the minimal sacrifice of individual liberty and freedom of choice. We must develop new incentives to encourage net change in desired directions while retaining a maximum of individual choice. For example, forms of selective taxation could be developed to accomplish needed improvements in central cities. A graduated property tax could be devised to make it unprofitable to allow deterioration of business or residential buildings. Alternatively, we could impose a personal property tax with a minimum tax base for home and lot if within walking distance of place of employment, and graduated tax base increasing with the distance between home and place of employment. Such a step should rapidly reduce the traffic congestion in metropolitan areas. Elimination of income tax exemptions for children and a graduated tax on increasing family size would provide a positive stimulus to family planning and reduced rate of population growth.

The United States can easily maintain a rate of population growth commensurate with its food production. Unfortunately, the world regions which have the highest rates of population growth are the ones with the least prospect of increasing food and shelter production to meet the expanding needs (Berry). Central and South America, Africa, and the Asian subcontinent have the least responsive technological base and the highest birth rates (Fig. 3A) and population growth (Fig. 3B). The fantastically high rates of population growth in underdeveloped countries can be directly traced to technological triumphs of public health measures and sanitary engineering.

THE POPULATION EXPLOSION

The terrifying implications of a population explosion are widely recognized, not only in industrialized societies but in underdeveloped countries. However, the future need not be regarded to be as bleak as extremists would indicate, because a true population explosion occurred in western Europe during the last century and was largely rectified spontaneously

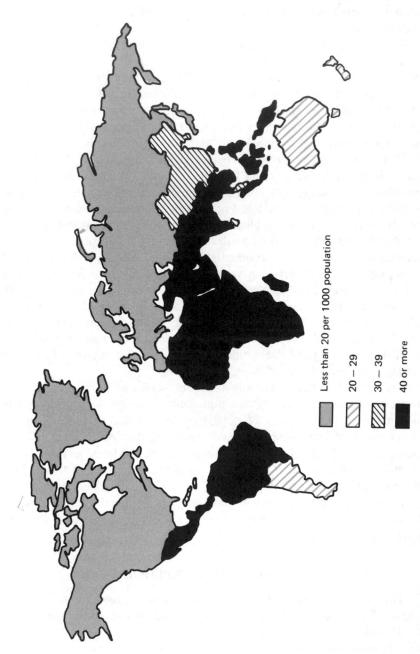

WORLD BIRTH RATES BY REGION

Less than 20 per 1000 population

20 — 29

30 — 39

40 or more

For 1967: *Source: United Nations*

3A

without our modern technologies of communication and birth control. Most of the countries in western Europe experienced a marked reduction in death rates over a period of some 50 years largely because of improved nutrition, environment, and affluence (Fig. 4). The population expanded greatly during this period but the growth was largely arrested by a reduction in birth rate owing to a number of shifts in social and economic factors such as delayed marriage and fewer children in each family unit, as though widespread fertility was depressed. A notable example was Ireland, where the average age of marriage was considerably delayed. The drop in birth rate has been sufficient to stabilize the population of France to a very small increment of growth per year, and in fact the French government has been known to express official concern.

Our present dilemma results from the fact that the reduction in death rates in underdeveloped countries has dropped so precipitously since World War II by control of epidemic diseases and improved nutrition that a major surge of population expansion is taking place. This population growth is occurring much faster than the birth rate can be depressed, even

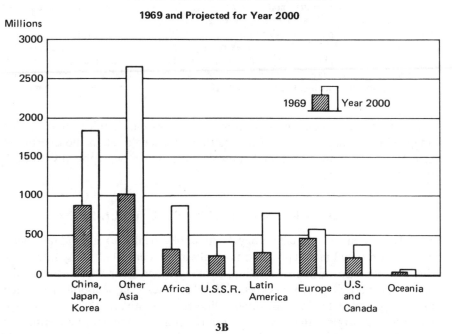

3B

Fig. 3. During the last century, death rates fell gradually and birth rates diminished spontaneously in Western Europe. Population growth is moderate and fairly stable in the northern hemisphere, but the recent abrupt drop in death rates in underdeveloped countries has not yet been followed by corresponding reduction in birth rates as illustrated in these schematic diagrams.

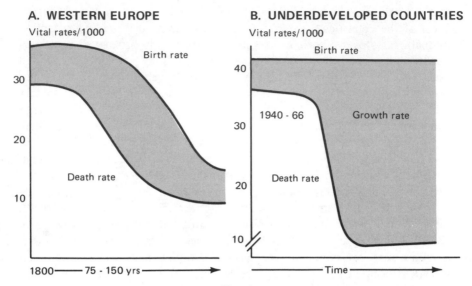

Fig. 4.

A) During the nineteenth century, the death rate diminished over several decades due to improved nutritional and living conditions and the birth rate declined spontaneously to restabilize the rate of growth.

B) Our current population explosion is most critical in underdeveloped countries where the death rate diminished extremely rapidly and the birth rates have not compensated rapidly enough. A sharp reduction in birth rate is conceivable, necessary, and may be possible through effective utilization of modern communication and medical technologies. It has happened before without them.

with our modern techniques of communication and fertility control. The adaptability of the human species may be sufficient to stem the exorbitant growth rates in underdeveloped countries if they can be supplied with both the will and the means.

HEALTH CARE AND EMOTIONAL WELL-BEING

The extension of technology from public health to individual health care has provided major progress not only in the control of many infectious diseases but also by the alleviation of many other types of functional disturbances, pathological processes, and deformities. The technologies which make it possible to diagnose many illnesses definitively and to introduce medical and surgical therapy have greatly improved the general health and life expectancy of the population. These technologies have become heavily concentrated in hospitals and medical centers accompanied by steeply spiraling costs of health care, which would be available only to the very wealthy without third-party payment mechanisms by means of insurance or federally supported health programs. The rising costs of medicine will be stemmed by improved efficiency and cost benefits through reorganization and application of management engineering, operations analysis, and other methods formerly the province of industrial engineering.

Paradoxically, at the very time when our greatest complication is the population explosion, modern technology can now support life indefinitely in previously fatal diseases with prospects of transplantation of vital organs. The most important single threat to future contentment, ego needs, and self-fulfillment is not disease or hunger or environment, but the debilitating effects of feeling (and being) unessential or superfluous.

Positive steps are required to reinforce the social needs, the ego needs, and self-fulfillment of these major segments of the population whose identity and self-satisfaction have been undermined, in part, by modern technology. For example, the Japanese previously had a tradition whereby the father retired from his job or business in his early fifties and directed his attention to becoming a scholar or even a philosopher. His eldest son assumed his responsibilities. The result was that the son had increased his status while his father would earn and deserve the respect of his family and peers for his wisdom and scholarly pursuits. Unfortunately, this tradition is being lost as the Japanese adopt or emulate Western "civilization."

PUBLISHING AND REPRODUCTION

With modern reproduction techniques, the finest and the worst of literature, art, and thought has been brought within the reach of virtually anyone interested. The color rendition of painting, the tonal quality of music, and even reproductions of sculpture, jewelry, and ceramics ever more closely resemble the originals. Photographic equipment has become so foolproof that the inexperienced novice can obtain consistently good pictures. The ready availability of all this wealth of cultural material may have somehow reduced its apparent value. Anyone can pursue his interests in the arts and sciences, politics, history, philosophy and ethics, but a glance at most book and magazine stands provides little evidence of interest in such matters. There seems to be an overwhelming tendency to discover the lowest common denominator in the offerings of publishers, motion picture producers, plays, and telecommunications. Modern man has not been prepared to reap the deeper benefits of modern technology and society. The publishing and reproduction industries respond to the tastes of the people, and these are not being adequately elevated by education.

TELECOMMUNICATIONS

Through newspapers, radio, and television, anyone can learn about the happenings around the world very promptly, not just once but many times a day. Modern telecommunications can bring into the home the best of the many cultural and natural beauties of the world. This enormous flow of information could be directed toward improving understanding between peoples, constructively approaching to the many vital problems facing mankind, and tapping creative genius of the best brains available. Instead, the verbal deluge incessantly emphasizes violence, crime, accidents, terror, and wars. Occasionally, positive accomplishments are acknowledged. Constructive approaches to problems are rare compared with the frequency with which crime and dishonesty are recognized. Much of the substance conveyed by telecommunications is inherently divisive when the need for cooperation and social consciousness was never greater. Again, the deficiencies lie not in the technologies but in the manner in which they are employed. This is the basic tragedy of the modern society which encompasses a myriad of missed or neglected opportunities to utilize products of human ingenuity fully while avoiding the unpredicted complications of technology.

CHANGING GOALS FOR IMPROVED QUALITY OF LIFE

The major sign of progress in industrialized society has been an increase in tangible goods and material wealth which necessarily tend to deplete resources and add to environmental deterioration. So long as industrial production remains the principal criterion of progress, our plunge toward creating a dying planet will continue. Technology and automation are currently increasing the number and proportion of the unemployed which are in turn producing stresses on our economic system. However, the younger generation is demanding a shift in emphasis and a change in life style designed to improve the quality of living. This is tantamount to a shift from a product-oriented society which demands massive expenditures of natural resources and capital to a service-oriented society which is primarily labor oriented. In short, the development of greatly expanded service functions for health, education, culture, art, communication, and other activities can be designed to improve the quality of life which could be accompanied by a contraction of unessential industrial production. The current trend toward planned obsolescence to maintain markets and employment could better be reversed by providing a much broadened selection of life styles which require above all else a rather profound shift in both national and individual goals and fundamental changes in the educational process. Clearly, this suggestion seems idealistic and unrealistic in the extreme, and yet continued expansion of our materialistic social orientation appears headed for disaster. It seems clear that a major change in direction is in order. For example, there are thousands of unemployed on welfare, while other thousands of handicapped and aged badly need kinds of help even untrained people could provide. With careful planning the growing group of unemployed could be constructively utilized in a human service-oriented society. An avenue of greatest importance would be communication services.

SUMMARY

Each of the major technological triumphs of modern society has been accompanied by complications and unpredicted threats. Accelerating technological changes have greatly increased the number and scope of the growing problems and reduced the time available for accommodating to the changes. The greatest defects lie in the human failure to plan and predict adequately and a serious deficiency in group wisdom to match the creative ability and drive of individuals in both innovation and production. We have more than ample human talent to solve most technological problems without additional knowledge. What is badly needed is sufficient mobilization of sound judgment which can prevail while overcoming the threats to modern societies.

REFERENCES

Berry, B. J. L. 1970. The geography of the United States in the year 2000. *Ekistics*. **29:**339–351.

Doxiadis, C. A. 1970. Man's movements and his settlements. *Ekistics.* **29:**296–321.

Huxley, A. 1958. Brave New World. New York, Bantam Books.

Morris, D. 1969. The Naked Ape. New York, Dell Publishing Company.

Population Program Assistance. 1969. Agency for International Development, Bureau of Technical Assistance, Office of Population, Washington, D.C. 20523.

Toffler, A. 1970. Future Shock. New York, Random House.

Wilson, I. H. 1971. The new reformation, changing values and institutional goals. *The Futurist.* **V:**105–108.

CHAPTER 17

CAUSES AND EFFECTS OF EXCESSIVE FEARS, ANXIETIES, AND FRUSTRATIONS

STEWART WOLF

Society has enjoyed a rich harvest of poetry, painting, scientific discovery, and all manner of human achievement when talented people have been under severe emotional pressure. A challenge to adapt can promote welfare and productivity. As Hans Vaihinger put it, "Man owes his mental development more to his enemies (adversities) than to his friends." Utter boredom would be the price of total immunity from fears, anxieties, and frustrations. When they are not balanced by a productive effort, however, such emotional disturbances may be accompanied by physical disability, disease, and even death.

THE BASIS FOR EMOTION

To experience fears, anxieties, and frustrations requires the complex integrative circuitry of the brain in the interpretation of life's events and encounters. The existence of an attitude or feeling state may in turn affect the processing of various kinds of information in the brain. Understanding of the relationship of emotion to bodily changes has been hampered by a lack of clear agreement as to what emotion is. Literally, the word implies movement of some sort. Many authors equate the term with a feeling state. To them, an emotion is a sort of sensation or at least an awareness which may be pleasant or unpleasant; for example, joy, satisfaction, hope, and appetite as well as fear, anger, and resentment fall into the category of emotions. Finally, some workers apply the term "emotion" to conscious or unconscious mental processes whereby events are interpreted in view of personality and past experience. In the latter instance, neural connections are made because of the significance of the event but without the process necessarily being brought to awareness.

INSTINCT AND INTELLIGENCE

Over the course of evolution there has occurred an extraordinary elaboration of the nervous system resulting in neuronal interactions that not only allow for the multitude of memories, associations, and interpretations that underlie emotional experience but also spell the difference between instinct and intelligence. Instinct is characterized by a fixed stimulus-response relationship. The caterpillar, for example, when triggered by environmental cues to build his cocoon, will not repair it if the bottom end is cut out, but will simply go on to complete it at the top, leaving a part of his body exposed. Intelligence, characteristic of higher animals, implies the ability to modify behavior on the basis of perception and interpretation of circumstances. The ability to exercise behavioral options, and thereby to make contingent responses, requires a circuitry for the processing of sensory cues far more complex than that possessed by the caterpillar. As the phylogenetic scale is ascended, the increasingly complex process of "interpretation" of experience has led to another important development, namely the identification of individual needs beyond those of nourishment, reproduction, and survival. Their satisfaction is sought through a wide variety of goal-directed behaviors.

WHAT IS BEHAVIOR?

The term "behavior" is often applied only to activity in skeletal muscles manifested in gestures, movements, and speech. The term should be extended to the functions of the viscera, however, since adaptive changes in organ function just as surely depend on the capacity of the nervous system to make fine discriminations among diverse cues. Thus, to respond appropriately to a changing environment with either skeletal muscles or with smooth muscles, blood vessels, organs, and glands requires a vast ramification of association nerve cells, or interneurons. These are by far the most numerous of man's nerve cells. The number of effector neurons, those that actually trigger behaviors of various sorts, amounts only to several millions, far fewer than the tens of millions of afferent neurons that bring information from the external and internal environment. Adding both afferent and efferent pathways together would still amount to only a fraction of the interneuronal pool, those tens of billions of nerve cells that process information and formulate responses. It is assumed that these highly specialized integrative neurons are responsible for our capacity to scan experience, interpret events, and determine the degree to which fears, anxieties, and frustrations are excessive, and whether or not disturbances in visceral or general behavior will accompany them (Fig. 1).

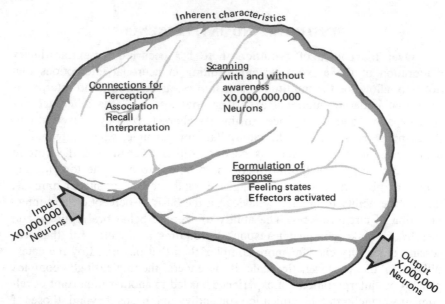

Fig. 1. The processing functions of the brain require vastly more nerve cells (neurons) than are needed to bring in information from the environment or to bring about various behaviors.

ADAPTATION TO SOCIETY

According to J. B. S. Haldane, progress in medicine depends on understanding how the human organism adapts to changes in his environment. The ability of individuals to accommodate to perturbations of all sorts depends on what has been called the plasticity of the nervous system; that is the ability to alter functional connections among association neurons and to select among alternate behavioral pathways. Being a social animal, man finds that many of the requirements for adaptation and for satisfying his needs stem from his relationships with his fellows. Unlike the ants and the bees, humans do not have a rigidly preordained role in society, but must continually select among a vast array of options that offer abstract as well as concrete rewards and punishments. Man must adapt to his social surroundings where relationships are largely based on verbal and other symbols. He must achieve nourishment of the spirit and satisfaction from activities while realizing his potential for love and for creativity. The quality and organization of the relevant processing mechanisms in the brain depend, of course, on the inherent characteristics of the individual, genetic and acquired, on previous conditioning experiences, and on myriad features of the setting, timing, and accompanying circumstances that surround an event. Each new experience plays some part in programming the brain to determine the ways in which subsequent experiences will be dealt with.

SENSORY OVERLOAD

The smooth operation of the biological computer may be disrupted in the presence of excessive sensory input. Thought is difficult in the presence of clanging bells or screeching sirens, or while looking at the confusing, rapidly changing kaleidoscopic images of a psychedelic experience. Too much sensation may be harmful.

SENSORY DEPRIVATION

Studies of very young animals and humans indicate that some sensory inputs are essential to the establishment of required circuitry by the nervous system. The classical studies of Harlow and Harlow demonstrated that the healthy development of an infant monkey requires that he have something soft to cling to. They found that, as a mother substitute, a turkish towel fixed to a frame was vastly better than nothing. Even better was a moving "surrogate mother," presumably because it stimulates development of vestibular and cerebellar systems. Totally deprived of a clinging experience, the infant monkey failed to develop the capacity for social relationships in play. Instead, he would simply sit in the corner immobile for most of the day, thereby resembling closely a patient with catatonic schizophrenia. Human infants appear to be even more vulnerable to sensory deprivation. Frederick the Great is said to have carried out an experiment in which he attempted to protect the health of infants in a foundling hospital with disappointing, indeed disastrous, results. It was the post-Pasteur era, and to many, at the time, prevention of microbial infection appeared to be the sole requirement for the promotion of health. The emperor, therefore, decreed that the nurses in one demonstration orphanage should wear masks and avoid touching the infants insofar as possible. Fondling was strictly prohibited. To everyone's surprise, nearly two-thirds of the infants died from undetermined causes, a mortality vastly in excess of that in the ordinary, less hygienic orphanages. An impressive documentation of the importance of human contact to the health of the developing infant was provided by Rene Spitz, who made a motion picture of infants in a South American foundling home. As described by Dennis:

> Although the hygienic aspects of the care these infants received was beyond reproach, overcrowded conditions rendered impossible any individual attention beyond routine feeding, bathing, and changing. The pictures show three-month-old infants who have lost their appetite, who lie inert, failing to smile or respond to the attendant. By the age of five months the "wasting away" process has set in with alarming acceleration. The babies look like wrinkled old men. Their expressions are vacant and weary. They show none of the interest in the world characteristic of normal infants of this age. It is as if the spark of life had long since flickered out, leaving only a grotesque physical shell.

Twenty-seven of these children died during the first year of life, seven more during the second. Twenty-one who remained in the institution but managed to survive showed such a drastic crippling of their emotional lives that it is doubtful if they could ever be classified as other than hopelessly mentally ill.

Although the need to be loved may be crucial to survival in early infancy, a similar need for symbols of social acceptance persists in most of us throughout life. Sudden unexplained death is a well-recognized consequence of complete social exclusion imposed under a variety of names by societies widely scattered over time and over the globe. The ancient Greeks wrote a rejected citizen's name on a shell and threw it out to sea, thus ostracizing him. Certain tribal societies even today practice bone pointing, voodoo, or make pouri pouri with the same objective. In contemporary American society, individuals are not formally placed beyond the pale. Moreover, our sudden unexplained deaths are, by convention, designated as myocardial infarction despite the fact that at autopsy pathologists fail to find evidence of infarction in upwards of 30 percent of the cases. It may not be coincidental that deaths attributed to myocardial infarction are encountered with special frequency among those who have been recently bereaved or are otherwise emotionally drained.

PATTERNS OF BEHAVIOR INVOLVING INTERNAL ORGANS

The path toward healthy development of a well-adapted human being is fraught with many pitfalls. The very multiplicity and potentially conflicting nature of human needs may result in their realization being hampered or blocked. As a consequence, uncomfortable emotions such as fear, anxiety, and resentment are engendered. Other consequences may be the disruption of general behavior or of visceral function, or both. The nature of the disruptions depends not so much on the accompanying emotions as on the significance assigned to the experience in the course of processing in the brain. The involvement of the internal organs in these responses is discrete, patterned, and similar to adjustments that are clearly purposeful. Thus, a frustrating experience may provoke in the nasal passages of one subject excessive secretion, swelling, and obstruction similar to that elicited by the inhalation of noxious fumes. In the stomach of another individual, interruption of digestive activity with nausea and vomiting might occur as it does following the ingestion of poison. In a third individual, the opposite gastric response might be brought into play, namely an outpouring of digestive juices and vigorous kneading movements such as normally accompany the ingestion of food or even the anticipation of eating. It is the capacity of organs of the body to react in anticipation that provides the basis for "psychosomatic" phenomena, disturbances in the organs of the body that occur in response to emotionally significant events. However inappropriate the behavior may seem, the person whose nose swells during an emotionally troublesome experience is behaving as if he were breathing in a noxious environment. The "stomach reactor" who becomes nauseated as his stomach ceases its digestive activity is behaving as if he were being poisoned. The one whose stomach behaves in the opposite fashion, pouring out quantities of acid gastric juice, is acting as if he were about to eat. The same parallels to protective adaptive reaction patterns can be drawn in the case of those who respond to meaningful situations with alterations in heart action, blood pressure, kidney, bladder, or colonic function, or other organ disturbances that the physician recognizes as the manifestations of disease.

THE STRESS OF CHANGE

The ability of the systems that regulate behavior to adapt to change and challenge without losing homeostatic balance depends not only on the quality and organization of the machinery of the brain and the rest of the body, but on the nature, frequency, and intensity of the demands for adaptation, often loosely referred to as stress. Holmes and Rahe have demonstrated the potential pathogenic nature of radical changes in life circumstances, even pleasurable and fulfilling life changes. They developed a weighted scale from which life change scores could be computed and demonstrated clearly that a high score was associated with heightened vulnerability to disorders and diseases of all sorts. Disease, therefore, appears to be not related so much to the nature of the accompanying emotions, but to the number and timing of changes and challenges and the degree to which the adaptive capabilities of the organism can deal smoothly with them. Our aim should certainly not be to eliminate the stress of life, but rather to concentrate on the cultivation of the self and specifically the organ of personality and adaptation, the brain.

TOWARD A SCIENCE OF MAN

From our slowly developing understanding of the circuitry of the brain and the way in which it is programmed by experience, it seems clear that in the pursuit of health the major effort should be directed toward the developing infant and child. We must be cautious in arriving at simple solutions, however, until systematic research yields far more knowledge and understanding, until we can truly find ourselves developing a science of man. The development of such a science will certainly require a synthesis of disciplinary approaches. Existing professional splits along both methodologic and conceptual lines have put us in the situation of the blind men trying to describe an elephant. The separation of sociology from biology has accentuated the problem. It was the biologists who brought us to our knowledge of the social behavior of the birds, the bees, and the ants. If biology is fundamental to their behavior, why not that of man? Social systems are based on complex communications involving symbolism, concept formation, understanding, and predictability, all requiring the processing of the biological computer and the effector functions of the neuro-endocrine system. The neurophysiology of drives, values, and goals has not been extensively studied, but must be pursued. Livingston has pointed out that as organisms, we build cultures and influence them; and in turn they deeply influence our perceptions and our behavior. An efferent system acts among the various afferent pathways to modulate perceptions strongly according to past experiences and according to the direction of attention and intention. Thus, cultural differences in language, custom, and human values may be deeply embedded in the mechanisms of central control of perceptual processes. According to Livingston, "we each wear an idiosyncratic physiological lens system that is invisible to us because it affects the very circuits on which we depend for knowledge of ourselves and the world around us. We have no other avenue for knowledge."

MAN'S NATURE AND HIS NEEDS

Medical science has been less concerned with understanding man and his interactions and interdependencies with the world about him than it has toward lengthening his life. Other social institutions have focused on reducing his workload and equipping him with prostheses such as automobiles with which to enjoy his leisure. The problem now is how to spend leisure time. In fact, we are faced with a crisis of leisure. Great numbers of people look forward to the day when they can retire and then, like Mr. Manette in "A Tale of Two Cities," they are uncomfortable with no last between their knees. Sometimes they just die. We need to apply ourselves to learning what fulfillment of man's spirit is all about.

Freud is one who made a major effort to understand man's needs and characteristics. He emphasized defects in the process of psychological development, but his work and that of many other thinkers leaves us with but a thread for the whole skein. Religions have been mainly concerned with influencing human behavior. Rather than telling us what we are, they have told us what to become. The Judeo-Christian tradition (but not necessarily the teachings of Christ) has held to a conviction that man is inherently "bad" and needs to be redeemed (changed). The anti-religious thinking of the "enlightenment" espoused a point of view not fundamentally different. The proposed means of "salvation," education, is different, but the need for change is made just as urgent. The search for truth, for freedom, for peace, and for ease and comfort have been vigorously pursued over the centuries with the aim of "liberating" man to express his own true nature. In each quest, dauntlessly pursued, we have neglected to learn what is the nature of man. Rene DuBos, among living savants, has given more thought to the question than most of us. He has pointed out the need for a new methodology, really a new science, if we are to begin to understand the distinctly human animal. He observes a reluctance to get on with the job and quotes to that effect the German philosopher and psychologist, Benno Erdmann: "In my youth, we used to ask ourselves anxiously: What is Man? Today scientists seem to be satisfied with the answer that he *was* an ape."

LEARNING MAN'S PLACE IN NATURE

Somehow, we have become deluded into thinking that mastery over the forces of nature is our proper aim. Therefore, instead of trying to define man's place in the world, we have been trying to engineer a sort of takeover by man. This has been remarkably successful. With the synthesis of a virus-like particle, man has come close to synthesizing life. The crowning achievement of our era may well be the ability to manipulate DNA. This will give awesome power to man, but so did the discovery of fire, of electricity, and of atomic energy. None of these discoveries has led along a very straight road toward man's better understanding of himself. The discovery of concrete, for example, gave man considerable capability to alter the face of the earth, but with it he made major manipulations of the seacoast in many parts of the world, converting marshlands to dry land, docks, and bulkheads. Thereby, he was able to interfere with a natural process, the consequences of which he did not understand at the time. One result was to reduce the supply of edible fish and mollusks by eliminating the nursing grounds of many life forms in the food chain. Up to the present, then, man has been able effectively to crowd out a host of other animal species and to eliminate them from the face of the earth as well as the seas.

Fortunately, there are many reminding us today that the mark of a healthy ecological unit is a diversity of species, and of a dying unit, a paucity of life forms. The old point of view, *"homo-sapiens über alles,"* was very recently espoused by Robert White-Stephens, a professor of biology at Rutgers. He wrote, "Conservation is directed primarily at conserving man, and those plants and creatures and areas that serve man: anything else is not conservation, but merely conversation." This is a strange statement from a biologist who must be aware that man often does not know, in fact, which creatures are serving him. Man is an enormous force in the world and, like all great forces, is potentially destructive. Forces like fire, water, and atomic energy become constructive when they are harnessed. It is not likely that the forces within man will be harnessed until they are better understood. In fact, without sufficient understanding, we have probably attempted too much harnessing already. With very little knowledge of man's nature or his needs, society has developed some pretty clear conceptions of how he ought to be; in fact, each culture has prescribed for man, attempting to regiment him toward an established "norm" of behavior. When he has deviated widely from this, be it in the manner of a psychotic, a criminal, or a genius such as Gallileo or Socrates, his culture has punished or even annihilated him. This rather Procrustean attitude is not likely to lead us to a greater understanding of man.

NEEDS FOR NEW KNOWLEDGE

What parameters, then, do we need to examine in order to develop a systematic knowledge of man? We already have a good grasp of the machinery of the body. Furthermore, we know that insofar as we are arms, legs, hearts, livers, and kidneys, we are all much alike. As persons, however, we are very different from each other. When the brain, the organ of personality, is damaged by senility or other causes, behavior becomes stereotyped. The person is essentially lifeless.

The very richness and almost unimaginable complexity of neuronal interactions involved in memory, learning, reasoning, and imagination have blinded us to the realization that the circuitry of the brain must operate according to an underlying set of laws. There must be definable requirements for the proper development and operation of the system. We know some of them, but we know them as we know the pieces of a jigsaw puzzle that have not been put together. A beginning is being made through the study of marine invertebrates. Their neurons are similar to those of man. So are their means of firing and the laws that govern depolarization and synaptic transmission. Some of the neurotransmitter chemicals that are responsible for conveying impulses from one nerve cell to the next are shared by man and earlier animals forms that came into being hundreds of millions of years ago. As the difference between rock music and Bach lies not in differences in notes of the scale but in the way the notes are organized, so the difference in brain function between mollusks and man, and the diversity among men, is a matter of neural organization and numbers, not so much a difference in materials.

What kind of background will young scientists need to begin to define the nature of man? One thing is clear: they must approach the problem by considering man in relation to other creatures. Interdependence is a very fundamental principle among living things. The realization of this truth may have been somewhat obscured by Darwin's emphasis on competition, the survival of the fittest. It is true, nevertheless, that interdependence is demonstrable in the very simplest of unicellular organisms. The top millimeter of the sea, for example, is occupied by a variety of microscopic forms, each separate and freely moving, but the product of one is essential to the life of another so that these unconnected cells are nevertheless very closely interrelated. Such interdependent aggregations must be the forerunners of tissues. It appears, therefore, that the process of nature has been differentiation, specialization, combination, and then differentiation again. There may be a great lesson for us in this story of interdependence. Perhaps cities are the tissue of human society. The mass of humanity on the face of the earth may be comparable to the organisms in the top millimeter of the sea. The interrelatedness of all life and hence the identity of life above and apart from individual identity is expressed by Teilhard de Chardin in his concept of the biosphere. In describing it he emphasizes that it is ever changing and evolving.

We are gradually learning that in the realm of conventional biology as well, the only permanent thing is change—change requiring ever new adaptive responses on the part of organisms, races, and species to serve their need to survive. Man's thinking brain has both aided him in his adaptations and created new challenges for him. Such challenges may engender fears, anxieties, and frustrations. Responses to the challenges may take the form of striving, creating, avoiding or destroying. Throughout, there has been growth in knowledge, increasing awareness and invention. Disability and death resulting from exposure to the elements were mitigated when man sought shelter and clothing; then the wild predators were fended off with arms and later the microbes with public hygiene and antibiotics. Now the prominent illnesses are those related to man's own activities and his relations with his fellow man. The creation of societies required that humans, especially males, learn to live together without destroying each other; now the survival of society requires that we learn to tolerate differences in people and their points of view. The stresses concerned with this step in development provide much of what is noxious in the environment of modern man.

REFERENCES

De Chardin, P. T. 1969. Human Energy. Translated by J. M. Cohen. London, Collins.

Dennis, L. B. 1957. Psychology of Human Behavior for Nurses. Philadelphia, W. B. Saunders.

DuBos, R. 1967. Man Adapting. 2d ed. New Haven, Yale University Press.

Haldane, J. B. S., and J. G. Priestley. 1935. Respiration. London, Oxford University Press.

Harlow, H. F., and M. K. Harlow. 1965. The affectual system. *In* Behavior of Non-Human Primates. A. M. Schrier, H. F. Harlow, and F. Stollnitz, eds. Vol. 2. New York, Academic Press.

Holmes, T. H., and R. H. Rahe. 1967. The social readjustment rating scale. *J. Psychosom. Res.* **11:**213–218.

Livingston, R. B. 1972. Neural integration. *In* Pathophysiology: Altered Regulatory Mechanisms in Disease. E. D. Frohlich, ed. Philadelphia, J. B. Lippincott Co.

Vaihinger, H. 1949. The Philosophy of "As If." Translated by C. K. Ogden. London, Routledge and Kegan Paul, Ltd.

White-Stevens, R. 1972. Pesticides: friends or enemies. *The Clipper Magazine* **12**:2.

Wolff, H. G. 1968. Stress and Disease. S. Wolf, and H. Goodell, eds. Springfield, Ill., Charles C Thomas.

CHAPTER 18

CAUSES AND MANAGEMENT OF CURRENT ANXIETIES AND FRUSTRATIONS IN UNIVERSITIES

Dana L. Farnsworth

During the last decade, a great majority of the young people in our high schools, colleges, and graduate schools have lost confidence in their elders, in themselves, in our system of government, and in the ideals and goals which had guided most of our people in earlier years. This has resulted in a profound disillusionment, shared to some degree by all people but expressed in quite emphatic terms by many of the more intelligent, idealistic, and impatient young men and women.

SOCIAL CHANGE IN MIDCENTURY AMERICA

This group of young people was brought up in the latter half of the 1940's and the 1950's when the majority of the people were reasonably well off and material standards were constantly increasing. At the same time, there were pockets of poverty, mostly in the centers of the large cities and in remote rural areas, which were also constantly increasing. Thus, affluence and poverty became visible because of their sharp contrast. Those who were poor and had ambitions became increasingly frustrated and disillusioned, and those who were affluent but possessed of a high degree of idealism became dissatisfied with the injustices they saw.

During this time there was also a constant increase in population, so that the acquisitions which were signs of affluence became more and more difficult to obtain or enjoy because of crowded conditions, particularly in the cities. And many of the goods and services thought to be essential for a more comfortable life became much more costly. Parents worked harder and harder to achieve their material ambitions; they had less and less time to spend with their children, thus losing the benefits of working together for common goals that were practically routine in earlier agrarian societies.

The extended family, comprised of parents, children, and other relatives living together or close to each other, began to diminish, while the number of nuclear families, consisting of parents and children alone, began to increase. With the father and often the mother out of the home much of the time, the children in school, and family members having no work in common, communication between the generations decreased, until the children were receiving most of their ideas about standards of behavior from their peers and from television rather than from extended contact with their own parents or other older people.

Peer group influences and influences from the mass media tended to be in a relaxed or over-permissive direction and were counteracted rather weakly by parents, teachers, and clergy. Young people felt a growing isolation, a lack of warm human relations with older people, and therefore resorted to developing ways of expression with one another which often did not take into consideration lessons learned from experiences of earlier generations. Many young people tended to discount the lessons of the past and devoted themselves in an increasing measure to making the most out of the immediate present, postponing planning for their futures as long as possible. This sense of concentrating on the present found a ready ally in marijuana, which also tends to minimize the effect of the past and concern for the future among those who use it extensively.

As standards for employment increased, more and more groups looked upon a college degree as a ticket of admission for the more important jobs. This stimulated increasing enrollment in the colleges and universities, which grew quickly in the past two decades. Coupled with this growth was a very rapid increase in knowledge within practically all fields, which resulted in increased difficulty and additional time to become competent in any particular field. Thus, maturity, commonly interpreted as being coincident with becoming financially and socially responsible for oneself, had to be postponed more and more. This prolongation of uncertainty gave many young people the feeling that they were marking time and that what they were studying was not relevant to what they might be doing in the future.

Since every occupation and profession demanded more competence, it became increasingly difficult for a person to change direction once he had advanced into any one field. Changing from medicine to law, or mathematics to social science, or business to the arts, was more and more expensive the longer it was postponed. Thus, the dilemma of choice was a profoundly troublesome one for many young people.

A growing dissatisfaction arose with the impersonality of government and large corporations, marked by feelings of futility regarding the power of any particular individual. Many persons felt that they really did not count and that the system was not responsive to their needs. Gradually this dissatisfaction became directed toward the universities, the courts, and to the basic value systems of the entire society.

The Vietnam war, which had been in an incipient, smouldering state in the late 1950's and early 1960's, began in 1964 to assume major proportions. The conflicts at all levels about this war resulted in a wide variety of disagreements and dissatisfactions which became so frustrating that there appeared to be no clear solution, no single enemy, culprit, or scapegoat. The disagreements thus fostered concerning national policy appeared to spread to many other areas of life, increasing the already strong tendency of many people to believe the worst of one another.

With the emergence of television as one of the greatest educational influences in the country, most young people became aware at an early age of the injustices, the inequalities, the acts of violence of human beings against each other; at the same time they became aware of the extremes of luxury and dire poverty in which many persons lived. This intense education in men's social and cultural conditions was heightened by the teaching many of them received at home and at school, that they should be critical, idealistic, and responsive to injustice everywhere.

Television not only had a positive function, it also became an instrument by which some groups could influence others for their own financial gain. It was not too difficult a step for groups to use television to exploit others, as is particularly obvious in advertising designed to create a demand in children that their parents buy certain products. The use of violence in programs designed to entertain or to explore human passions became commonplace.

Beginning in 1954 with the Supreme Court decision in the Brown case,[1] a renewed attempt was made in the United States to achieve equality for persons of all races, particularly the blacks. By 1960 this movement had acquired strong momentum and was further stimulated by President John F. Kennedy, resulting in increased hope on the part of underprivileged groups. With President Kennedy's assassination and the ultimate failure of the country to respond to the numerous liberal legislative programs of the Johnson administration, a period of disillusionment set in. This began after a series of demonstrations, particularly the Mississippi Summer of 1964 and the Freedom Rides, and the migration of the blacks to northern cities; it was further accentuated by the assassinations of Martin Luther King, Jr., and Robert F. Kennedy. Thus, the racial conflicts brought out into the open resulted in considerable progress but also polarization in

---

[1] *Brown vs. Board of Education of Topeka,* in which the old doctrine of separate but equal educational facilities was overthrown.

some localities of moderate against militant blacks and whites against blacks.

Quite often dissatisfactions of black college students resulted in protests that became confused in most people's minds with the demands of white students. In the last few years, the development of movements designed to change the status of other groups seen as oppressed (particularly those grouped under the general term of Women's Liberation) has added a new dimension to the general confusion.

Early in the 1960's, Timothy Leary and Richard Alpert at Harvard University, in combination with a variety of people from other parts of the country, began to publicize their experiments with psychotropic substances, particularly the psychedelics, which were alleged to be helpful in opening up new areas of consciousness, often described in terms parallel to the exploration of outer space. As psilocybin and LSD rose in popularity, the use of cannabis preparations (marijuana) began to spread from its formerly circumscribed manifestations among lower socioeconomic groups to the middle and upper classes. From the mid-1960's until the present time there has apparently been a gradual increase in the number of persons who have used marijuana and the number who continue to use it regularly. This increase is much more marked among high school and college students than among any other group in our society.

At the same time, the use of all kinds of drugs began to increase, notably the amphetamines ("speed" being a term used to denote intravenous use) and the barbiturates. A disturbing number of persons adopted a life style centering around the use of practically any drug available. Heroin became a problem in many colleges and universities, but an even greater one in the crowded sections of urban areas. The use of drugs practically always incites strong feelings on the part of those who disapprove, and marijuana, which was among the least dangerous of these drugs (National Commission), became a symbol of dissatisfaction with a wide variety of social conditions.

Soon a rapidly changing set of standards, life styles, customs, attitudes, and goals began to emerge. Rock music festivals became a kind of romantic expression of these changes. Shifts in sexual attitudes and behavior were soon manifest in newspapers, magazines, song lyrics, the movies, and theater. Many of the old values appeared to many young people to be outmoded and ineffective, particularly because they observed so many of their elders who did not live up to the ideals they professed. This rapid change in standards created much confusion among older persons as to which of their values were really essential and which were temporary. Faculty members, particularly the younger ones, and many parents adopted various aspects of this new counterculture; many persons in the advertising, fashion designing, and entertainment industries adopted them almost completely.

RAPID CHANGE, CONFUSION, AND DISILLUSIONMENT

The result of all these events was that many of our young people became disillusioned with previously workable and acceptable goals, developing feelings of discouragement, depression, hopelessness, and a sense that it didn't really matter, after all, what they did. Because they felt that they had had many things misrepresented to them, they tended to reject all ideals of the past, and their behavior then led older people to condemn them uncritically rather than to work with them in a close and friendly way toward the achievement of changed values that would be mutually acceptable. In an attempt to find some kind of rapport with their fellows, they changed their hair styles and relaxed their speech and sexual caution. But they were still unable to find warm and rewarding relations with any others than those in their own special group, and thus they became more and more isolated, while their conformist tendencies led critics of college students to overestimate the significance of their behavior. The net result has been that colleges themselves became targets of bitter criticism, complicating the task of raising funds which are so necessary to meet ever-increasing costs.

Students who felt deeply about the injustices observable on every hand, unable to work directly toward their removal or to influence those who might be able to do so and noting the growing lack of opportunities for many of those who held advanced degrees, often developed attitudes of cynicism and confusion. Having been trained to be idealistic, critical, and confident that good ideas and good will should enable them to solve problems, their frustration turned to anger and finally to an attempt to find dramatic but simplistic solutions.

In the early 1960's, a few groups began to arise among young people which were devoted to stimulating discontent. The majority concentrated their efforts on weakening those influences which they felt were contributing to the growing impersonality of society. They appeared to be taking action to increase personal liberty, develop means of establishing warm relations between human beings, relieve oppressed peoples, and further the goals that had been professed by large numbers of Americans. In practice, however, many of these organizations sought the achievement of their goals with such single-minded intensity that they eventually polarized groups against one another more than they united them toward achievement of common goals.

Various techniques of protest arose, coming to an early peak in 1964 during the disorders at the University of California at Berkeley and continuing to the present. Such activities were frequently concentrated in those colleges and universities that had attracted highly qualified students whose attitudes were basically liberal. Hence, the majority of the severe disruptions occurred in such universities as Stanford, the University of Chicago, the University of Wisconsin, Harvard, Yale, and Columbia and other New York City institutions.

THE EFFECTS OF VIOLENCE

As disillusionment, dissatisfaction, and hostility began to be expressed in terms of violent protest, bombing of buildings, and other measures unacceptable to practically everyone, a turning back toward methods of collaboration between the young and the old became obvious. At present, the more extreme proponents of violence have lost a great deal of prestige and respect and find themselves increasingly isolated. Many of those who were very active in the 1960's are now engaged in constructive work designed to minimize the injustices they deplored. A few of the more active protest leaders committed acts of violence which caused them to go underground, a condition in which some of them have lived for several years.

Probably the tragic events at Kent State, Jackson State, and the University of Wisconsin following the invasion of Cambodia in 1970 were a turning point in the struggle between students and the Establishment. Younger students, having seen what was happening to their older colleagues, have tended to adopt a more conciliatory and constructive set of attitudes, realizing that it was their future which was being endangered. During the past two years there appears to have been a slow return to opinions, attitudes, and practices that are consistent with maintaining academic freedom and with keeping colleges and universities as free places for the exploration of any ideas.

This apparent return to less violent forms of protest should not be construed as a loss of idealism or determination on the part of students. Relatively isolated attempts to provoke violence have usually met with failure, but much of the credit for this goes to the restraint practiced by police and administrative officials, who have realized that arbitrary policies applied with a show of violence provoke still further violence from students. The temporary increase in anti-war sentiment during the spring of 1972 was characterized by less violence than in 1970. This was in part due to fatigue and frustration, but it also embodied the belief that misdirected efforts against relatively helpless institutions produced strong disapproval on the part of many citizens who were themselves opposed to the Vietnam war but were even more opposed to internal violence. Christopher Dawson's warning seems to have been taken to heart by many:

> But our generation has been forced to realize how fragile and unsubstantial are the barriers that separate civilization from the forces of destruction. We have learnt that barbarism is not a picturesque myth or a half-forgotten memory of a long-passed stage of history, but an ugly underlying reality which may erupt with shattering force whenever the moral authority of a civilization loses its control. (Dawson, p. 24.)

If one were to judge the way society is moving by the changing attitudes of students, it might be possible to underestimate the gravity of our present situation. Their confusion, anxiety, and frustration have been shared in varying degrees by most citizens, compounded by constant evidence from mass media and entertainment industries that standards of behavior are becoming less and less inhibited. Old standards are being threatened, and new ones involving equal or greater responsibility have not yet emerged. A moderate degree of pessimism about the future seems quite appropriate—especially if that pessimism is expressed in such a way as to stir large numbers of people to seek favorable change.

THE UNIVERSITY'S RESPONSE

Dealing with a syndrome so vast as the current set of anxieties and frustrations calls for massive efforts by large numbers of people. Probably the most important element in keeping sullen discontent from erupting into destructive action is the composite attitudes of faculty and administration members, especially in their relations with students, in groups or individually. Any actions that suggest imposing the will of that group on the students will be met with stout resistance. On the other hand, vacillation between indecision and temporary displays of force will bring about the same result. A reasonable consistency of policy, based on sound principles which encourage the greatest amount of freedom for everyone but do not result in injustices to individuals and small groups, appears to be effective in creating a climate of opinion in which people of widely varying opinions can work together.

This sounds fine in theory, but in practice a number of complications arise. For example, in most faculties a few members have not worked through their own maturational problems and see in unrest a way of achieving some of their goals by playing off students against the administration. Others need the good will of students, to the point of adopting student customs and viewpoints in the hope of ingratiating themselves. When communication between these faculty members and their more conservative colleagues becomes strained, polarization of issues becomes accentuated. To many of us, the rigid stance of the confirmed radicals has a remarkable similarity to the attitudes of those who resist change at all costs. Each of the extreme groups contains many persons who are prisoners of their own beliefs and are not able to remain flexible in the face of rapidly changing social conditions. The result is that they become stereotyped, dated, and ultimately left behind.

The energies, ideas, and ideals of our unhappy but concerned students may eventually be one of the most conservative forces in our society—if *conservative* is understood in its positive sense, the conservation of values which we and they both prize. But this can only happen if all citizens work together in defining and furthering those values.

Counseling services, including the psychiatric departments of college health services, have a particularly important role to play in helping students deal with their frustrations. Not only do they have the task of trying to prevent the loss of student effectiveness from self-defeating reactions, but they also have a responsibility to aid students to work effectively in achieving the social reforms necessary. Social protest must not be equated with psychiatric disorder (Farnsworth).

THE WEB OF MORALITY

The task facing our colleges and universities is largely that of helping students regain self-respect, mutual confidence between themselves and their elders, and the ability to apply their enormous energies to the solution of the problems facing all elements of society. Basically, this means that students need to develop moral controls to replace outer controls and to train themselves and others to study and respect those standards, customs, attitudes, and practices that enhance the dignity and equality of opportunity for all individuals. The discrepancies between their ideas and their practices are fully as great as those they protest in the conduct of their public servants and industrial, business, and union leaders; yet their ability to recognize them seems slight.

It is no exaggeration to point out that the signs of decay in our civilization are not unlike those seen in many previous civilizations. The Roman Empire fell because of economic crises, deterioration in governmental skills, declining morale, and widespread immorality. The contrast between the wealthy and the poor was vast indeed. Attacks from without, aided by widespread passivity exemplified by the "bread and circuses" mentality within, combined to bring about its gradual dissolution.

The similarities between the causes of decay at that time and the social, economic, and political conditions at present are so great as to be shocking. The vital questions are: Can we develop the restraint, self-control, and discipline to prevent history from repeating itself? Can we learn to strengthen the web of morality which enables society to perpetuate itself?

A prime goal of college education is to develop young men and women who are observant and critical but who are at the same time constructive in their criticism. We need have no complaint that during the past few years our students have become passive or apathetic, but there is much convincing evidence that criticism has become so strong and lacking in specificity that our colleges and universities are being seriously weakened. Not only are the conditions under which college administrators work becoming less and less tolerable, but the public is increasingly reluctant to support institutions that appear unable to govern themselves responsibly.

From the viewpoint of many idealistic, sensitive, but critical students, the present political system seems to be too powerful and not responsive to their needs. In seeking objects through which they may express their feelings of powerlessness, cynicism, and despair, they naturally tend to strike out against those institutions near at hand, which are themselves practically defenseless against violence. Through the relatively helpless colleges and universities they can express their hostility toward those institutions that are strong—the federal government, the courts, and business and industrial organizations.

What measures can an individual educational institution adopt that will be both responsive to and respectful of the genuine dissatisfactions of concerned students and faculty, and at the same time be consistent with the atmosphere of freedom that characterizes the true university?

A first principle is that there should be open channels for discussion of all kinds of issues that are of concern to the college community: between administration and faculty, faculty and students, or any other communication. Free communication should also be maintained between members of the administration, counseling staffs, health personnel, and those who deal with the intimate problems of students, although at the same time great care must be taken to see that the privacy of no individual is violated.

In general, any policies or customs that seriously impair the physical condition of top officials and hence interfere with their judgment should not be encouraged. Obviously, no single person, particularly not the president, can make himself available to every person who wants to see him about specific issues as they arise. He can, however, arrange for periodic appearances to discuss any or all of these issues, and he can get the opinions of many individuals through one or another of his associates. He may also authorize one or more officials of the institution to speak for him during periods of crisis when he cannot be available to all who want to deal with him directly. Responsibility for institutional policy has to be shared by several persons if scapegoating is to be avoided.

Each institution should have the goal of evolving policies that have a clear consensus of support from faculty and student opinion leaders, the elements of which can then be discussed in greater detail by the various groups. When feelings are running high and extreme demands are made, such as the demand to sever all connections with groups or agencies whose activities evoke strong emotional reactions, there should be firm rejection of actions that are quite probably detrimental to the institution. Policy measures of grave importance can seldom be decided fairly when emotions of various groups are at a high pitch. A continuing educational effort should be made to distinguish between those issues which can be supported wholeheartedly by all members of the institution, such as the principle that free speech and academic freedom should be protected at all times, and those which of necessity call for different solutions and hence need various approaches. A corollary to this might be that the right of dissent does not include the right to force assent. The rights of individuals should always have high priority so long as the exercise of those rights does not deprive others of their rights.

Administration, faculty, and students should have representation in the maintenance of discipline, along with provision that the rights of the entire institution and its surrounding community should also be taken into consideration. When a student or faculty member is suspended, the institution should have the authority to enforce his suspension. Expulsion for the more outrageous types of behavior is both necessary and desirable. Any student who has been suspended or even expelled once and who compiles a good record of reliability for the next one or two years should have another chance. But a student who violates such a probation, or who is readmitted and repeats his behavior of the past, should have his connection with the institution severed permanently.

When buildings are occupied or other types of violence occur, there should be as much reliance on the courts as possible, but at times it may be necessary to take more immediate action if the offenders are violent or destructive. A combination of careful and deliberate court action accompanied by waiting out occupations when the participants are peaceful seems to be a formula with considerable merit.

It is most important that any police who are involved in disturbances around colleges or universities be well trained in both firmness and restraint. Violence should be kept at a minimum and should not be directed toward injuring individuals unless there is absolutely no alternative.

The much-discussed theme of student representation is an important one. As I view it, students should be represented in practically all of the considerations that concern them, but they should not be in control. The well-governed institution, in fact, is one in which no faction has absolute control except in occasional legal decisions, which are made after full consultation with all parties involved.

When dealing with students and others in times of crisis, it is quite important to make a clear distinction between those who are sincere and genuine in their activities and those who seek action for devious personal reasons and who have become more or less fanatic in their activities. The former will respond to logic, reason, and sincere attempts at cooperation. The latter ordinarily do not.

Another principle deserving of consideration is that no promises should be made that cannot be fulfilled and no threats should ever be made that cannot be enforced. At any time during a crisis when some individual becomes adamant and provocative in his fixed point of view, the chances of trouble are greatly increased. This is true of the chief administrative executive, the student leader, or any person with significant authority and responsibility.

The Cox Commission, which investigated the troubles at Columbia University in 1968, observed that, "A university is essentially a free community of scholars dedicated to the pursuit of truth and knowledge solely through reason and civility" (Crisis at Columbia, p. 196).

Following a long and detailed analysis of a controversy that had adversely affected one of the Harvard graduate schools for three years, two members of the Harvard Corporation, who had been on a committee to investigate and settle the disturbances, commented at the end of their report:

> Finally, the committee notes with regret the intermittent failure by people involved in this controversy to abide by the conventions of civil discourse. Those conventions, in the academic world as elsewhere, help to contain the rhetoric of debate so as to keep disagreement from fostering antagonism. If students are to participate in academic processes, they must learn to temper their language, oral and written, and to speak to issues rather than personalities. In the petition of 1969 they failed so to do. Even more does the committee lament similar failures on various occasions in the relationship among faculty members and between faculty and administration at the School. It is perhaps too much to hope for spontaneous, reciprocal charity in the relationships among members of an academic community. In those relationships, however, it is not too much to expect an unvarying and disciplined civility. (Harvard University Gazette.)

The colleges and universities cannot afford to shrink from the task of developing standards by which men may live with one another in peace and with a minimum of conflict. Likewise, they must constantly work toward an observance of those minimal but essential restraints that will achieve the greatest amount of freedom for everyone, even though much study will be necessary to determine what those minimal restraints should be. Educational institutions, working in harmony with the family, the churches, schools, and the wide variety of other voluntary organizations devoted to human betterment, can reverse the trend toward dissolution and decay if only they can generate the will to do so.

REFERENCES

Bell, D., and I. Kristal, eds. 1969. Confrontation: The Student Rebellion and the Universities. New York, Basic Books.

Crisis at Columbia. 1968. Report of the Fact-Finding Commission Appointed to Investigate the Disturbances at Columbia University in April and May 1968. New York, Random House.

Dawson, C. 1958. Religion and the Rise of Western Culture. Garden City, New York, Doubleday (Image Books).

Farnsworth, D. L. 1970. College mental health and social change. *Ann. Int. Med.* **73**:467–473.

Foster, J., and W. Long. 1970. Protest: Student Activism in America. New York, Morrow.

Handlin, O., and M. F. Handlin. 1971. Facing Life: Youth and the Family in American History. Boston, Atlantic-Little, Brown.

Harvard University Gazette, January 7, 1972, p. 6.

Heirich, M. 1970. The Beginning: Berkeley, 1964. New York, Columbia University Press.

Hook, S. 1970. Academic Freedom and Academic Anarchy. New York, Cowles.

Keniston, K. 1971. Youth and Dissent. New York, Harcourt.

Kennan, G. F. 1968. Democracy and the Student Left. Boston, Atlantic-Little, Brown.

Lee, C. B. T. 1970. The Campus Scene: 1900–1970. New York, McKay.

Mayhew, L. B. 1970. Arrogance on Campus. San Francisco, Jossey-Bass.

Metzger, W. P. 1969. Dimensions of Academic Freedom. Urbana, University of Illinois Press.

National Commission on Marihuana and Drug Abuse. 1972. Marihuana: A Signal of Misunderstanding. Washington, Government Printing Office.

Schlesinger, A. M. Jr. 1961. The Crisis of Confidence: Ideas, Power and Violence in America. Boston, Houghton Mifflin.

Schwab, J. J. 1969. College Curriculum and Student Protest. Chicago, University of Chicago Press.

Smith, G. K., ed. 1968. Stress and Campus Response: Current Issues in Higher Education. San Francisco, Jossey-Bass.

Taylor, H. 1969. Students Without Teachers: The Crisis in the University. New York, McGraw-Hill.

Wallerstein, I., and P. Starr, eds. 1971. The University Crisis Reader: The Liberal University under Attack. New York, Random House.

CHAPTER 19

THE SOCIAL AND PSYCHIATRIC ASPECTS OF PSYCHOTROPIC DRUG USE

DANIEL X. FREEDMAN

INTRODUCTION

Men use drugs to enhance their purposes. But cultural norms, social regulations, peer groups, and the family differ in the purposes which they value and the permissible means for their expression. We are condemned to private experience but designed to be linked with this range of tutoring agencies. These agencies give our private experience a certain meaning, regulation, and negotiability. We cannot be born alone or become human alone; yet in our limited span of life we alone must endure, decide, or acquiesce and generate, accumulate, and exchange experience with others. We regulate ourselves and in so doing are regulated.

The point to emphasize is that the regulation of the giving and getting of drugs is closely linked to self-regulation—the regulation of the self and its purposes. Further, the range of person to person, societal, and ideological tutoring systems have powerful effects that determine not only the use of drugs but also their consequences. In this linkage between the self-regulation (of anxiety and private, personal, peremptory wishes for control of mortality, morbidity, and moment-to-moment comforts) and social regulation of such needs, one of the powerful governing social systems is the doctor-patient transaction. It is my belief that an appreciation of the links among beliefs, social systems, and private experience are important if one is to thread his way through the variety of complex, often bewildering discussions labeled "drug abuse."

SOURCES OF IRRATIONAL DRUG ATTITUDES

We can manipulate our own intentions and seek retreat and comfort with or without the aid of chemicals. We can dream while awake and attend to voices no others have heard. All men are anxious about their mortality and vulnerability, the limits of their capacity to control either what they experience or what occurs in reality. The need both to transcend the moment and to have some sense of control and predictability over what life brings—the governance of our search for comfort, novelty, pleasure, and avoidance of pain—is a dominant motive in the various patterns of psychotropic drug usage, from ritual and recreational drug consumption to the various patterns of self-administration and misuse.

No society is comfortable when quite private purposes and meanings can be given to common social events. While in the Darwinian scheme of things most of us seem to be designed for consensual experiences (for social engagement, for sufficient vigilance to achieve reproduction, survival, and nurturing of the young), it is also true that individuals may use "the cover" of socially sanctioned activities to pursue a variety of quite personal or idiosyncratic aims. We not only can revise public meanings in our private experience but also can skillfully implement either shared or megalomanic and retreatist goals. These facts generate a gradient of anxiety about retreat and pleasure seeking beyond social bounds—a concern of parents and others as to whether their tutoring works. The fact that drugs simultaneously affect both private experience and public behavior, that their use provokes value judgments about performance and pleasures, means that there is always anxiety about the control and predictability of expected behaviors—of just what a person is capable of when intoxicated or medicated.

Drug use, misuse, and dependence impinge, then, on belief systems, and these systems serve to link the personal and social. Basically, we all recognize the power that drugs give to the consumer—the power magically to obliterate pain, to ignore social consequences, change the world in a single gulp, and privately revise its meanings and demands. Thus, whether we can control expected or feared behaviors is at issue—whether drug-taking individuals will respond reliably to the social signals and to the cues by which we normally influence and regulate each other. Most societies believe there are good occasions and bad occasions for the consumption of drugs; the social sponsorship and purpose of drug consumption (whether by self-administration or prescription) is always an issue—generally fraught with tension and passion.

We never forget the deep irrational roots underlying our attitudes about what we consume in the way of substances. For, from our very origins, we are deeply ambivalent. The mother's food is given with the attitude of "it is good for one"—for pleasure, growth, strength, or relief of pain. Other substances are bad. Chemicals and drugs are either "chicken soup" helping us to transcend a variety of ills and ails—bringing potency, power, and control over events of the moment; or they are poison—a threat to our potency. Fads for and phobias against foods and chemicals are the visible consequence of this inevitable heritage.

When a drug or potion is more or less accepted, we deny many of our fears. In medicine we observe that physicians and/or patients can often practice drug giving and drug consuming too freely—it becomes pill dispensing; once a medicine has an established place we tend to ignore the complexities and cautionary rules for weighing the risks and gains. The medicine is useful as a "device," a "simple" means to go about getting what we want in life; we can have relief when we want it.

The other side of the coin is the fact that we endow the drug giver with great power. A visible substance can be transformed into a powerful internal agent and this can always create awe both in the giver and consumer. In the consuming of substances we do not explicitly monitor and track the sequence of events that we know to take place in physiological fact. We simply feel. We are tutored in what to expect and how to interpret our feelings. But it is true, when we cannot explicitly monitor and track events, that attitude and customs will tend to regulate our approach and bind anxieties.

Accordingly, rational drug management is somewhat astonishing, given the deep irrational roots of our experiences with consumed substances. Indeed, if we look at the extent to which rumor and fad have governed the physicians' behavior with medicines, the extent to which toxicological drug effects are greeted with sensation and panic before the rational basis for, or validity of, such reports are investigated, we can appreciate the anxiety and emotional power that lie behind even a rational approach to pharmaceuticals—not only by politicians (who minister to beliefs) but by professionals.

THE SOCIALIZATION OF DRUG USE

The social and psychological factors of drug use are crucial, from the very definition of what chemicals are considered fit for consumption and who should consume and provide drugs, to the occasions appropriate for this and the tasks to be performed in the drug state and following it, to the definition of harm and good of tolerable and intolerable uses and degrees of acceptable dependencies. I know a French chemist who is quite ready to recognize ethanol as a drug, but not of wine as an instance. No usable drug represents either pharmacological original sin or pharmacological original perfection; nor should we conceive of originally evil people (vulnerable as some may be to unwanted effects). As physicians we must recognize that persons seek to enhance their ideals and values, sometimes with and often without the use of drugs.

Recreational drug usage shifts our attention from the day's constraints to a different order of events, of communion and community. This shift of attention alone can provide a brief holiday, an exultation and release

of energy, as in a hobby or at a theater, or simply a change of scenery
The beer or the cocktail party, an aperitif on a promenade—these are socially sanctioned events for many which mark a change of pace. A religious
question asks, "Why on this night we drink this wine?" And the father
answers, citing tradition: the wine is used simply to dispose one to regard
the occasion in a special way, to put one in a different frame of mind,
to share an unstated but understood communion, and the content is provided by the story of heroic survival and escape. Similarly, in subgroups
or cliques of young adults drugs become symbolically meaningful. If they
do not mark a special occasion, they are the shared means to achieve an
identity—to belong and "be with it." The unstated subjective experience
that the drugs induce in the members—the fact that each of the group
partakes of it—creates a sense of community and distinctiveness without
any necessary regard as to whether there is actual commonality of experiences or even an elaborate myth to elevate and bind the group beyond
the life of drug taking. The induction of members into drug-taking groups
entails different dynamics than sustaining of membership, but the climates
of fashion or ideology are characteristic.

The way the *consequences* of drug intake are anticipated is crucial
to the experience. American Indian sages note that their legendary vulnerability to firewater is believed by the Indian—who is, in a way, "drunk"
prior to starting his weekend binge. He fulfills the white man's prophecy
(as do many addicts and children of whom the worst is expected), an
expectation that in a certain sense is shared. For the Indian, to drink at
all is to have "had it." It is the time to "let go," and the consequences
of alcohol are frequently violence and deep inebriation, rather than
courtly pleasantries. While there may well be genetic differences in the response and capacity to tolerate alcohol, these psychosocial expectations
are crucial. Similarly, the consequences of intoxication are socially defined;
whether after a noisy drunken spree one is subsequently accepted or ostracized is critical. Whether the event is disapproved of but tolerated and
accepted as a part of what occurs in life, or whether those who succumb
and show loss of control are considered pariahs, helps to determine the
meaning of drinking and the uses made of drink in a society. And what
to do about tissue dependence can also be socially influenced; whether
one takes more alcohol for a morning hangover or resorts to stoic en-
durance, for example. Thus, within obvious dosage limits, it is the way
we hope to manage the effects of drugs and the personal and social uses
to which we and our reference groups put drugs that lend definition and
shape to the pattern of drug effects, whether this is called drug use or
misuse.

Informal social systems can define the way events are to be interpreted and managed during the drug state. When one is intoxicated, the

bridge to reality lies in the customs of the group, as internalized by the individual and interpreted by the occasion. In the Peyote religious ceremony held by American Indians, one sees the family: parents, grandparents, children, and neighbors with the sacramental guides (called "road chiefs"). Enormous quantities of the sacramental drug are consumed. The substance is not designated as a drug; it has a religious meaning. The communicants are told to ignore the perceptual effects of the active ingredient (mescaline) and to let their mind be caught up in the ceremony and its purpose, echoed in the ritual drum beats and droning of prayers. They are taught to yield the activity of deciding what to attend to—the task of coping with detail—and "to be in the mind of God." "Bad trips" are interpreted and treated with group prayers and instructions in order to capture and divert attention away from evil and disturbing thoughts. Competitive and aggressive feelings (for which many drugs can be used) are thus contained and shifted. The ceremony is given a special place in a sequence of life events. The entire procedure is circumscribed and defined by ritual. Thus, the individual is guaranteed a regulated journey through a period of diminished capacity for self-regulation, by the ethic and tutoring of the group, which in turn is empowered by belief that transcends the egocentric and idiosyncratic impulses of any one member.

THE MEDICAL SOCIALIZATION OF DRUG USE

Similar tutoring occurs within the medical system. We give drugs to aid the individual in his regulation of the self and its purposes. For example, if a physician diagnoses a truly disorganizing tension and anxiety, and treats with pharmacotherapy, he is helping the patient to manage the effects of the drug for a specific situation and time-limited purposes. Or, if morphine is given for analgesia there is an agreement—generally tacit: doctor and patient agree that the drug is being used for pain. In a sense, they "agree" not to exploit the euphoric effects of a narcotic analgesic, even though such effects may to some degree be present. In general, the patient tends not to notice these effects and, in any event, to localize the entire experience to the medical occasion for use.

A physician's patient who receives (or even wants) pharmacotherapy is attempting to regulate his feelings, his aches and tensions, and that odd psychosomatic mixture that expresses dys-ease (dys = abnormal, ease = comfort). He does this to enhance his personal purposes and to get his job done. He may wish to have aid in enduring his pain while living and coping with office or household or family tasks or situations of stress. He may need to shift his attention from neurotic inhibitions that paralyze his personal effectiveness. But in general—and recent national studies both of prescribing behavior and the attitudes of patients bear this out—medication is sought for a limited period to achieve a specific task. This is not to say that either physician or patient will not exploit—consciously or unwittingly—the use of drug for other purposes, but in general this is not the norm, publicized and sensational beliefs to the contrary.

The medical management of drug use, of course, always may borrow from powerful wishes for a superior agent to relieve discomfort, and once again tap into the infantile roots of our experiences, our magical thinking and wish for transformation. Effects of drugs then may be more than purely pharmacological. Nevertheless, the use of drugs can also be managed as a kind of collaboration between patient and physician. When the heroin addict agrees to the methadone therapy there are some important shifts in definitions. In some sense the patient shifts *his* power to use the drug and to manipulate his own feelings. He may also shift his attention from hustling for drugs in the streets to more socialized interests. This can probably best be done if the approach is not simply "pill-dispensing." The patient somehow alters his drug taking from the street definition of purpose to that of "treatment." This psychosocial fact may be a powerful rehabilitative force to the extent that pharmacological treatment is useful (assuming that treatment and rehabilitation are indeed available). A society that can constantly rather than episodically facilitate re-entry and resocialization provides a key factor for successful therapy of the addict. Given the intransigence of many confirmed narcotic addicts in their dependencies, the politicized and transient concern of the public and public agencies, this is a most difficult attitude to sustain.

The point here is not to detail the problems in treatment of narcotics addiction but to indicate the power of the social system in redefining the terms in which drug effects are to be experienced. We suspect that antianxiety and tranquilizing effects of narcotics, as well as the avoidance of withdrawal, are important in "medically socializing" the addict's drug taking; despair, loneliness, and rage may be less readily perceived and their disorganizing effects less likely to supervene because of pharmacologic effects. But what is important is that the management of one's feelings and the treatment of one's ills and ails can be socialized either in the outlets and tutoring provided in healthy development or in special treatment situations, with or without the use of drugs.

The medical profession must count on the fact that both customs and social functions, including religion and recreational drugs, help people to solve, redefine, or contain some of their problems and impulses. We could not as a profession adjudicate every anxiety to which people are prone. An individual must learn to diagnose his own condition, learn to tolerate and interpret pain, and to find some relief through extramedical resources. At some special and reasonable point they may seek special help. Intelligent—or wise—self-medication has a social role. The function of modern medicine is to find a way of rearticulating our contact with our clientele and thus to tutor in the appropriate uses of medication, whether prescribed or self-administered.

CURRENT IDEOLOGICAL CONFUSIONS

In today's climate of renewed concern over values and uses of the products of nature and technology there has been a lack of explicitly informed focus on what is required for appropriate and reliable administration of drugs. On the one hand there is the stern demand that the "crutch" of medication be avoided and withheld. But there is also a strident clamor that each individual has the right to experience *whatever* he wishes, and sometimes, *whenever;* and sometimes with the added codicil: as long as it is private and does not harm others. The fact that one's "civil" right to drug-induced experience can hardly be private seems to elude examination (as does the fact that in infancy similar intransigent demands are properly dealt with by empathy and respect for feeling but tutoring in restraining action). For one to have his drug of choice means that there must be a market and availability of the product. Drug seekers must come to some position about regard for rights versus the inability of others to consume drugs reliably and reasonably. They rarely tutor in wise drinking or consumption of marijuana, nor help to put boundaries on appropriate usage. Ex-addicts and others who work earnestly to rehabilitate victims are often unreasonably furious at those who do not abolish the drug which they "fight"—not regarding whether this is feasible or on target: for the human desire for the drug is also a problem. Such debates and intransigencies were in part involved in our prohibition experiment in which the idea of temperance was lost and urban values were pitted against rural virtues; one sector of society claimed that another was ruining it.

And so today we see verbal young individuals who feel they can manage their marijuana with skill and for personal pleasure; at the same time they require of government that any legitimate medication receive a guarantee of absolute immunity from error. Forgetting that individuals regulate individuals, there are many who blithely pass medications (or a drink) to a friend without any regard for whether the friend is able to consume it reliably or whether they, the friendly passers, can vouch for the purity of the drug. We see a new "authoritarianism": one's own experience is sufficient for judgment. At the same time, it is apparently possible to adjudicate risks of medicines in the press or in the halls of Congress with little more preparation than distrust of power and confidence in the superior power of righteous advocacy to diagnose ails.

It is often forgotten that there are psychotropic medications (lithium for manic-depressive psychoses, the phenothiazines for psychoses and schizophrenias) that are used to dampen abnormal intensities of experience and to enhance the individual's capacity to select and choose. As indicated earlier, this may (or may not) apply to methadone's tranquilizing and anti-anxiety effects in helping addicted individuals manage otherwise disorganizing effects. The good physician, of course, does not—if he is wise—medicate to enhance habits of avoidance and escape but rather to help the individual gain mastery. The effective use of amphetamine in children with multiple disorders and a syndrome in which control over attention and motility is grossly deficient dates to the late 1930's. Yet the empirical and research observation of efficacy was challenged on a variety of grounds: prejudice against amphetamines, belief that exuberance rather than inability to control was the target, and so forth. The "amotivational syndrome" seen after extensive and intensive psychedelic and other psychotropic drug use in some persons was similarly mistaken for laziness or a commitment to Eastern antimaterialistic philosophy. It eludes the educated that inability to deploy attention *at will* is entailed (either to inner or outer concerns), and that such states are abnormal in Eastern as well as Western culture. Information is not identical to the ability to decide and analyze data, nor are slogans substitutes for a grasp of operative processes.

If we really respect the individual differences among individuals (in their capacity to organize their perceptions selectively), we cannot be innocent of the consequences of their particular state in relation to the goal of achieving gratifying function. In spite of an enormous amount of sociological mythologizing there is no way of "un-naming" disorders by calling them mythical. There is a group of individuals who are variably at risk for profound and incapacitating disorganization of mental and behavioral skills. We call them the psychiatrically ill; we do not confuse these dysfunctions with the miseries of everyday life; we do not deny their need for learning, love, respect—nor their need for a clear and accurate grasp of their ailment.

There are other medical areas, however, where ethical issues are primarily involved: when the physician is asked to use anabolic hormones to enhance muscle mass, or sedatives and stimulants to improve athletic performance or to diminish tension so that overtaxing work can be performed; or thyroid not for glandular disease but for heightened energy. The "pill" is a good example of the interface of the availability of pharmaceuticals and social values. With the psychotropic drugs it is clear that we do not wish to deprive individuals of the chance to gain strength and experience in managing the stresses of life. But in our judgment of the nature of man we need to recognize his fallibilities and his limitations.

Patients often govern drug giving and getting with sanction from these—often educated—subcultures; asking for penicillin rather than for a diagnosis. We must learn from and share values with our patients—but not surrender our special function. A part of the tutoring functioning of an overworked professional practice is to demonstrate "problem solving" through good diagnosis, the giving of care, and ongoing assessment in a continuity of care. Professional practice requires sensitive social and ethical judgment as well as keen appraisal of problems and limitations of men. In his commitment to individuals it is important that the physician be able to assess them, their situation, potential, *and* capacity on the one hand, and at the same time, to recognize that there are quite appropriate and manageable occasions for the prescription of a period of psychotropic medication.

INTRINSIC FACTORS IN DRUG MISUSE

Finally we should come to an understanding of some of the intrinsic psychiatric factors that endow the self-administration of drugs with such power and intransigence. What is it that makes treatment so difficult? What are some of the resources that we can use? We should look forward to a far more reliable appreciation not of *the* motive, but of the *various* motives subserved by drugs. While it appears virtuous to discern the root cause and not treat the symptom, it is essential to focus on the sustaining motivations of drug taking and of contemporary stress contingent on it. Behavioral effects sought through drugs may be simply for a change of normal state, but also, for some, a different disposition toward a task, or toward the self and others. Drugs of widely different specific effects can enhance any number of purposes, especially when taken under the regulation of clique, fad, and fashion.

We do not understand why some drugs tend not to be used or misused in self medication—tricyclic antidepressant drugs, the monamine oxidation inhibitors, lithium, and the phenothiazines. And there are effects from specific drugs which can serve (too well) special purposes. For example, to achieve indifference to anxiety and the environment, the opiates may be chosen; alcohol and barbiturates may tend to lower inhibitions and allow a spurt of social, sexual, agressive, or self-aggrandizing impulses. In addition, those who want a passive experience in which reduction of aggression and anxiety and euphoria may be sought may find marijuana serves (while tranquilizing, attention is turned inward, sometimes not only revealing the "TV show in the head" but also "revealing" special meanings of the environment in a paranoid way). At times, LSD can be used either for an internal experience of vividness without the exertion of effort or for a wish to see old things in a new way or at times to achieve insight. For treatment of poly-drug use and sustained alcoholism, a period of drying out is most often instructive in revealing motives and is the first task; for narcotics, a stabilizing of the habit—bringing it under control—can equip some individuals to cope, choose, reflect, and learn. In any event, one must be wary of routinely ascribing motives to the drug user and instead ponder why *he* does so. Essentially the order of experience produced by LSD is instructive if it brings a lack of boundaries to the control of effects and perception, so that the utility or familiarity of an object or a thought or image is no longer as important as an aspect of it. When intensities (for example, color) are somewhat detached from their usual contexts they gain a special meaning; this is often felt as an uncanny sense of significance—one which can *never* be explicated but "feels" impellingly important. The private sense of meaning and truthfulness is enhanced but not the disposition to test the truth of the senses! There has been the speculation about the various motives enhanced by specific classes of drugs, but there is much evidence that the private exploitation of magical thoughts and illusion is generally appreciated, whether through the waking dream (or nightmare) of LSD or other changes of mental and bodily states.

We find novelty in manipulating our own minds and bodies; children swing and delight in changing their feeling state—within bounds! To control—or command—a change of state (to be out of the ordinary state) is an enormously powerful human motive that can tap our most private perserving, primitive, and peremptory wishes. The power of denying risk to transcend reality is awesome. Observing from the outside, we often forget that the drug-dependent patient gains something in achieving this immediate and private change. While drug dependencies may objectively appear terribly costly (especially when the individual can be judged to be truly out of control of his habit), we must acknowledge he does indeed gain something.

To specify the gain is difficult. It is clear that he has some sort of comfort which is somehow within *his* power to achieve; he cannot often correctly perceive what it is that he is gaining, or what the costs are, even though they are acknowledged. Obese people, for example, often do not perceive satiety; they require help and training to do so in order to begin to exercise control. Yet, even though they must be miserable with their fat, they believe in their own experience—of relief, of corporal importance, or avoidance of depression, or comfort. Some are compelled (by unnamed panic or urge) to binges; some are at it consistently.

The power of the self-administration of drugs to manage uncertainty is probably critical. The principal of familiarity or constancy is, at the phase of dependency, impressive. The extent to which we ward off not only challenge but also moment-to-moment change by ritual is at issue. The cigarette addict can become aware that the cigarette is a familiar experience for him. He exerts control over what immediately to expect; a thin gray veil of comfort lies between him and external stimuli and acts as a token barrier against intrusion and the unexpected—a private mastery. The smoker has the assurance of a familiar private experience in his response to the nicotine and to the ritual of the cigarette. These barriers, comforts, and reassurances are regulatory functions that, for the infant, are performed by the mother. All men have an enduring need for them in one form or another.

Many addicts simply do not feel like "themselves" without the familiar state produced by the drug. They learn through the drug experience ways of relating to others and to stresses. They need only see, think, or encounter these conditioned signals to once again remember their power, their small mastery while functioning in the drug state. Thus, part of the relapsing character of narcotic and alcohol addiction has to do not only with internal needs but also with the external signals—human events woven into the fabric of life which reevoke a craving for the drug state. Again to take a familiar example we need only watch cigarette smokers; as one lights up another tends to. After a time he has experienced so many events under this state that he automatically reaches for a cigarette in the presence of the stimulating occasion—be it a person, moment of tension, or whatever. His capacity to interpose a delay between himself and the world and have an assured experience combine to provide a powerful motive.

Many alcohol or narcotic addicts are "treating" themselves—phobias and disorganization, even schizophrenia. Some manage to be productive with such self-medication; for them the only issue is the price; for example, the heavy drinker who thereby socializes and is less inhibited in getting his work done with this consolation. Some patients fight depression with amphetamines and gain a sense of power with the access of energy and focused attention.

In all drug-dependent individuals the importance of magical wishes and demands is clear. They may, on the surface, be exceptionally self-demanding and shy (many alcoholics are). They are governed by requirement for some kind of perfection—an uninterrupted and unchallenged serenity. This, of course, cannot be achieved in reality. Some of these individuals transfer their notions of power and perfection to the physician—or other idols to whom they ascribe a sort of eternal presence and power. They then become angry and crushed with slight disappointment in themselves or the other. They engage in magical manipulation of supplies and needs, and this is often socially evident as charm or blarney as the addict expresses his preoccupation with bringing others into the ambit of his control and inflated self-esteem. Characteristic of these individuals' behavior are rage and frustration over failure and the lack of assured protection, and the inability to perceive how others manage their imperfections (this includes the inability to perceive the doctor's limits and imperfections or a destructive test and search for them). All these factors refer to the same eternal problem: that man is indeed limited; that his capacity to perceive of perfection is not identical to the prescription for real life. And in all of this, the actual power to take the drug (no matter how this fact is masked) is crucial. As one youngster said when thinking over his loneliness, shyness, and inability to feel confident, "I can turn on as good as the next guy."

The power of belief is enormous in sustaining addictions as well as in overcoming them. We are all aware of some of the cures of alcoholism with religion (which seems as potent as any therapeutic drug). Belief can supersede detail and habit and arrange all events under a guiding attitude that is protective. One can then view the events in life as designed for ultimate good. Ritual also is a device; it can capture attention and divert one from brooding uncertainty. Thus, one can either ignore detail or focus upon it to put bounds around anxieties. We can see both factors operating in sustaining drug use but also in overcoming it. Self-help groups are powerful.

What is the power of the group? In general, any surrendering of the coping, tracking, decision-making problems can provide enormous relief if we share the functions of decision-making with others. It is the sharing of painful autonomy, the relaxation of internal tension which many experience in decision-making, a certain loss of the self (and self-centeredness can indeed be painful as well as compelling) that is characteristic of many of our shared group experiences.

The group not only helps to induce and socialize drug experimentation and/or recreational drug taking but also to permit some yielding of the infantile version of and the wish for unblemished autonomy. In such situations a self-help group need not produce violent authoritarian conflicts. All are sinners, and rather than weakness being perceived as a taunting imperfection, it is either shared or, as in "confrontation" groups, excoriated by those who confess their own imperfections.

This is not to say that all self-help groups are well-managed or can readily accomplish what we would assess to be the most authentic self regulation—any more than can conversion experiences. But one may have to choose between the tyranny of a habit such as drug taking and a less damaging dependency on the analyst, group, or conversion. For many ex-addicts intransigent attitudes toward drug consumption are an important defense against relapse.

Many of the self-help groups and "rap sessions" that are common among adolescent drug users fail to recognize their limited use. Such groups (and spontaneous groupings) can support self-pity and dependency and be used to make certain that there is not sufficient tension and challenge to promote growth. What is striking about many of the more successful self-help groups is the extent to which the temptations to addiction are literally comprehended in all their specific detail; the evasions and tactics of the drug user are all readily spotted. Physicians can learn to do this, but require experience so that the detail can be properly evaluated; seductive and manipulative patients whose drug subculture is unfamiliar to the physician can readily evade a solid and real therapeutic engagement. Physicians can learn to reach adolescent patients without either indulging them (by unnecessary agreement) or challenging and alienating them by unnecessary aloofness—whether this is evidenced in attitude or in lack of flexibility. "Operation Outreach," which is common today, often deprives young people after a time of someone who really knows better than they who has the advantage of hindsight and foresight—is comfortable in tolerating differences in values while being receptive to exchanging them. Tolerance for deviant behavior in our culture has led also to a remarkable indifference to "one's brother," to the dangers of suicide and self-destruction.

Since we cannot here describe the details of therapy, what we should fully grasp is that in the context of shared experience, learning can take place if there is a design for it. Again when tutelage in self-regulation is coupled with regard for others, the medical treatment ethic flourishes. In disease, we seek optimal physiological function through a variety of medical devices, allowing natural forces to operate at their optimal level. This seems to be the most viable aim in our psychological and rehabilitative interventions.

PREDICTION OF RISK

Who is at risk? In general the longer a psychotropic drug is prevalent in a subculture, the more the initial mythology surrounding it loses relevance and the more the drug becomes "institutionalized." When this happens some people may learn how to use a drug well. This can be done even with heroin or opiates, although these are the most seductive of drugs and loss of control for occasional use is frequent and highly likely. But in general, we must expect a "constant reservoir" of people who will get in trouble and a constant volume of people currently in trouble with drugs. There is about a 6 percent chance of alcohol-related problems. This results in appallingly large numbers of people in trouble but is a relatively small risk considering those who manage alcohol well. People move in and out of the category of having drug and alcohol problems. But those who are treating internal fragmentation, depression, and phobias probably are recruited from a special population. There is growing evidence that children born of schizophrenic parents (and even those reared separately) have a higher incidence not only of psychoses but also of a whole range of deviant behaviors seemingly based on the difficulty in integrating pleasure with reality. Such studies indicate a relatively high incidence of alcoholism and homosexuality in the offspring. The point is that there are some people who may be much more vulnerable than the majority; they will be unable, even if they wish to integrate around reality engaged behaviors, to do so without fortune or guidance. The developing young also should be thought of as at risk; less has been experienced and settled, so to speak, and hence chemically induced distortions of reality may not lead to sound learning or useful probings of risks and limits.

Finally, drugs bring their own problems. There is learning under the drug and, more often, unlearning of psychological skills. Frustration tolerance diminishes with the learning that frustration can be avoided. The therapeutic task is not to solve our curiosity about why drugs are taken, or how family constellations may predispose (a useful topic for research), but to help the individual to come to grips with some of the elements in his life that he is avoiding and that he may, with therapy, begin to master.

CONCLUSION

The use of drugs provides, then, a striking metaphor to think of man and his purposes, to perceive the discontinuities and links between private experience and public behavior. Their use also can illustrate the mediating mechanisms from molecular to the psychosocial whereby the effects and consequences of drugs are defined and structured.

I have often wondered whether the fact that drugs rarely sustain their initial allure and promise was a mischievous and malevolent trick of nature. Whatever the problems of nature's design, there do appear to be intrinsic biological and biosocial limits on the extent to which the chemically induced moment of pleasure can be sustained and woven into a fabric of viable social life. We can readily give up our lease on reality, but apparently it is difficult to gain ownership of paradise! One can surely find better myths and parables to express men's striving and pain than drug experiences—especially when the power to use them well and wisely is within our grasp.

CHAPTER 20

CAUSES AND MANAGEMENT OF CRIMINALS: PSYCHIATRIC ASPECTS

W. WALTER MENNINGER

The first man born on earth killed his brother and became a criminal. His punishment, he said, was greater than he could bear. But he was not executed and his descendants became great musicians, artisans, and herdsmen. How would it have turned out if Cain had killed Abel in West Virginia last month?

The criminal tendencies of mankind have been one of our compelling interests since that day in the Euphrates Valley so many centuries ago. We still don't know how to protect Abel and we still don't know what to do with Cain; whatever we do seems to be wrong. Crimes increase, but most of those who commit them are never caught. Those who are caught seem to get caught over and over again and are given the same unprofitable treatment.

> —Karl Menninger, M.D., in his Foreword to
> *Psychiatry and the Dilemmas of Crime,* 1967, by
> Seymour L. Halleck (New York, Harper & Row).

It is axiomatic that when man encounters a problem he cannot solve, he will repeatedly struggle with it. He will work at it, put it aside, then come at it again from another direction, and try, try again. So it is with the eternal struggle to understand and deal with criminals. Volumes have been written on the subject, some much better than others.* Throughout all the discussions, certain critical themes persist, and this chapter attempts to review some of those themes from a psychiatric perspective.

In the area of causation, the themes are (1) The Definitional Problem, (2) The Dilemma of Understanding, (3) The Wish for a Simple Explanation, and (4) Mental Illness and Crime. In the area of management, the themes are (1) The Atrocious Nonsystem of Corrections, (2) Principles of Correctional Management, (3) Effects of Institutionalization,

---

* For further reading, searching discussions of this chapter's topics are provided in Halleck's *Psychiatry and the Dilemmas of Crime,* Karl Menninger's *The Crime of Punishment,* and Mulvihill and Tumin's *Crimes of Violence,* which is a three-volume Task Force Report to the National Commission on the Causes and Prevention of Violence.

(4) The Incorrigible Few, (5) Outside the Walls—The Role of the Community, and (6) The Role of Science.

CAUSATION—THE DEFINITIONAL PROBLEM

What is a criminal? In the common parlance and understanding, a criminal is defined as one who breaks the law; but there are many different kinds of criminals, just as there are many different kinds of crime—simple, complex, minor, major, nonviolent, violent, crimes against property, crimes against persons, victimless crimes.

From a psychiatric standpoint, criminal behavior can be placed in a context of the life-long struggle of every individual to adapt to his environment. Criminal behavior is one kind of effort to adapt, albeit an effort that is socially undesirable and unacceptable, or "maladaptive," as defined by society's rules. The criminal behavior may be the best attempt possible for the offender in his efforts to adapt, and it may reflect his inadequacy to achieve a successful adaptation in his world. It is also quite possible that the individual may not perceive his adjustment as unsuccessful. Yet, when it violates the rules established by society, codified either by courts of law or legislative bodies, it is clearly "criminal."

Crime and criminals have always been subjects of considerable fascination. At the same time, "law and order" issues in recent years have prompted great anxiety in the United States. There has been much public attention to crime and violence, and at least six recent national commissions have studied and reported on some or all aspects of the problem. There has been considerable publicity attending each announcement of the FBI detailing an increase in crime rates. For most of us, the statistics make us ever more fearful of our fellow man and prompt us to a continuing search for safety, a part of which is directed toward the causes and management of criminals.

We tend to think of crimes as being committed by others; but the subject of crime is fascinating, in part, because crime is a universal temptation. To a greater or lesser degree, we all have violated the law at some point in our lives, and the vast majority of people continue to do so. The point of differentiation is not so much the breaking of the law, but the judgment of when one can break the law and get away with it. It is knowing when one can speed without getting caught, or which tax deductions will get by, or what offense is too trivial to warrant attention.

To maintain one's self-esteem, there may be considerable resistance to looking at one's frailties and a wish to deny any wrongdoing. Indeed, part of the difficulty in addressing the causes and management of criminals is related to our inner feelings and guilt. We strive to overcome our potentiality for criminal behavior and deny the universal temptations to wrongdoing. We do this through internal psychological mechanisms reinforced by external social controls. The internal mechanisms are feelings of anxiety or guilt which seek to keep unacceptable impulses in check. The social reinforcement comes from formal rules of law, institutions of law enforcement and corrections, and religious institutions with their moral suasion.

Whence cometh our potentiality? One need look only at the behavior of the infant and small child. The infant has no commitment to rules or laws aside from a basic motivational force to find pleasure and relief of tension, and to strike back in response to being hurt or frustrated. Society has the challenge of teaching these self-centered, irresponsible creatures to tolerate frustration and respect the rights of others, in order to maintain an orderly society. As the individual matures, the social institutions of the family, school, church and law are all involved in the socialization process. All these institutions play a role in both the causes and management of criminals, for within every individual there remains a infantile "core," covered to varying degrees by a veneer of "civilization."

CAUSATION—THE DILEMMA OF UNDERSTANDING

There is often a good deal of resistance to rationally approaching the subject of criminality. Many people give lip service to wanting to understand criminals; but they do not really want to know, because reason limits their freedom to respond emotionally. It is much harder to be angry and retributive to someone who has done something "bad" when a rational formulation is presented to explain the "bad" action. The emotional preference is to be free to turn loose one's anger and vengeance when confronted with some senseless or brutal act against society. The intensity of this human response is repeatedly illustrated in real life and fiction, whether in the "one British soldier to be killed for every Catholic martyr" in Northern Ireland, or in the struggles in organized crime as exemplified in *The Godfather* (Puzo).

Understanding is a constraining force, and there is the wish not to be so constrained. Beyond this, there is often an implied equation, namely that understanding or explaining is tantamount to approving or condoning a crime. This false logic pervades the thinking of a good number of citizens who seem to say, "Don't confuse me with the facts; my mind's made up!" Yet unless we can understand more of the "why" behind human behavior, we cannot develop reasonable and effective plans to prompt change in individuals and to manage criminals.

"The great secret, the deeply buried mystery of the apparent public apathy to crime and to proposals for better controlling crime lies in the persistent, intrusive wish for vengeance." Thus does Dr. Karl Menninger identify the resistance to understanding in his *The Crime of Punishment*. Nearly every religion emphasizes the forgiveness of sins, and yet when put to the test of vengeance, society rarely seems to turn the other cheek. As he discusses further the concept of vengeance, Dr. Menninger observes:

> We are ashamed of it; we deny to ourselves and to others that we are influenced by it. Our morals, our religious teaching, even our laws repudiate it. But behind what we do to the offender is the desire for revenge on someone—and the unknown villain proved guilty of wrongdoing is a good scapegoat. We call it a wish to see justice done, i.e., to have him "punished." But in the last analysis, this turns out to be a thin cloak for vengeful feelings directed against a legitimized object.

So, today we have penitentiaries that have little or no similarity to the original institution of that name established by the Quakers in the early years of the Colonies as a place where offenders could be placed to meditate and gain penance for their wrongdoing.

CAUSATION—THE WISH FOR A SIMPLE EXPLANATION

The eternal wish in studying phenomena is for a simple, linear cause-effect explanation, which then makes it perfectly clear what has to be done to bring about change. This is certainly true in the search for the causes of crime.

As everyone knows, the problem of juvenile delinquency is too much permissiveness! The real answer to containing the high incidence of crime by young adults is discipline and firmness. Thus go the simple explanations for the cause of criminal behavior. However, no scientist has been able to draw such sweeping conclusions. Rather, the scientist refers to "multiple and interdeterminate variables" in causation. Interestingly enough, studies to compare such factors as strictness or permissiveness in relation to behavioral problems of youngsters discovered that the critical factor was neither one extreme nor the other. Rather the critical factor in parental management was consistency, so that the youngster could accurately anticipate the parental response and maintain a consistent behavior accordingly. The problem children were those whose parents were inconsistent; one time they might be permissive; the next, strict and rigid.

The unfortunate reality about human behavior is that it results from multiple causal factors, and solutions must generally take into consideration the multiple factors. The crime problem will not be solved by simply hiring more police, judges, lawyers, and correctional officers. Rather, as noted by the National Commission on the Causes and Prevention of Violence, the solution requires a reordering of our national priorities "to improve the conditions and opportunities of life for all citizens and thus sharply reduce the number who will commit violent acts" (Eisenhower et al., 1969).

Despite the awareness of multiple causal factors, investigators pursue the search to identify principal causes of crime, to simplify the complex.

In a recent overview of crime causation, sociologist Don Gibbons noted: "Although both genetic and situational factors are implicated in criminality, . . . the latter may well be more important and more frequently encountered than many criminologists have acknowledged to date." Predictably, the sociologists tend to emphasize the sociological factors, and the psychologists and psychiatrists emphasize individual factors.

Historically, biological or constitutional factors were sought to explain criminality. The constitutional theories of Cesare Lombroso (1876) contended that criminals had simply not advanced as far as normal men along the evolutionary scale. Ernest Hooton surveyed 11,000 prisoners in the 1930's and emphasized inherited biological inferiority; and William Sheldon studied body shapes before associating one type with delinquent boys. Heredity, mental deficiency, endocrine abnormalities, and neurological disorders have all been studied in relation to crime. A survey by the National Institute of Mental Health (Brown and Courtless, 1968) of mentally retarded prisoners found an unusually high incidence of the incarcerated mentally retarded were convicted of crimes of violence; yet the study could not causally link mental retardation and crime.

A biological characteristic more recently alleged to have some relationship to crime has been an abnormality in the sex chromosome in males, the XYY aberration. Yet the findings are still inconclusive, as summarized in a report of a conference also sponsored by the NIMH (Shah, 1970):

> Several XYY cases studied in institutions for criminal violators do demonstrate a variety of endocrinological, neurological, and other abnormalities which appear related to their deviant behavior. However, many XYY individuals display no such abnormalities. . . . The widespread publicity notwithstanding, individuals with the XYY anomaly have *not* been found to be more aggressive than matched offenders with normal chromosome constitutions. . . . It appears that premature and incautious speculations may have led to XYY persons being falsely stigmatized as unusually aggressive and violent compared to other offenders.

Presumably, physical factors and inherited biological traits exert a significant influence on human behavior patterns, but it is extremely difficult to distinguish which factors may be associated to a high degree as opposed to an actual causal linkage with criminal behavior.

In recent years, sociology has made a major commitment to the study of criminality. In general, the sociological approach searches for the social processes that tend to direct human behavior along certain patterns, as exemplified in the work of Wolfgang and Ferracuti, *The Subculture of Violence*. The tenet is that criminal or antisocial behavior is learned from the environment, and is not related to any innate antisocial forces within the individual. Other sociological studies have examined specific types of offenders, such as Sutherland's classical study of "White Collar Crime," or Einstadter's investigation of armed robbers. In the sociological assessment of significant social influences, surroundings and economic factors are relevant to the concept of "anomie." This concept is used to explain some of the criminal behavior in the poor; it refers to the sense of being deprived or "without" when others have material goods; thus an individual may feel deprived unfairly and justified in taking goods from others.

The psychiatric perspective reflects the focus of the psychiatrist on the individual; criminal behavior is related to predisposing and precipitating factors which affect the individual. The early environmental influences and developmental experiences of the child are critical, particularly as they affect how much the child learns to trust people and to establish meaningful relationships with other people. Adolescent stresses present the inevitable struggle to gain emancipation from a childhood identity and gain an independent adult identity. For some individuals, criminal behavior is the predictable result of a characterological development over many years. For others, criminal behavior is a reaction to some stress, and therefore symptomatic of a kind of "decompensation" from their usual functioning. In any case, the criminal activity represents an adaptational effort. Its resolution, as far as the individual is concerned, must depend upon an understanding of the adaptational process.

Insofar as some understanding of causal factors is important in determining the management of criminals, a balance is needed in understanding biological, sociological, and psychological factors. Social planning must take cognizance of social factors that contribute to crime; at the same time, individual offenders must be considered individually. One might compare this approach to the practice of public health and preventive medicine preserving the health of the public at large through sanitation, water purification, immunization, etc., while the individual practitioner of medicine deals with individual patients and their specific needs.

CAUSATION—MENTAL ILLNESS AND CRIME

Reference has been made to the psychiatric perspective of human behavior as a function of the personality-environmental struggle for adaptation. Criminal behavior is one kind of maladaptational effort; illness is another. And mental illness is a kind of maladjustment that may or may not be associated with criminal maladjustment.

Various statistical studies assess the relationship of mental illness and crime. The findings are sometimes confused by an inexactness in the psychiatric labels. While Healy and Bronner noted that 91 percent of the delinquents they examined had deep emotional problems, most investigators do not report that high a frequency and are more specific in their diagnoses. Guttmacher and Weihofen reported that 1.5 percent of the criminal population is psychotic, 2.4 percent mentally defective, 6.9 percent neurotic, and 11.2 percent psychopathic. A study of 10,000 men in

Sing Sing prison in New York State divided the population into 1 percent psychotic, 13 percent mentally defective, 20 percent psychoneurotic, 35 percent psychopathic, and 31 percent dyssocial criminals. A survey by this author of a federal reformatory population (age 18 to 26) found 2–3 percent psychotic, 3–4 percent mentally deficient, 3 percent psychoneurotic, and the remainder with personality disorders of various types. The highest incidence of any personality type was the passive-aggressive personality, followed by schizoid, infantile, emotionally unstable, and sociopathic types.

Actually, relatively few criminals are psychotic, although there are a good many of individuals who might be characterized as having a "borderline" condition. The statistical studies do not find any higher incidence of mental illness as now defined in the criminal population than in the general population, with the exception of the so-called character disorders, especially the antisocial personality. Further, with rare exceptions, neither statistical surveys nor individual case studies suggest any causal relationship between mental illness and crime.

In a discussion of the relationship of mental illness and violence, the Professional Advisory Council of the National Association for Mental Health prepared a statement which emphasized:

(1) The popular idea that the mentally ill are over-represented in the population of violent criminals is not supported by research evidence.
(2) Generally, persons identified as mentally ill represent no greater risk of committing violent crimes than the population as a whole.

There is a further fallacy in considering criminals "sick," beyond the reality that their behavior and condition in most cases does not fit the psychiatrist's diagnostic categories of "illness." Many offenders actively reject the idea of being "ill," especially mentally ill, as they see illness as an alien concept. They prefer to be "bad" and have a negative identity, rather than be "sick" with an identity of not being mentally in control of oneself. To maintain a self-concept of integrity, they will actively resist efforts to be treated as "ill." Similarly, most psychiatrists and mental hospitals are not prepared to treat individuals who cannot accept an "illness" identity and who do not want to be treated.

MANAGEMENT—THE ATROCIOUS NONSYSTEM OF CORRECTIONS

Various study commissions have repeatedly emphasized the problems of managing criminals in a system of justice that is really not a system, with a corrections component that is similarly inadequate to the task. As expressed in the Task Force Report on Corrections for the National Commission on Law Enforcement and the Administration of Justice (Katzen-bach, 1967):

> The American correctional system is an extremely diverse amalgam of facilities, theories, techniques, and programs. It handles nearly 1.3 million offenders on an average day; it has 2.5 million admissions in the course of a year; and its annual operating budget is over a billion dollars. . . . Most [jurisdic-tions] lack capacity to cope with the problems of preventing recidivism. . . . Some fail even to meet standards of humane treatment recognized for decades.

Or, as stated by the Joint Commission on Correctional Manpower and Training (Bennett et al.):

> Correction today is characterized by an overlapping of jurisdictions, a diversity of philosophies, and hodgepodge of organizational structures which have little contact with one another. It has grown piecemeal—sometimes out of expedience, sometimes of necessity. Seldom has growth been based on systematic planning. Lacking consistent guidelines and the means to test program effectiveness, legisla-tors continue to pass laws, executives mandate policies, and both cause large sums of money to be spent on ineffectual correctional methods.

> The public and their legislators must understand that there can be no solution to the problem of recidivism as long as harsh laws, huge isolated prisons, token program resources, and discriminatory practices which deprive offenders of employment, education, and other opportunities are tolerated. They must also expect that as long as there is a predominance of low-paid, dead-end jobs in corrections, the field will continue to be burdened with a poor per-formance record.

Finally, a most thorough indictment is leveled by a Violence Commis-sion Task Force (Mulvihill et al.), which concluded:

> Existing features of the correctional response to crime in the United States reveal a condition that undeniably needs serious revision and improvement if an effective rehabilitation of offenders is to be achieved. In all major features of the system, there are drastic shortages of material and human resources. Public attitudes are hostile, and public support of needed innovations is absent or ineffective. Lopsided imbalances in the allocation of resources to institutions versus community-based programs seem to persist without much change. Efforts at individuation of treatment are hampered by lack of understanding, sympathy, and attentiveness to the present outcomes.

> The failures of the present system, however visible and chronic, seem to be preferred by both the lay public and its elected officials to the costs of change. Those who violate criminal codes are, on balance, treated as undesirable discards who "deserve" whatever fate they incur, and whose rehabilitation is a matter of little consequence. At the same time, persistently high rates of crime and recidivism are deplored, while little thought is given to the probable intimate relation between inadequate correctional response and offender repetition.

Some of the problems in the management of offenders are highlighted by comparing the management of criminal maladjustment with an illness maladjustment. In the processing of the criminal through the judicial sys-tem, the case finder (law enforcement), diagnostician (court), treater (correctional institution), and the renderer of after-care service (proba-tion) all function separately, with little interagency communication or co-operation. The judge, for instance, passes sentence (prescribes treatment) with little or no knowledge of the institution to which he is referring the offender for correction. The contrast of the above with the referral and treatment process for an ill individual should be obvious.

MANAGEMENT—PRINCIPLES OF CORRECTIONAL MANAGEMENT

In the course of our history, various themes have dominated correctional philosophy. In the order of their emergence, correctional goals have been identified as retribution, deterrence, and rehabilitation. As exemplified in the attitudes today, these same themes might be referred to as punishment, custody, and treatment. Roughly speaking, punishment and retribution were the main correctional themes in the eighteenth and nineteenth centuries; deterrence and custody in the first half of the twentieth; and rehabilitation and treatment in the last three decades.

While there have been various rationalizations to justify each of the management goals, questions persist. To what extent is retribution justifiable? Does hate cure? How much is the "punishment" dictated by our emotional need for vengeance rather than by any rational program for correction? Thus, capital punishment remains controversial, and clearly, pressure for long sentences stems as much from a reaction on the part of the public to certain heinous offenses as to any rational expectation that the offender will be changed by the length of time he is incarcerated. There is no evidence that hate in human relations does anything other than to provoke a counterresponse of bitterness and hate.

The concept of deterrence has likewise been the subject of considerable debate, whether one considers the special deterrence to the individual who has already been convicted and sentenced and who is subject to further punishment, or the general deterrence to prevent the public at large, including the criminals in it, from committing criminal acts. In a careful and detailed review of the concepts of deterrence, Franklin Zimring concludes that it is extremely difficult to generalize the effects of deterrence. There is rather an overwhelming specificity of findings from the research on the subject. He observes that, "A particular legal threat involves a mix of factors—communication, enforcement, type and extent of threatened consequences, type of behavior, social attitudes—and the mix will be different for different threats."

In its survey of the effect of longer sentences on recidivism, the Task Force on Crimes of Violence of the Violence Commission found little evidence that longer sentences are more deterrent. William J. Chambliss reviewed some empirical data on the types of deviance and the effectiveness of legal sanctions and found evidence that some punishments clearly do not deter crime. The determining factors as identified by Chambliss are the commitment of the person to a criminal way of life, and the meaning of the criminal act to the person who commits it. An individual with a high degree of commitment to the criminal life and who is least concerned about the criminal act is least likely to be deterred—a drug addict, for example. An individual with a low commitment to criminal life and whose criminal act is for material gain is most likely to be deterred—the shoplifting housewife, the parking violator. The emotional impulsivity involved in the commission of the crime represents another element which complicates the assessment of the deterrent effect.

Custody and preventive detention represent one specific kind of deterrence, for a person in custody cannot at the same time commit another offense except within the confines of an institution. The Crime Commission concluded that preventive detention is the major activity of corrections, because there is little positive treatment in most institutions, especially in jails, and there is much less individual treatment of particular offenders. The whole concept of preventive detention bridges constitutional issues and prompts considerable reaction from civil libertarians. It has also been the subject of intense discussion in the area of involuntary commitment of mentally ill patients. Yet, the continuing concern for what is to be done with "dangerous" persons puts psychiatrists on the spot, since they are supposed to be able to make some kind of reasonable prediction of dangerousness—even though this is rarely possible.

The goal of treatment and rehabilitation is no less subject to controversy, since there is limited evidence that current techniques are effective. And there is no agreement as to what is treatment. The concept of treatment in a correctional institution is far broader than in other traditionally therapeutic settings, and all too often, philosophies of treatment are equated by old-line prison personnel with "molly coddling" and permissiveness, as if to polarize the issue and contrast punishment and discipline with treatment and permissiveness.

Yet the persisting challenge, sounded over and over again in studies of the correctional system, is to individualize the correctional response, insofar as possible. This can be effectively implemented only if there is a commitment to studying each offender in a total sense, and developing a treatment program that will best meet his or her needs and prompt a change in that individual's life syle from criminal adaptational efforts to efforts more socially acceptable.

MANAGEMENT—EFFECTS OF INSTITUTIONALIZATION

What are we "teaching" in prisons? Three prominent elements are actually antitherapeutic—dependency, violence, and dehumanization. Individuals are placed in an institution which is structured so as to remove from them any need to make independent decisions. Regimentation is a major means of management, and the inmate is completely dependent upon the institutional policies and programs as implemented by the correctional officers. It is not surprising that the rate of recidivism is so high when so many offenders are released from prisons without effective preparation for returning to independent functioning. It is quite a transition to go from a situation where room and board and all expenses are paid and where work and leisure time are programmed, to the "streets" where the situation is just the reverse. Indeed, a study of Indiana State Reformatory inmates found that the longer the armed robber spends in prison, the higher is postrelease recidivism for any kind of crime.

The problem of dependency has prompted a host of developments in recent years with halfway house and transitional programs for offenders to be managed in the community. When the Federal Bureau of Prisons first gained legislative permission for such a program with "work-release" provisions, only the inmates who were the best risks were selected to participate. As the programs have become more established, more and more offenders have been referred to the centers as a stepping stone toward independent functioning. These community-based correctional programs are filling a vital need for a total treatment program for offenders.

Violence is a second antitherapeutic influence in prison. John Conrad wrote, "Violence is the lingua franca of the prison. Its disciplined use is the basis of order. The officer in the tower and his colleague on the gun walk in the cell block exemplify the use of violence to gain objectives as surely as the robber with his pistol. Violence is the language which everyone in the prison speaks; for some it is the only means of reliable communication." These observations are particularly true in institutions that are either understaffed, so that the inmates serve as the controlling force within the walls, or in institutions where the correctional personnel are so inadequately paid and trained that they must rely on brute force instead of knowledge of modern techniques for inmate management. These are the lessons in human relations and how to get along with one's fellow man in most penal institutions.

Dehumanization is a special kind of violence, aptly described by Paul Keve, who wrote to the Violence Commission:

> It is my feeling that correctional institutions generally have contributed to violence in exactly the same way that ghettos have made their contribution: through all the demeaning characteristics of the ghetto or the institution. The correctional institution takes people who are particularly in need of a sense of self-pride, self-respect, and self-identity and, instead of providing opportunity for growth of these personal characteristics, it regiments, represses, and demeans the individual in countless ways.

Thus, an individual becomes a number, wears uniform clothes, may correspond with only a specified list of friends, may receive only one package at Christmas, may receive a hometown paper only if so permitted, etc., depending upon the various institutional regulations wherever he may be situated. One may quite reasonably ask, "How we can expect to develop in any offender a new sense of respectability by placing him in such a dehumanizing setting?"

MANAGEMENT—THE INCORRIGIBLE FEW

The Violence Commission found that offenders arrested for major crimes of violence or burglary generally have long criminal histories, and their careers are predominantly filled with offenses other than the most serious of violent acts. Further, they found that a relatively small core of offenders is responsible for a high proportion of all offenses, particularly serious acts of violence.

A University of Pennsylvania study of Philadelphia males—9,945 boys born in 1945 who lived in Philadelphia at least from ages 10 to 17—found that approximately one-third were contacted by the police for delinquent acts over that time span. Of the 3,475 boys contacted for delinquent acts, 55 percent were one-time offenders, but they accounted for only 16 percent of all the delinquent acts. In contrast, 6 percent of the group were "hard-core" recidivists, accounting for 52 percent of all the delinquencies, 53 percent of all assaults, 71 percent of all robberies, and 62 percent of all property crimes (Mulvihill et al., 1969).

Thus it is that an inordinate amount of energy, time, and money must be committed to the task of dealing with a small percentage of individuals in the correctional process. The strategy for management must have two directions. A first-priority resource allocation should be given to preventing the first offender from recidivism, with emphasis on community programs. Remaining correctional resources need to be concentrated on the hard-core repeaters. This group will require a mix of institutional programs with community treatment where appropriate. And some may require confinement in a controlled environment for a lifetime.

MANAGEMENT—OUTSIDE THE WALLS— THE ROLE OF THE COMMUNITY

The theme of the 99th Congress of Corrections was, "The Wall, built to keep people in. It has served just as often to keep people out. But crime will not be effectively controlled until the public becomes knowledgeable and concerned about corrections; not until our many walls are breached and the public becomes a part of correctional programming." The thrust of public concern has been increasingly focused on corrections in recent years, in part the result of violence both inside and outside of prisons. A high point was achieved with President Nixon's calling the National Conference on Corrections in December, 1971, attended by a wide range of correctional administrators, law enforcement personnel, interested pro-

fessionals, and concerned citizens. Penal reform has also been the theme
of such organizations as the League of Women Voters, Mental Health Associations, the Junior Chamber of Commerce, and others.

A movement of increasing strength in recent years has been the volun-
teer court movement. Originating in situations like the municipal court of
Royal Oak, Michigan, programs like Volunteers in Probation, Inc., have
been developed to involve citizen volunteers in probation programs, working with all kinds of offenders (Morris, 1970). The first national conference of volunteers in courts held in Detroit, Michigan, in 1970 attracted
some 500 people from across the country. A second conference in Mem-
phis, Tennessee, in 1972 was attended by more than 1,000 formal dele-
gates and 200 observers.

A firm conclusion of the Violence Commission was that communities
and justice systems must plan and act together. A Violence Commission
Task Force Report, *Law and Order Reconsidered* (Campbell et al.), put it
this way:

> Constructive citizen action on the local level can be a powerful force for
> criminal justice reform. There are simply too many important aspects of the
> private citizen's duty to expect local government to solve the crime problem
> all by itself.
>
> The private role begins with each citizen responding individually when called:
> reporting crime, appearing as a witness, serving as a juror, hiring the
> exoffender. . . .
>
> Beyond individual action, the private role requires group participation. By
> and large, citizens fearful of crime are uninformed about the problems of
> criminal justice administration. They are too often unread in the literature
> of crime commissions, uninvolved in efforts to improve the system, and over-
> loaded with myths and scapegoats. All too many citizens continue to advocate
> simple solutions to complex crime problems. Those who dig deeply almost
> always change their minds.

MANAGEMENT—THE ROLE OF SCIENCE

From the perspective of physician, psychiatrist, scientist, one of the
major developments of the future of corrections must be the degree to
which science really has an opportunity to get involved and does so in
the management of criminals. One aspect of the involvement is utilizing
the scientific method to separate the emotional aspects of the problem.
It is clear that for the most part in our society, emotions are a key force
in determining the course of corrections. The task of the scientific commitment will also be a more effective evaluation of the individuals who manifest the criminal "maladjustment." We ought to be able to better identify,
classify, and diagnose these individuals; to predict those in whom we can
anticipate change and those who are more resistant to change. We must
improve our capacity and techniques to bring about change.

No one profession may be expected to have all the answers in achieving new developments in the management of criminals. Rather, the answers will come through a team approach, with a sharing of knowledge and perspectives by several disciplines. All too often, psychiatry is looked to for the answers, but it may be that the role of psychiatry will be as much to identify the critical questions which must be the subject of joint research and practice. In corrections, the major commitment must be to bringing about change—and in the management of criminals, it means that the line personnel who work most with the offenders will need to be trained to be agents for change.

The Violence Commission Task Force delineated a host of guidelines for actions and research, in a framework that is based on the concept that justice insures safety. Thus, an effective approach goes far beyond "control" measures to address some of the basic injustices of our society. As part of that, the restructuring of the correctional response is not just a function of humane considerations; but rather, "the best research suggests that the factors which produce recidivism are similar to those that induce new criminal activity by undetected and unpublished populations" (Mulvihill et al.).

Certainly the average citizen seems to prefer some loss in justice to criminals for the possible improvement in his own safety. Most view the need for safety as a first-priority issue. But it is also clear that this narrow perspective may prompt actions that provide safety in the short-range, but that are counterproductive in the long run. Thus, a wholesale practice of preventive detention can so embitter innocent individuals that they later increase the danger to the public at large. It is imperative for leaders in the community to take into account both the longer reaches of time and the broader ranges of the population in formulating policy decisions.

At the same time, what is the role of psychiatry? It is no better expressed than by Halleck who sums it up with these thoughts:

> Because our society cannot afford to redefine crime as illness, criminology will not and should not become a subspeciality of psychiatry. Still, the suffering of the criminal and the havoc he creates throughout the community will often call for the services of the psychiatric profession. Psychiatric resources thus far have been spent in the wrong directions. Efforts to redefine criminals as patients are socially damaging and wasteful. The usefulness of the psychiatric criminologist will ultimately depend upon his ability to find a rational means of integrating his individual-oriented philosophies and practices into a correctional system that is rarely sympathetic to individual needs. He must begin by helping his community to understand the unreasonable aspect of deviant behavior, and by demonstrating that techniques which help the mentally ill may also help the criminal. . . .

> The usefulness of any helping profession is severely impaired if the community is uninterested in humane and rational treatment of offenders. Unfortunately, . . . when crime has become one of America's major problems, our society seems to show little enthusiasm for rehabilitating criminals. New government programs in crime prevention and detection have created interest in the total problem of crime, but this interest seems to terminate abruptly once

the offender is apprehended. The apprehended offender is still exposed to a system of correctional justice that is inconsistent, cruel and irrational. Society errs when it attempts to fight crime while failing to treat the criminal.

REFERENCES

Bennett, J. V., and M. Rector, et al. 1969. A Time to Act. Final Report of the Joint Commission on Correctional Manpower and Training. Lebanon, Pa., Sowers Printing.

Briley, J. M., et al. 1970. The Criminal Offender—What Should Be Done? The Report of the President's Task Force on Prisoner Rehabilitation. Washington, D.C., U.S. Government Printing Office.

Brown, B. S., and T. F. Courtless. 1968. The mentally retarded in penal and correctional institutions. Discussion by W. W. Menninger. *Amer. J. Psych.* **124:**1164–1170.

Campbell, J., J. R. Sahid, and D. P. Stang. 1969. Law and Order Reconsidered. A Staff Report to the National Commission on the Causes and Prevention of Violence. Vol. 10. Washington, D.C.

Chambliss, W. J. 1967. Types of deviance and the effectiveness of legal sanctions. *Wisconsin Law Review*, 686–719.

Conrad, J. P. 1966. Violence in prison. *Ann. Amer. Acad. Pol. Soc. Sci.* **364:**113–119.

Eisenhower, et al. 1969. To Establish Justice, To Insure Domestic Tranquility. Final Report of the National Commission on the Causes and Prevention of Violence. Washington, D.C., U.S. Government Printing Office.

Gibbons, D. C. 1971. Observations on the study of crime causation. *Amer. J. Soc.* **77:**262–278.

Halleck, S. L. 1967. Psychiatry and the Dilemmas of Crime. A Study of Causes, Punishment, and Treatment. New York, Harper and Row.

Jeffery, C. R. 1967. Criminal Responsibility and Mental Disease. Springfield, Ill. Charles C Thomas.

Katzenbach, N., et al. 1967. Task Force Report: Corrections. Washington, D.C., U.S. Government Printing Office.

Katzenbach, N., et al. 1967. The Challenge of Crime in a Free Society. Report by the President's Commission on Law Enforcement and the Administration of Justice. Washington, D.C., U.S. Government Printing Office.

Kerner, O., et al. 1968. Report of the National Advisory Commission on Civil Disorders. Washington, D.C., U.S. Government Printing Office.

Menninger, K. A. 1968. The Crime of Punishment. New York, Viking Press.

Miller, H.J., et al. 1966. Report of the President's Commission on Crime in the District of Columbia. Washington, D.C., U.S. Government Printing Office.

Morris, J. A. 1970. First Offender. New York, Funk & Wagnalls.

Mulvihill, D. J. and M. M. Tumin, and L. A. Curtis. 1969. Crimes of Violence. A Staff Report to the National Commission on the Causes and Prevention of Violence. Vols. 11–13. Washington, D.C., U.S. Government Printing Office.

Puzo, M. 1969. The Godfather. New York, G. B. Putnam's Sons.

Shah, S., ed. 1970. Report on the XYY Chromosomal Abnormality. National Institutes of Mental Health, PHS Publication No. 2103. Washington, D.C., U.S. Government Printing Office.

Wolfgang, M. E., and F. Ferracuti. 1967. The Subculture of Violence. London, Tavistock Publications Ltd.

Zimring, F. E. 1971. Perspectives on Deterrence. NIMH Crime and Delinquency Series Monograph, PHS Publication No. 2056. Washington, D.C., U.S. Government Printing Office.

CHAPTER 21

THE CRIMINAL JUSTICE SYSTEM: CRIMES, CRIMINAL PROCESSES, AND SENTENCING

JOHN M. DARRAH

In the monumental study *The Challenge of Crime in a Free Society*, published in 1967 by the President's Commission on Law Enforcement and Administration of Justice, it was noted that a large volume of crime is not reported to or detected by the police. Much detected crime is not solved, and much that is solved does not lead to prosecution or, if prosecuted, does not end with a conviction. If this is true, our criminal justice system may be irrelevant or ineffective with respect to the overall crime picture. The study also showed that by the time nine out of ten have reached adulthood, American males have engaged in conduct which, if successfully prosecuted in adult court, would brand them as felons. Would it be fair then to say that 90 percent of all males are criminals? If one rejects this characterization, it must at least be admitted that "criminal" is a very selective or equivocal label.

Perhaps more disturbing to us is the ineffectiveness of the "corrections system." With varying degrees of precision (and honesty), information is being amassed to indicate not only that prisons have no benefit for the prisoners inside, but also that they have a strong negative effect. The men who are locked up to be "corrected" are returned to society several years later more bitter, no better able to exercise responsible choices, and wiser in the ways of criminal techniques.

Without surveying the full range of details and procedures in the criminal justice system, let us examine some of the more critical questions related to the treatment of people: What conduct is prohibited and penalized? Are the procedures by which violators are identified relevant and fair? Is the treatment or punishment applied to such violators appropriate?

WHAT IS CRIMINAL CONDUCT?

General agreement exists in the United States, as in virtually all civilizations, that certain forms of aggressive, acquisitive, or dishonest behavior are unacceptable and therefore prohibited. Included are murder, assault, arson, larceny, and the like. Essentially, unacceptable conduct is that which substantially interferes with the person or property of another. In addition, we have inherited from puritan England a tradition of having the criminal system deal with acts that are mainly of moral significance. Such acts have included at various times in our history all manner of sexual relations outside marriage (and some within), sex for hire, homosexual relations, sex for reading or viewing, gambling, abortion, alcoholic beverage usage, tobacco usage, and marijuana usage. Many prohibitions continue to the present time. Also, as our society has changed from rural to urban, legislative bodies at all levels have proscribed various acts on the basis of health, safety, or welfare, all of which are crimes to be dealt with by courts.

While all proscribed conduct is labeled "criminal," the moral crimes and the health, safety, and welfare crimes are dealt with half-heartedly by the law.[1] Both categories of crimes clog the criminal process, making difficult its timely attention to serious matters. Laws relating to gambling, prostitution, alcohol, and drug use have been unevenly enforced, which has caused periodic corruption of the police and the political process in virtually every section of the country. Also, the disrespect with which law enforcement is consequently viewed by lower economic groups hurts the effectiveness of the justice that the courts mete out.

THE PROCESS OF LABELING A CRIMINAL

Societies have produced two basic approaches to the identification of persons as criminal violators. One is our own, the adversary system, inherited, again, from England, in which the court and jury are impartial arbiters of a struggle between the prosecution (including the police) and the defense. The alternative, most developed in continental Europe, is the inquisitorial system. Here the court conducts an inquiry, gathering evidence against the defendant without the impartiality of the adversary system.

Within the adversary system the courts apply constitutional limitations upon the investigative techniques of the police and the conduct of the trial. The interpretations vary considerably with changes in court personnel and with the shifting attitudes and expectations of the public. Nonetheless, the basic approach has continued with little change.

---

[1] See Herbert Packer, *The Limits of the Criminal Sanction,* Stanford, Stanford Univ. Press, 1968. This scholarly examination concludes that the criminal law cannot effectively deal with behavior which is not regarded by virtually the entire public as unacceptable.

One of the system's more important aspects is the way it deals with mental illness. The threshold issue for the court is whether a person is mentally competent to stand trial. The test is usually whether he is able to understand the charge against him and able to assist his attorney in the preparation of his case. Before the advent of drug therapy, the practice of sending incompetent defendants to hospitals for long stays was dismal, indeed. The right to speedy trial might be ignored completely and many years elapse before the defendent was confronted by his accusers.[2] Drug treatment, by controlling hallucinatory or psychotic symptoms, has greatly reduced the need for commitment before trial. Still, one study (Rosenberg and McGarry) conducted jointly by members of psychiatric and legal professions found a surprising lack of understanding of the issues by the defense lawyers, the examining psychiatrist, and the committing judge. The consequences, of course, are tragic for the defendant.

More difficult is the issue of whether, and at what level, mental irresponsibility should excuse otherwise criminal conduct. Existing law requires that a person be proven sane before he can be held criminally responsible for his acts. It therefore sets standard tests ("irresistible impulse," "inability to know right from wrong," "mental disease rendering the defendant unable to conform his conduct to the norm," or some other) for the jurors to apply after hearing the testimony. Psychiatrists tend to chafe at the role thrust upon them by the law as witnesses on the sanity issue and tend to question the relevance of these tests to the problems that humans struggle with.[3] On the other hand, because of our vengeful and inappropriate corrections system (which is discussed further below), defendants and their lawyers cling to these traditional tests, searching for a defense and seeking ever to broaden the scope of tests. Tremendous amounts of time, energy, and money are expended on the sanity case and appeals. While there is as yet no consensus to this effect, good arguments have been advanced for the elimination of insanity as a defense. The trial of any person, insane or otherwise, would then determine whether the defendant committed the act other than by accident. If he did, it would be the court's task to decide what should be done with him.

The determination of who has violated the law may be looked upon as a labeling process. Most of the protections built into the system by the constitution and laws may be bypassed by the defendant if he wishes to admit guilt. He may plead guilty and short circuit the lengthy pretrial and trial procedures, thus labeling himself a criminal. Thus, the felony label can, by statute, prevent a person from entering a particular profession,

[2] Thomas Szasz, *Psychiatric Justice.* New York, MacMillan, 1965. Dr. Szasz documents the inappropriate use of the law to hold people without trial on the assertion that they are incompetent to stand trial.

[3] Karl A. Menninger, *The Crime of Punishment.* New York, Viking Press, 1968, p. 112 *et seq.*

business, or trade. For example, in Washington State, an ex-felon cannot be a barber because, presumably, he might let his razor slip. Businesses may have a policy of not hiring ex-felons, and most citizens, particularly those who make hiring decisions, have little or no acquaintance with the labeling system or the people who pass through it. Consequently, a person labeled a criminal carries that label through life, often with disastrous results for his employment opportunities. These results are unjustified and counterproductive in terms of any rehabilitation goals. Because of this, judges, at the behest of defense lawyers and with the acquiescence of the prosecutors, have devised ways of avoiding the label. One method is to defer or put off sentencing. After guilt is admitted, the court defers sentencing for a specified time and places the defendant under probation supervision. When the period of time is over and the defendant has not misbehaved, the judge brings him back to court, permits him to withdraw the plea of guilty, and then dismisses the charge. If he has misbehaved, the judge may impose a prison sentence or any other appropriate punishment.

Variations on this theme exist throughout the country, but one of the most extreme is found in New York. Here, a project of the Vera Foundation of Justice plucks defendants out of the criminal process (with the prosecutor's agreement), works with them closely on personal and employment problems, and stays with them until their living patterns have stabilized at a healthy level. The program's success rate is outstanding by any measure. The importance of this example is not simply in its success, as virtually any traditional probation procedure could accomplish the same short-run goals with an infusion of money and fresh manpower. Rather, it is in the recognition that the justice system may be so ponderous and inappropriate to people problems that public officials are willing to circumvent it almost entirely in order to achieve the desired results. It is significant that one of the desired results is the avoidance of the label of conviction.

Should we move toward a system where no labeling goes on? For those who contest their guilt and wish to avoid being labeled a criminal, the labeling process cannot be abandoned. It is the protection for every accused against arbitrary action by the state.

More important, however, is changing the laws and practices which made the label significant for anyone other than the sentencing judge. Laws barring offenders from jobs or careers should be eliminated, and questioning about arrests or convictions should be forbidden for persons or businesses hiring for routine or nonsensitive work. Questioning should be permitted only in certain specified occupations. For instance, day care centers should screen out child molesters and banks should screen out larceny offenders. The label, however, should be only a red flag leading to further inquiry and not an immediate end to the job application.

SENTENCING THE CRIMINAL

Once a person has been established as a law violator, it must be determined what should be done with him, how he is to be sentenced. The several states vary widely in their legislative prescriptions for sentencing dispositions. Statutes generally set outside maximums for incarceration. However, the maximums possible in most states are far in excess of any reasonable justification, e.g., 20 years imprisonment for the forgery of a $10 check. Crimes of violence, including murder, should receive a maximum prison term of 15 years.[4] This would permit long-term psychiatric or other treatment for the more difficult cases. For larcencies and other nonviolent behavior, two years at most should be available to a judge, but only as a backup for other programs. For example, a young, unskilled offender might be deprived of his liberty long enough to cover schooling or training which would enable him to obtain a good job upon release.

In no event should mandatory penalties or minimum sentences be prescribed by the law. The judicial selection process must be sharpened to get the very best people into this sensitive position. Once this is done, the fashioning of a program for the offender's future must be done individually in each case by judges and not by legislative fiat.

Even if the statute sets appropriate maximum sentences and no minimums, it must still be asked how much of the decision in each case should be with the judge and how much with the parole board or other agencies. Should the judge control only the terms and duration of the probationary or other nonprison disposition and not those of a prison sentence? Many feel that sentencing should be taken out of the hands of judges and given to a panel of specialists in fields such as corrections, social work, criminology, or psychology. Laws currently providing for sentencing require the judge to prescribe a maximum term and only recommend a minimum term. The actual time served is determined by the parole board, commonly made up of persons with social work or police backgrounds. Various possibilities exist for a probation violation. The defendant might be handled in one state by a judge and in another by the Board of Probation and Parole. For a crime committed in prison, the punishment decision might be made by a judge, jury, parole board, or the prison warden. Suffice it to say that no agreement exists on an optimal system.

The setting of standards for sentencing or other decision making on incarceration or prison discipline is of great importance in making the criminal system operate properly. Standards cannot be tailored for mechanical application; they should be based on a philosophy of corrections

---

[4] The Model Penal Code, proposed by the prestigious American Law Institute, and adopted now in half a dozen states, adopts a classification of crimes along this approach.

and indicate factors which may be considered by the decision maker. Such a statement of philosophy might be as follows:

> Jailing or imprisonment has been found to be ineffective in influencing the behavior or attitudes of prisoners in positive or healthy ways. Incarceration is not acceptable as a disposition except in the case of a person who has shown himself to be a danger to other persons or has repeatedly engaged in the theft or destruction of property of substantial value, and is unlikely to respond to supervision or resources available.

The implementation of such a philosophy depends in part upon the behavior of the defendant who has admitted his guilt or been proven guilty. Far more, however, it depends on the more subjective judgment as to how responsive he will be to available help. There appears to be no way to lessen the subjective factor, but at least certain guidelines can be provided. Thus, in deciding the defendant's potential for growth or change, the court might be directed to consider such factors as emotional maturity, mental illness, use of drugs and alcohol, and particularly the extent to which he has responded to appropriate help in the past. The court should be directed to consider every reasonable alternative to prison and consider appropriate resources in other localities if they are not available within its own jurisdiction.

Perhaps the most difficult problem society faces is the substance of the "correction" or "rehabilitation" to be imposed by sentence. The lawyer commenting on the process of the system walks on thin ice when he gives his opinion on the type of treatment needed. In recent years, however, judges have begun to demand from defense lawyers an advocate position on what the sentence should be. As light has been shed on the failure of the prison experience, the defense lawyer has begun to search diligently for community resources which he can recommend as the basis for proba-tion. Such resources include psychiatric and drug counseling, half-way houses, education or training programs, and employment situations. The hope is that some combination of these resources might provide the serious offender with the basis for changing his life style or coping with his emo-tional problems in order to avoid a repetition of the offending behavior.

Defense lawyers tend to be skeptical about the value of psychiatric counseling for most offenders. Generally, the defendant has no background for respecting the "head shrinker" or his art, and he tends to lack motiva-ion over any extended period of time to confront his emotional problems. Society simply does not prepare the American male to look to this source for help. On the other hand, most offenders have a very low opinion of themselves, are lacking in self-confidence, and could profit by the self-awareness and self-acceptance a psychiatrist would seek to bring out. Looking at the broad picture one doubts that either the psychiatric man-power or the public purse would permit any significant amount of services in this area. More plausible is the provision of therapy groups under the leadership of trained social workers or others.

CONCLUSIONS

The result of studies of the effectiveness of even the best programs of rehabilitation either within or outside the prison leads to pessimism that the answer lies in "corrections." Perhaps the reformer must be satisfied with a prevention approach rather than a cure. Once an individual has developed a strong antisocial pattern in his life or a deep-seated emotional illness, the prognosis for change is poor. The obvious long-range approach is the development of institutions, services, traditions, and the like which tend to support the family and help provide the young growing child with love and care.

The criminal justice system, like any other institution or process, is a reflection, however imperfect, of the needs of the society creating it. It is perhaps fanciful to expect truly fundamental changes in the attitudes and habits of residents of our complex culture such as to cause a withering away of the criminal process or a change to a no-fault or similar plan. On the other hand, there is a very real possibility that social systems will stabilize. While the corrections system has little prospect of correcting, preventive measures such as qaulity day-care centers for children of working mothers and more responsive educational programs can help to reduce the human deficits that underly criminal behavior. With crime reduced in such ways and, with it, the fear of crime, prisons could well become museums for future generations to behold with wonder.

REFERENCES

Skolnick, J. 1966. Justice Without Trial. New York, Wiley Press.

Morris, N., and G. Hawkins. 1970. The Honest Politician's Guide to Crime Control. Chicago, Univ. of Chicago Press.

Rosenberg, A. H., and L. McGarry. 1972. Competency for trial; the making of an expert. *Amer. J. Psychiat.* **128:**9.

CHAPTER 22

SOME MAJOR GUIDES FOR LAWS

LUVERN V. RIEKE

THE RECOGNITION OF A PROBLEM

In 1971 the U.S. Senate resolved that a National Advisory Commission on Health Science and Society should undertake a "comprehensive investigation and study of the ethical, social, and legal implications of advances in biomedical research and technology. . . ." The commission was specifically directed to include in its study an "analysis and evaluation of laws, codes, and principles governing the use of technology in medical practice. . . ."[1]

The Senate resolution reflects a serious concern. The survival of human beings, it seems, has always been conditioned on continuing adjustments needed to restore the balance between man and his environment and between human societies and the individuals who make up those societies. Essentially "natural" controls—evolution and the market place, for example—have until now made these adjustments. Only in our day has man claimed the prerogative and asserted the capacity to determine his own affairs. Medical science, in particular, has upset the "natural" balances and we all sense that we are now deeply involved in activities that have far-reaching, probably irreversible, consequences.

While man has demonstrated his scientific power to alter the course of nature, he has not yet shown that he possesses the capacity to govern the forces he has unleashed. It is therefore urgent that we ask how we are to manage the amenities, the quality, and the continuance of life.

Presumably it was considerations such as these that prompted the Senate to adopt the resolution quoted above. When the Senate spoke of "laws and codes" it undoubtedly had in mind a set of rules. Many scholars think of law as being essentially a body of rules; others insist that law

---

[1] Senate Joint Resolution 75, 92nd Congress, 1st Session, 1971. The adoption of this Resolution did not signal swift action on the part of Congress. From the Senate, the proposal went to the House Committee on Internal and Foreign Commerce. A half year has passed since the Senate action, but the House, so far, has done nothing with the proposal.

is a process in which specific rules are made, used, amended, and finally replaced by other rules. No one would deny that the rules are an indispensable part of law and that law is the expression of man's attempts to govern his own affairs. How a rule is formulated, who decides to adopt it, and upon what basis the decision is made, are critical inquiries. A more precise question, and one that is the threshold for the subject discussed in this chapter, is: What are the major guides that influence the articulation of the rules (laws) concerning health care? Are the rules really the announcement of what we have discovered by scientific investigation or are they the product of political activity? Or put yet another way: Do these rules control us or do we control them?

For reasons that will be examined in detail, rules used in the legal system are normally tentative and often are essentially value statements. These characteristics distinguish rules of law from scientific pronouncements which are usually deemed to be demonstrably accurate and relatively value free. The necessity, in law, to decide issues without having scientifically conclusive proof accounts for the cautious, conservative attitude of most lawyers. On the other hand, the assumed certainty and value-free quality of scientific fact encourages the scientist to plunge boldly ahead without extensive pondering about the social impact of his work. The unspoken premise had been that scientific knowledge cannot harm anyone—it must in fact be good—and that the use of such knowledge remains within society's legal control. The easy confidence of this dichotomy is now in question. It is true that the *facts* that the atom is not an ultimate unity and that genetic factors determine the condition of a man do not terrify people; however, the ability of man *to divide* the atom or *to manipulate* the gene is another matter. Gradual awakening to the potential social consequences inherent in the power to manage these phenomena has evoked a burgeoning interest in ethical matters among scientists who, a short time ago, regarded such questions as being substantially alien to their work. The interest is commendable. The danger is that the scientist may conclude that his procedures, excellent for his problems, are also valid for problems of law. However, the good life does not lie simply in the discovery and definition of things. Things must still be allocated. Good things—even the ministrations of medicine—have a price and may not be available to everyone. What is desirable for the individual may be undesirable for the group. We dare not presuppose a world without conflict or a world in which one man does not stand in opposition to others.

The need to allocate resources, to redress social imbalance, and to manage trouble requires law to function at a number of levels. We should, therefore, expect the "guides for rules" to come from a number of sources. To understand how these sources contribute to the formulation of rules, it is necessary to examine the nature and purpose of the process in which the rules are used.

WHAT LAW DOES

A legal system is expected to accomplish a variety of objectives. Law is a catalyst in social organization; a mechanism for the identification, implementation, conservation, and transmission of ethical values; a means of distributing the benefits and burdens of society among persons. In these processes, law establishes, or at least identifies, social positions. Responsive to these positions people claim, or are assigned, varying shares of wealth or poverty, power or impotence, health or illness, and accordingly a lengthened or shortened span of life. Such claims and allocations often occasion disputes. This is especially true when the members of a society do not share religious, political, or ethical structures of sufficient strength to produce common perceptions of how these problems ought to be resolved. Unanticipated decisions appear "wrong" and invite resistance. Resistance can and does produce violence and destruction. History illustrates all too graphically man's propensity for violence, including the destruction of human life. It is, therefore, understandable that a basic expectation of the legal process is that the taking of life be minimized, rationalized or, if possible, avoided. The demand is addressed not only to the destruction or erosion of the quality of life resulting from such terrors as war and homocide, but also to similar consequences that may result from socially approved activities, including the provision of health care.

"Thou shalt not kill" excels as a point of beginning in law, but its generality precludes utility in most disputes. The reason for the impotence of this or any other general rule is that a dispute that results in formal legal action involves, always, a question with respect to which persons differ even when they are reasonable, honest, and well informed. Where accepted knowledge provides "scientific proof" of disputed facts and when values held in common indicate "proper conduct," there is no need for litigation. Only when the "right answers" are actually, socially, or economically unknowable must there be resort to the "opinion" or "judgment" of the legal system. This is why lawyers can only present "arguments" to the court or to the legislator. By definition, formal disputes in law, including questions of life and death, are those in which the reasonable, honest, and informed members of the community disagree on how to apply the rule that allegedly governs the dispute. Obviously some procedure beyond acknowledgement of general principles is mandatory.

What system can resolve the unresolvable?

One way of examining the legal process is to define, rather arbitrarily, the tasks the system is expected to accomplish, study each task independently, and observe how the tasks are sequentially related. Understanding of the law tasks will suggest how rules are developed at each level of operation, and why these rules are applicable to specific issues such as those that arise in the provision of health services.

Among the fundamental tasks we expect law to accomplish, ranked from the most obvious and simple to those of greater obscurity and complexity, are the following:

1. *Resolving disputes*—with minimum violence and as little other social cost as possible.
2. *Managing trouble*—by identifying danger areas and providing alternative routes around such difficulties.
3. *Reconciling technology and ethics*—by keeping the innovative surges of science and the value-conserving quality of society in constructive tension.
4. *Promoting goal attainment*—by the purposeful manipulation of rewards and penalties.
5. *Reformation of values and goals*—the establishment of new criteria of legitimacy and acceptance.

Merely naming these law jobs illustrates the indivisibility of the system. Each level blends into and partly determines the next; they build from the simple and obvious need to maintain peace to the complex and obscure task of restructuring the values of the society. The legal sequence finds an approximate counterpart in medicine. That system may also be divided, for discussion at least, into a sequence of operations that begins with the highly visible task of treating the specific ailment of a given patient and proceeds through tasks of increasing complexity until the final level of abstraction, the theoretical inquiries of the experimental scientist, is reached. As already suggested, there will be some law applicable to each level of medicine. However, the need for legal control has been much more apparent at the application end of the scientific spectrum and much less visible with respect to the activity of the research scientist. The explanation of this is that law reacts to harm that has been realized or is at least imminent. Science has, therefore, enjoyed the greatest freedom at the theoretical level; the area that has seemed most remote from human impact.

All of this is changing. The temporal distance between discovery and application has narrowed dramatically in recent years. The technological capacity to translate theory into practice rapidly has, in fact, created problems of great importance. Velocity is so marked that suspicion is inevitable: Was there adequate theoretical understanding before thalidomide was used? Did the researcher know much about rejection mechanisms before the first heart transplant? Will genetic manipulation continue before more than superficial attention has been given to the consequences? The pressure on the other side of this problem is equally great: Must the expense of developing new treatment be so great in time and money? Can a governmental agency make adequate professional judgments? Should persons in need of treatment be given greater opportunity to offer themselves as experimental cases?

Stated in this fashion, the decisions might appear to be ones that could properly be left to the practitioner and his patient, but they are not that finite. The problem is not simply the speed with which basic research is translated into treatment; there is also the dimension of scale. The magnitude of potential damage associated with error in modern science is awesome: the malformed child of the thalidomide user; the emerging capacity of genetic engineering to alter radically what has been known as human; the possibility that cloning might put man into an inescapable evolutionary cul de sac. Given this context, the exertion of legal control can no longer be deferred until damage has occurred. Somehow the evaluation of impact and the exertion of social control must be expanded from the end stage of application back into earlier levels of scientific inquiry without, however, destroying the freedom requisite for scientific endeavor.

These considerations lead to certain hypotheses about the "guides for laws." Because the legitimate interests of individuals, the public, members of the profession are different at each level of the legal and medical sequences, it follows that the rule-making process should also vary. One would anticipate, for example, a substantial input from the medical professional at those levels where the legal task is to decide on the technical competence of a physician but a lesser contribution when the essential task is to change a social goal. However, no level of either sequence is exclusively a private, public, or professional concern. The formulation of rules emerge from dialogue among the parties. The need to balance the competing demands and to remain open to continuing adjustment remains dominant.

HOW THE RULES ARE FORMULATED

The dialectic between medicine and law that produces rules related to health care must be seen by posing specific problems at each level of the outlined sequence of law tasks. For our purposes it will be most convenient to work from the most complex, Task 5, to the most basic, Task 1.

Reformation of Values and Goals

Thomas Kuhn, in *The Structure of Scientific Revolutions,*[2] has explained that our measures of validity presuppose a recognized paradigm. When enough exceptions—inexplicable under the paradigm—to this presupposed truth have been observed, there is no alternative to rejection of the old paradigm and the articulation of a new "truth." This rejection of the old and the articulation of a new paradigm is, of course, the scientific revolution of which he writes. So it is with the historic demand that medi-

[2] T. Kuhn, The Structures of Scientific Revolutions. Chicago, University of Chicago Press, 1970.

cine shall struggle unconditionally to preserve life. Population statistics, however, seem to demonstrate that (for the first time in history) preservation of man depends upon less, not more, life. Humane and economic considerations seem to argue for termination, not prolongation, of some lives. Discussions concerning genetic deterioration appear to suggest suppression, not augmentation, of some family lines. But each of these activities may oppose the basic rule which forbids killing. The Hippocratic Oath is generally understood as a requirement that the doctor strive unflinchingly for the life of his patient.

The historic value has served medicine well. Unquestionably, physicians have mastered valuable procedures that, lacking an absolute ethical demand, might have been abandoned as hopeless. The confidence felt by most patients in the decisions of the doctor depends essentially upon the conviction that the doctor's sole objective is the preservation of life. Society has rewarded the profession unstintingly, providing it with the wealth and freedom indispensable to professional progress because the basic ethic of medicine has correlated precisely with the fundamental value of our culture.

Can medicine, responding perhaps to changed social circumstances, reject that ethic? It should not try, because law can provide a better alternative. The process is, in fact, under way. "Thou shalt not kill" is being refined into "thou shalt not murder," the explanation being that such was the original and true meaning of the rule anyway. The words "life" and "death" are also under scrutiny. Yielding to the new evidence of science, law is abandoning the once adequate position that a person is either alive or dead and that the transition occurs at a given instant. The emerging rule acknowledges that death of "all that which comprises a person" is a process spanning hours, perhaps days, and that there may be persuasive reason to acknowledge death at different times for different purposes. The outlines of this process may be clearly discerned in the provisions of the Uniform Anatomical Gift Act and in the well-known *Harvard Medical School Report* dealing with brain death and irreversible coma.

The historic rule of law and the usual reading of the Hippocratic Oath require the surgeon contemplating an organ transplant to inquire, "What are the odds that the physiological life functions of this patient will continue?" The guide for a new rule suggests that the question may become: "What is the chance that human benefit will be realized if physiological function is continued?" The two questions will often elicit different answers and require different behavior. The questions presuppose different paradigms. Since, as Kuhn informs us, it is not possible to move by logic from one paradigm to another, the restating is a task for law. The guides for the new rule should come primarily from the perspective of the society and the patient, not from the professional. The question is not one of technology.

Promoting Goal Attainment

It is clear that our civilization has reached a stage where the coordination of work being done in various disciplines may no longer be delayed. People working in isolation often are dangerous. Dramatic illustrations of this danger can be seen in the field of interest currently called ecology. How much lead poisoning has resulted because the designers of automobiles have not talked with environmental scientists? How much mercury is ingested because operators of factories seem oblivious to the needs of fishery interests and water users? Is there any mechanism in operation, or that can be established, to protect society against comparable harm arising from the absence of coordination in medicine? Have the benefits of private enterprise been overstated and have they become detriments in health care?

Persuading ourselves that we cannot afford the immense waste resulting from uncoordinated activity should not be too difficult. However, it seems equally apparent that the hope for reward at the stage of production and distribution has provided the major encouragement for the development of technology, the compensation for work of the applied scientist, and even the funds which support the basic sciences. We have been content to permit the unseen hand of economics to guide, confident that anything that can be developed and sold is a gain, and that gain is good. Until recently we scarcely noticed that the costs of private gain are frequently hidden in the pollution of air and water, or in the destruction of esthetic and cultural amenities. Indeed there is reason to ask whether gain in one area has not often been offset by considerably greater loss in another. Furthermore, these unrecognized costs are often directly related to health. How much emphysema, for instance, can be traced to inadequate attention to purity of air resulting from poor design of automobile exhaust systems? Should the health practitioner use his expertise affirmatively, through the development of new laws, as a variety of preventive medicine? How will he, or someone else, be able to measure cost-utility if we elect to depart from the historical operation of free enterprise?

The requirements can be specified: we need rules that will assure us of *net* gain after the costs have been reckoned, and the assessment must come *much* before the crisis level of recognized harm resulting from the application or consumption that occurs at the end of the process. Ideally, this social assessment should be made *before* any form of encouragement is given to discovery or, at the very latest, before newly discovered knowledge begins to be moved from the basic science toward ultimate utilization.

This need exists as much, or more, in health research as in any other area.

Some examples of what these generalities mean in the health care field have already been stated: thalidomide, organ transplants, genetic engineering, and cloning. Other examples come to mind: Does medical science have the capacity to arrange for advance assessment of the ultimate social impact of a given piece of basic research? Does medicine even attempt to measure collateral consequences—such things as impact upon employment, pollution, family organization—that may result? Perhaps the individual scientist occasionally does wonder what will happen when the genie is out of the bottle, but the rule to which we seem to be resigned is that what can be learned must be learned, what can be done must be done. That rule needs changing. What guide is there for the change?

Our earlier statement of this law task comes nearer to finessing the issue than to answering it. The proposition is that law must reward movement toward *desired* goals. The job description does not say how to decide what goals are desired. That issue, however, is only another way of saying that value choices must be made, and it has already been suggested that the controlling rule concerning value should require an inquiry on whether the proposed activity will enrich the quality of life. Assume that the value question has been resolved; the problem now is whether the legal system can manipulate available contingencies in a fashion that will effect coordination of effort and will stimulate movement in the direction of a defined goal.

No claim can be made that the law is now adept in long-range planning and goal implementation. There are encouraging indications however. The National Environmental Policy Act, to refer again to ecological concerns, offers a model that may prove useful. A portion of that act requires that federal agencies, in making recommendations and in their own actions, shall "utilize a systematic, interdisciplinary approach . . . in decision making . . ." and shall "insure that presently unquantified environmental amenities and values . . . be given appropriate consideration . . . along with economic and technical considerations. . . ." The act further provides that before an agency recommends action affecting environmental quality, it shall prepare a detailed statement indicating:

1. The environmental impact of the proposed action,
2. any adverse environmental effects which cannot be avoided if the recommendation is implemented,
3. alternatives to the proposed action,
4. the relationship between short-term and long-term productivity, and,
5. any irreversible and irretrievable commitments of resources which would be involved.

What success could be expected of legislation that authorizes appropriate agencies to delay developmental work in basic health sciences until similar study and reporting had been accomplished? Considerations of public welfare and health, which motivated enactment of legislation for protection of the environment, must also require the coordination and control of developments in such areas as pharmacology, artificial insemination, and euthanasia. To date, however, legal controls over the latter subjects have been quite feeble, usually after the fact, and often misdirected. We need rules requiring early assessment, evaluation against social goals, and informed management of sanctions.

Reconciling Professional Technology and Societal Values

It has just been asserted that the members of one discipline—here the experts in health—cannot be trusted to assess adequately the long-range impact of their own work. Their scientific paradigms test only technical issues. Seldom does the scientist think through to the remote ethical implications of his work, nor will he often attempt to draw up a social balance sheet of the consequences of his discoveries. The tendency toward introversion ends, however, when the activity of another scientist has observable effect upon the work the first researcher has under way. So the heart specialist may not be much interested in addiction control of itself, but he will pay close attention if persuaded that addiction significantly affects treatment of the heart. This phenomenon is understandable enough; interest accompanies expertise. Does the combination of interest and expertise mean that professionals, even if not the best judges of long-range goals, should be allowed to guide the choice of rules governing their immediate practice?

The hazard in this proposition has been indicated in the statement of the third law task. The practitioner is a man of technology, and technology has a corrosive effect upon the concept of law as a process designed to benefit human beings. Jacques Ellul, writing in *The Technological Society*[3] (p. 297) has made the point: ". . . whatever a technician believes to be true must be made into law. . . . His analytic spirit leads him to perceive, understand, and affirm strictly localized truths; and thus strictly delimited, they then become the objects of the law." If law is to express choices concerning value, the decisions must not be determined purely by functional utility. On the other hand, it is obvious that the professional must have a major voice in structuring his own activity.

The necessity for a dialectic between medicine and law at this level is visible enough so that the participants are aware of what is occurring. The practitioner who has developed, for example, a safe procedure for terminating pregnancies can state "medical" reasons why his skill should be available to a distraught minor. A rule requiring parental consent is, to him, an interference with "good medicine." The lawyer, reasoning from some historically derived indications of the value of family solidarity, may regard the medical opinion as gratuitous meddling. The opportunity for useful cooperation is evident.

<hr>

[3] J. Ellul, The Technological Society. New York, Knopf, 1964.

Legal rules applicable to patient care are usually (and quite properly) negative; i.e., what the medical practitioner may not do. To the extent that the prohibition of abortion arose out of lack of technical capacity at some earlier date (the danger of infection, lack of adequate technique, etc.,), medicine can now demonstrate justification for change. Such argument does not reach the family solidarity point, however. Perhaps the medical profession will next offer reasons, possibly based upon newly discovered genetic facts, that provide reasons for pregnancy termination never before known. If a persuasive case is made for repeal of abortion prohibition in general, the special problem of consent by a minor—the reason for the family rule—still remains unsettled. Even with respect to this last aspect of the problem, medicine can voice an informed opinion about how the operation will affect the quality of the patient's life. In short, a dialogue can test the assumptions upon which the existing rule was developed and perhaps show that modification of the law is appropriate, but that showing must involve both technical and social considerations.

When the dialogue arising from the collision of new technology and old laws has resulted in a more or less generally held belief that the time has come to change a rule, the problem of rule-adjustment mechanism still remains. The choice of mechanism depends upon the purpose in mind.

If all that is sought is protection of the private practitioner, a test case may suffice. The outcome will depend largely upon professional testimony, but the lawyer will be in obvious control of the proceeding. When a broader purpose, say a type of public legitimation, is sought it may be essential to resort to legislation. Here the medical professional can be as effective as, or even more effective than, the lawyer. A modern legislative body is more comfortable with the language of science and with the consideration of immediate, practical matters than it is with the moralistic and ambiguous problems of culture preservation. If the purpose is broader still, if the practitioner wishes protection, legitimacy, and maximum freedom, he may seek to have the rule changing done by a statutorily established administrative body, preferably one composed of fellow professional experts. In this context, contentions based upon technology are most persuasive of all. Indeed, as suggested earlier, technological considerations may in that setting become the law.

Managing Trouble

We now reach those law tasks most directly applicable to the individual practitioner. The issue is no longer reconciliation of the technology of the medical profession with the values of the society, but rather the avoidance and, when necessary, the resolution of trouble between the individual practitioner and his patients. How do we get rules for these tasks?

Trouble occurs when things have not worked out as anticipated. The more clearly possible consequences are defined, the greater the probability

that the parties will have foreseen and agreed upon the handling of disappointment. Rules for avoiding trouble, then, are usually those that provide the practitioner with such devices for predicting and limiting his liability as insurance, waivers and consents, and exemption from the criminal
law. Keeping abreast of the major current trouble areas is not difficult.
Courtroom trial calendars enable the professional to distinguish those situations that actually produce trouble from those in which trouble is only
theoretical or, though real, is already well-controlled.

Some criminal law troubles do exist for physicians. Like other persons, doctors are forbidden to murder, maim, or take improper liberties.
As a practical matter, however, a medical practitioner is much less likely
to be found guilty of any of these offenses than another defendant, given
the same circumstances. The cases in which a physician has been indicted
for criminal conduct in his practice often involve the withdrawal by his
colleagues, for some reason or other, of their collective mantle of protection. The selective enforcement of the criminal laws regarding abortion,
birth control, venereal disease treatment, narcotic alleviation, and care to
minors without parental consent is quite revealing. Clearly a medical practitioner can do things that, if done by a nonprofessional, would result in
prosecution. The explanation, of course, is that the physician is assumed
to be acting for his patient's benefit—even when the act is forbidden—and
to be without guilt or criminal intent. The distinction is patently unsound,
as good intentions do not justify prohibited acts and the practitioner undoubtedly means to do what he does in these cases. Perhaps the results
will be different when (and if) a prosecutor elects to indict a doctor for
an act of euthanasia; it depends largely upon the facts, the community,
and the people involved. It is probable, however, that the medical profession can pretty well write the criminal law in this area to suit itself.

The situation is less clear with respect to planning around civil liability in dramatic situations—euthanasia, for example. The case will usually
arise under a wrongful death statute where the plaintiff will be the next
of kin or the personal representative of the estate of the deceased. It is
at least arguable that permission for the doctor to terminate life-sustaining
care, given by such prospective plaintiff, would preclude the bringing of
a damage action. But the case need not arise that way. There are situations
in which the death of one spouse before the other, or postponement of
death until an adoption has been arranged, or the occurrence of death before a divorce can be obtained, will have very substantial economic consequences and will, accordingly, cause great disappointment to someone who
may argue that the physician has interfered with an advantageous relationship. These risks are as yet largely uncharted and protective measures have
yet to be developed.

In situations not involving death, the trouble will normally be between
the physician and his patient. How much exemption from liability can be

arranged? The doctor will probably continue to exert dominant influence in defining who can consent to what and under what circumstances. The current conflict centers on the issue of "informed" consent. The law says that the patient must be "fully informed" of the risk he is to assume, but the definition of what that requirement means will be largely written by those in the medical profession, not lawyers. There are, to be certain, some sharp limits on what hazards can be consented to and what rights against the physician cannot be waived. One cannot protect the physician from criminal liability by consenting to one's own death, nor may one authorize the death of a relative—especially if the person purporting to give the consent is one who may profit from the death, as is frequently the case when a relative is involved. Legislation is of course important in these special instances.

To successfully circumvent areas of high risk, the medical practitioner must avoid the appearance of self-interest. Sensitivity to this requirement is demonstrated by the section of the Uniform Anatomical Gift Act that provides that the physician who attends the donor at death, or who certifies the death, "shall not participate in the procedures for removing or transplanting a part." Professionalizing the issues and remaining free of conflict of interest are the important keys to trouble avoidance. To the degree that the practitioner persuades the judges, legal and social, that decisions about living, dying, transplanting, and other health care activities are in fact technical questions to be resolved by asking what the majority of competent physicians do in such cases, he will retain management of his hazards of practice.

Resolving Disputes

Little need be said here about this last task of the law. The literature dealing with medial malpractice is so extensive that comment here is unwarranted. Our only interest is to inquire about the development of rules by which liability is determined.

Dispute settlement is certainly significant for the medical practitioner, but the process of trial in his case is not unusual. Concerning this activity, the lawyer has become the man of technology, striving to have his discoveries about functional efficiency incorporated into procedural rules, while the medical practitioner has assumed the role of the consumer of services who speaks as any other layman. He may question the social value and the morality of the paradigms under which the legal process operates, but when he does this he is addressing himself to a law task further up the scale of abstraction than that occupied by the basic job of settling disputes. Because formalized dispute settlement is the peculiar function of the lawyer, he must also bear the responsibility for its technology. Whether his procedures are too costly, too cumbersome, or otherwise socially unacceptable is a value judgment. Evaluation of that issue would necessitate another trip through the law task sequence, this time asking a new set of questions.

CONCLUSION

Law, as a system, incorporates both procedural and substantive rules. Procedural rules are largely matters of technique. Substantive rules are those that indicate the value choices of society. Both types of rules are constantly being revised. Changes in technique develop within the legal profession, but amendment of the substantive rules should result from an ongoing discussion between legal professionals and the nonlegal consumers of law.

The provider of health services is a law consumer. So is the recipient of such care, as are other persons who constitute the society in which the provider and recipient live. The special needs of all these persons must be recognized and accommodated. This recognition and accommodation guides the development of new rules for the legal system.

The legal system applies to almost every human activity, but the visibility of each law element varies from one level of abstraction to the next. Parties who are less conscious of the legal ingredient of their activity tend to make fewer contributions to rule development, and the suggestions that are made are often not as good or appropriate. However, the levels of activity are inextricably linked and a ripple effect cannot be avoided. To obtain maximum advantage from the legal system, users should understand and participate in the operation of law formulation as well as in its implementation.

The capacity of persons engaged in health services to aid and to harm others has increased geometrically in recent decades. This increase in capacity has made increased legal control desirable and inescapable. Professionals in the health care field can contribute significantly to the shaping of these legal controls.

CHAPTER 23

PSYCHOSOCIAL AND RELIGIOUS ASPECTS OF MEDICAL ETHICS

E. MANSELL PATTISON

"I will not permit consideration of religion, nationality, race, party politics, or social standing, to intervene between my duty and my patients."
Declaration of Geneva
World Health Organization, September 1948.

I. RELIGION AND MORALITY

Background

The Second World War convulsed the world both physically and morally. In the aftermath came a determined attempt to assess a world moral order. The Nuremburg war crimes trials were the focus of this reassessment in which two opposing moral positions were brought face to face. The defendants argued that they were implementing the laws of the land; the prosecution argued that certain basic human rights and responsibilities were self-evident and inviolable. The issue was clear: Are there universal norms of human morality or does each society construct its own relative system of morality?

The issue was not new. Philosophers had struggled with the issue until the turn of the twentieth century, only to give up the task and turn to analytic and process philosophy—to analyze *how* men make moral decisions. Social scientists, especially anthropologists, had brought in a multitude of competing social moral systems from other lands and peoples. Sigmund Freud and the pioneers in psychoanalysis had demonstrated the vagaries and inconsistencies of personal moral conduct. But all this work did not directly challenge the world and popular thought until the cataclysm of war, ghetto, and concentration camp made the moral confrontation inescapable.

The issue was made more pointed by the growing realization after World War II that the historic Christian church institutions had not sus-

277

tained a viable morality for contemporary civilization. In their postwar studies on prejudice, Adorno et al. discovered that the ideologies of the Christian church actively fostered anti-Semitic hostility. This was confirmed and extended in the 1950's and 1960's by a multitude of psychological and sociological studies that demonstrated that traditional Christian morality was not only inconsistent but more tragically fostered bigotry, authoritarianism, dogmatism, and anti-humanitarianism. It appeared that rather than contributing to the welfare of man, traditional Christian morality had a negative and dehumanizing influence on Western man.

Not only was traditional morality bankrupt and found wanting in terms of the past. The world was in flux. New decisions had to be made. How were we to decide? Women no longer were dependent on men, divorce became socially feasible. The pill arrived, and pregnancy was no longer a Sword of Damocles. The black man in America rose to claim his humanity and found himself barred from the doors of the community church. Children in an affluent age found that the self-ratifying and self-congratulating pose of success in a God-blessed America had covered human misery of a corrupt and oppressive society that poorly tolerated dissent. The traditional moral answers of conventional religious institutions seemed only to perpetuate the status quo and to provide no platform for reform and reassessment.

It was in this context that theologians began the serious task of crafting a "new" morality. A reassessment of religious moral conventions. An analysis of the new ethical dilemmas posed by a changing society. Bishop John Robinson brought out *Honest to God,* soon to be followed in America by Joseph Fletcher's *Situation Ethics*. The debate was on! Robinson, Fletcher, and fellow travelers were seen as agents of a moral anarchy soon to devastate the country. As theologians they had betrayed God, man, and country. But perhaps the polemics were hasty as well as ill-advised. For the issues Robinson and Fletcher struggled over came closer to home, with the polarization over the Vietnam war and the civil rights struggle. The moral dilemma has invaded almost every significant area of contemporary life.

Personal versus Social Morality

Much of our thinking about morality has been formulated in personal terms. We are fond of quoting Martin Luther: "Here I stand, I can do no other." The individual conscience pitted against the forces of a society. Yet this misconstrues the essential nature of morality, which is simultaneously a personal and social concern.

Clyde Kluckhohn, the late famed Harvard anthropologist, summed up the issue well:

> There is the need for a moral order. Human life is necessarily a moral life precisely because it is a social life, and in the case of the human animal

the minimum requirements for predictability of social behavior that will insure some stability and continuity are not taken care of automatically by biologically inherited instincts, as with the bees and the ants. Hence, there must be generally accepted standards of conduct, and these values are more compelling if they are invested with divine authority and continually symbolized in rites that appeal to the senses.

No society then can function without a specific morality. Morality, therefore, is not a question of merely prohibitions or musts, but rather the values and definitions of appropriate behavior by which man governs his behavior and protests against social mores and injustice. For too long, however, we have seen the morality of a society in static terms. Morality must be a process, for society is always in a process of change, and new moral decisions for human relations must be negotiated.

This on-going process of moral decision-making is highlighted by sociologist Philip Rieff:

> To speak of a moral culture would be redundant. Every culture has two main functions: (1) to organize the moral demands men make upon themselves into a system of symbols that make men intelligible and trustworthy; (2) to organize the expressive remissions by which men release themselves in some degree from the strain of conforming to the controlling symbolic, internalized variant readings of culture that constitute individual character. The process by which a culture changes at its profoundest levels may be traced in the shifting balance of controls and releases which constitute a system of moral demands.

This view of process morality is an explicit recognition that a social morality not only can but must change with time and culture. To some this might appear as if all values and morality are relative. In part this is so, but it may be more accurate to say that all morality must be relevant. Hence, we must look at different categories of values and moral decisions to see how a process view of morality must take into account both absolute and relative concepts of morality.

First, we can arrange "values" along a continuum from the most relative to the most absolute in the following hierarchy:

1. Idiosyncratic values—held only by one person in the group under consideration, i.e., personal preferences.
2. Group values—which are distinctive of some plurality of individual, whether this be family, clique, association, tribe, nation, or civilization.
3. Personal values—private form of group values.
4. Operational absolutes—values held by members of a group to be absolute in their application for them.
5. Tentative absolutes—those operational absolutes found to exist in all societies.
6. Permanent absolutes—assumptions that may be asserted but unknowable in any scientific sense.

Now anthropologists no longer hold to the radical cultural relativism of a quarter of a century ago. Rather, there is a growing consensus that tentative absolutes do exist—a rough parallel to the Mosaic Decalogue. This is not at all at odds with the emphasis of the new morality as the ethic of love, for the Ten Commandments are negative defintions of love. That is, the Decalogue spells out some, but not all, conditions of nonlove.

Thus, we can affirm an ethic of absoluteness, whether from a scientific base that affirms a certain uniformity of morality, or from a Judaeo-Christian base of affirmation of man's relationships to God. But this affirmation of absolute moral norms does not help us in dealing with life's problems, for our absolute moral norms are broad general principles. Specific interpersonal pieces of behavior are not self-evident, but vary with time, place, and culture.

Let us look at a few examples. Stealing is violation of human relationship. The use of a neighbor's car, without his knowledge, in a farming community may not be defined as stealing, whereas it probably will be defined as stealing in the city. In certain South Sea Islands, people leave their coats outside their huts in case a passerby needs a coat, but one would be upset if a stranger took one's coat from the cloakroom at the opera. To shoot a horse-thief was appropriate moral behavior in the Old West, but not the new. In other words, we are faced with the task of defining what the conditions shall be of love or the Decalogue in our time, in our place, in our society. And we will have to assume a sense of moral authority for our behavior until such time as we reevaluate our moral stance.

Let me put it in brief theoretical terms. We have to apply our absolute moral norms in a manner relative to the society at hand. However, that relative definition must be treated as an absolute standard. Several examples may clarify the principle. In my town today, we must define what behavior shall constitute stealing. Having agreed on a definition, we all must live by it until we redefine what shall constitute stealing. Another example is the action of the Supreme Court. To it are brought moral issues. The court makes a ruling as to the most appropriate moral resolution in the light of available evidence. We must act according to that ruling until the same dilemma is brought to the court for another evaluation and moral ruling. It is recognized that the Supreme Court is not handing down a "final" decision, but rather the best decision that men can make at this time. In terms of school segregation, the "separate but equal" doctrine of the 1860's was the best moral decision that could be achieved in that context, but 100 years later a reevaluation of school segregation produced a new moral doctrine to be followed. We can expect that the whole issue will be reevaluated in the decades to follow. It is important to note here that the Supreme Court still follows a set of moral absolutes—the Constitution. The moral problem is not one of absolutes, but how to apply the absolutes of the Constitution within the framework of society.

The relationship between personal and social morals can also be looked at in terms of moral development. The child first learns morality as a very personal, idiosyncratic set of behavior and only later begins to develop a more generalizable and universal set of values. Lawrence Kohlberg has constructed a scale of moral development that consists of six stages:

Stage 1: Obedience and punishment orientation. Egocentric deference to superior power or prestige, or a trouble-avoiding set.

Stage 2: Naively egoistic orientation. Right action is that instrumentally satisfying the self's needs and occasionally others'.

Stage 3: Good-boy orientation. Orientation to approval and to pleasing and helping others.

Stage 4: Authority and social-order maintaining orientation. Orientation to "doing duty" and to showing respect for authority and maintaining the given social order for its own sake.

Stage 5: Contractual legalistic orientation. Duty defined in terms of contract, general avoidance of violation of the will or rights of others and majority will and welfare.

Stage 6: Conscience or principle orientation. Orientation not only to actually ordained social rules but to principles of choice involving appeal to logical universality and consistency.

It has been shown by Kohlberg and his colleagues that the majority of people sampled in the United States consistently operate in terms of the first few stages of morality. This produces much confusion because our general social institutions such as the courts and our fundamental ethical theology are written in terms of Stage 6 morality. Put in another way, much of the everyday Christian morality has been framed in terms of the lowest levels of morality (avoidance for fear of punishment) rather than in terms of the highest levels of morality (commitment to responsible application of principle).

Milton Rokeach, one of the foremost research psychologists in the area of values, comments on this problem:

> If religious institutions taken as a whole are indeed, at best, irrelevant and, at worst, training centers for hypocrisy, indifference, and callousness, it is unlikely that those who are part of the Religious Establishment will voluntarily initiate the program of radical change that seems called for. . . . If a way can be found to reverse the emphasis between proscriptive and prescriptive learning, children can be taught that salvation is a reward for obeying the "thou shalts" of the Sermon on the Mount, rather than the "thou shalt nots" of the Ten Commandments. Such a simple shift of focus, however, would probably require a profound reorganization of the total social structure of organized Christian religions. And if such a reorganization turns out to be too difficult to bring about because or rigidity, dogmatism, or vested interest, the data presented here lead me to propose that man's relations to his fellowman will probably thrive at least a bit more if he altogether forgets or unlearns or ignores what organized religion has tried to teach about values and what values are for.

Such a pessimistic evaluation is based on the fact that expression and acting out of Christian ideals is itself a culture-bound phenomenon. The social institution of the Christian church is a time and place phenomenon—yet one which readily became encrusted with a sense of permanence and "rightness." Thus, the church and its morality readily becomes a defense of the status quo. One of the traditional roles of the church has been that of definer, sustainer, and enforcer of moral values. In primitive societies, religious institutions represent the major social embodiment of the morality of the culture. The same was true for much of the history of Christianity in relation to Western society. But that is no longer true for our society. That in itself is not necessarily cause for dismay. But the fact that the churches of America have come to be bastions of defense of the status quo is cause for dismay. Overlooked is the need for challenge and change in morals, not merely the maintenance of morals. The church in Western society has become primarily an agent for the maintenance of outmoded moralities and has lost its function as a creator of new moralities. Thus, it has lost half of its relevance as a moral agent. The "new morality" movement then can be seen as a renaissance attempt at reclaiming the role of moral innovator in society.

The Christian institutions of our culture have participated in this culturally clouded process of moralizing. Thus, it has appeared that moral decisions had some intrinsic sense of rightness and self-evident validity about them. But now we face a new world in which cultural innocence has been lost. We can no longer plead ignorant of the fact that moral decisions are not self-evident and that as a culture, as church institutions, as individuals, we ourselves, we humans have constructed our day-by-day moral codes.

The reaction to this awareness in the first half of this century was to proclaim a universal relativism. No man might lay moral claim to any other man's behavior. However, no society has or could exist in such moral anarchy. We now face a profound opportunity to accept the freedom to craft moral decisions for our time and place. To craft moral decisions that do justice to universal and absolute norms of human integrity. Yet with the realization that the moral decisions that we make today will be outmoded tomorrow and that we shall have to again reconsider our moral decisions. We shall have to craft moral decisions today as the best possible means of implementing universal norms, yet with the humility that as we learn and grow, our knowledge tomorrow may force us to reconsider them. Finally, we shall face our moral decisions with integrity. If the consequences of our moral decisions turn out to be undesirable, we shall deal with those consequences and not punish ourselves for not having been wiser. We cannot accurately forecast the consequences of our moral decisions, but we can commit ourselves to deal with the consequences with the same integrity with which we made the decision.

What has been outlined here is a revised concept of morality that is not static but process. Morality becomes a question of how we make moral decisions, apply our decisions, and deal with the consequences. It is a morality that takes into account both the absolute and relative nature of morality. It is a morality that takes into account that moral decisions are both personal and social (Pattison, 1968).

It should be clear that the new morality is not a new permissiveness, nor is it moral anarchy, nor is it untutored relativism. The new morality is not an attempt to escape from responsibility or integrity. However, it should be noted that these are all perversions that can be observed in our contemporary society.

This brief description of the nature of morality stands as a reminder that medical ethics involve the whole society. Our approach to ethical issues invites and demands a participation by the medical profession, by the patient and his family, and by the community at large. Further, moral issues, ethical issues, are not solely or primarily the concern of the church or the religiously minded. They are *our* corporate concern.

II. THE PRIEST AND PHYSICIAN

In primitive society the healer was the shaman, the witch doctor, the priest-physician. Mind and body were one. Sin was sickness, and sickness was sin. The shaman was simultaneously the healer of the spirit and the body. By the performance of healing acts and rituals, the spiritual problem was resolved, and the body was healed. The shaman, the priest-physician, was effective, not because of what he did but because of who he was. (Compare for example, the parent kissing the cut on the finger of the child to "make it well." The parent is an effective "healer" because one is a parent, not because of the therapeutic potency of kissing fingers.)

As societies became more complex the shaman, priest-physician, role became more complex. Illness came to be defined less as a personal spiritual problem and more as a natural phenomenon. And so the shaman came to be defined in terms of technical skills: what he could do, rather than who he was. As this trend progressed the spiritual and technical roles of the shaman were separated into two divergent professional roles: the priest role and the physician role. And the concept of healing was separated into a spiritual healing of the soul (person) and a technical healing of pathology (body).

In some ways we see a great polarization of these two processes today. For example, certain aspects of the priestly function do not depend on personal skills, but upon the role (sacramental rituals, baptisms, confessionals, last rites, etc.). Here the technical competence of the priest is not at issue. He is effective because of who he is, namely a priest. But on the other hand, we tend to evaluate a physician not on role, but in terms of technical competence, i.e., what he can do. Yet it is obvious that this is a distortion. For the priest (minister, rabbi) is expected to acquire competency in a variety of human helping and ministering skills. Conversely, much of the physician's effectiveness is dependent on who he is, rather than what he can technically perform. Both the priest and physician are concerned with healing of the person, and the professional healing role continues to retain some combination of both who the healer is and what the healer can do.

The separation of the healing role into priest and physician in our society is not an absolute necessity, but represents two major accommodations:

1. A matter of convenience in a complex society, because the technical requirements of being both a priest and a physician make it difficult to prepare for both roles and to spend the required time to fulfill the requirements of both professional roles. Separation of roles is a practical convenience.
2. A matter of necessity in a pluralistic secular society where all patients and doctors do not necessarily share the same religious systems. Therefore it is impossible for the physician to always fulfill the requirements of priest.

Consequently we have formal distinctions and limitations for the priest and physician. Yet I want to emphasize that these are not mutually exclusive but rather overlapping and complementary roles. That is, both professions are concerned with the wholeness and health of the patient who can only arbitrarily be divided into physiological, psychological, or spiritual parts (Pattison, 1969).

The priest who perceives his task solely as the saving of souls inevitably fails when he ignores the emotional, social, and physical needs of his parishioners. Likewise, the physician who perceives his task solely in terms of restoration of physiological function inevitably fails when he ignores the emotional, social, and spiritual needs of his patient. Note that I said *ignored* rather than met the needs of the parishioner or patient. For neither priest nor physician can always meet the needs of his client. But awareness of the needs of the whole person allows the priest or physician to collaborate with the other to provide the help he himself cannot personally provide. Thus, the priest and physician serve as mutual consultants to each other. But beyond these complementary roles there is an overlapping of roles. People do not have just spiritual problems or just physical problems. Rather they have "problems in being." For example, birth control, a mentally retarded child, and a chronic terminal illness are problems in life that involve a person's spiritual attitude as well as technical medical issues.

There is an aphorism attributed to Oliver Wendell Holmes that sums up the point: "The physician's task is to cure rarely, relieve often, and comfort always." This aphorism highlights the overlapping role of priest and physician, in that both professionals deal with people who come with problems of living for which there is rarely a specific spiritual or medical cure. Both priest and physician overlap roles in "comforting always," and partially overlap in "relieving often." Whether a person seeks a priest or physician for comfort and relief is perhaps a rather arbitrary and artificial choice. If a person defines his "problem in living" in symptoms of anxiety, guilt, or feeling bad, he may seek a priest. Yet he may just as well define his "problem in living" in symptoms of chronic pain, a stomach upset, or dysmenorrhea and seek a physician. Both the priest who dismisses the person with a prayer or the physician who dismisses the person with a pill may have ignored the needs of the person.

Arthur Shapiro has aptly noted that only in the past 50 years has the physician had much in the way of specific medicines or techniques to offer the patient. Yet the physician has been successfully helping patients for centuries. The curative factor is in the personal relationship. And for this reason, priests, ministers, rabbis, teachers, even philosophers and faith healers often "help" people more than the physician! Of course, this has resulted in physicians sometimes defining medicine solely in terms of its scientific content: the treatment of body pathology. That may be science, but it is not medicine. For as Peabody noted in his famous Harvard lecture: "The treatment of disease may be entirely impersonal . . . but the care of the patient must be completely personal . . . the secret of the care of the patient is in caring for the patient." In similar vein, Erik Erikson notes that: "Clinical arts and sciences, while employing the scientific method, are not defined by it or limited by it. . . . The healer is committed to a highest good, the preservation of life and the furtherance of well being . . . pre-committed by basic propositions while anticipating what can be verified scientific means."

These wise elder statesmen are not deprecating the science of medicine or suggesting that the art of medicine take preeminence. But rather I interpret them to say that the practice of medicine is a social enterprise in which the scientific methods are used as part of the process of helping people in distress. Therefore, it seems ill-advised to advocate, as some have, the training of a general practitioner who would be a less rigorous scientist than the specialist or researcher. We need more science in medicine, not less. But that science cannot be construed as medicine, for medicine is ultimately the care of human beings.

Parenthetically, it should be noted that science is a humanistic enterprise. And the humanistic basis of science is part of the nonspecific basis of medicine. In his Harvard Gay Lectures, Blumgart notes: "Pure science prided itself on its non-ethical and amoral character . . . yet science contains within its domains social values and social responsibilities requiring affirmation . . . from the always underlying humanistic criteria. . . ."

My proposition then is that the priest and physician continue to share overlapping roles in caring for people in distress. This "healing of the person" is basically a humanistic and nonspecific spiritual enterprise of interpersonal help, whether defined as the nonspecific art of medicine or the nonspecific spiritual needs of mankind. Either priest or physician may fulfill the "healing" professional role. Any further attempt to separate the overlapping professional role is impossible and would result in the destruction of both the physician's and priest's "healing" role in society. This does not overlook the specific contributions each profession can make. There are specific and unique spiritual healing functions and medical healing functions. But these unique contributions are in addition to the general functions of healing of the total person.

The evolution of the shaman, witch doctor, into separate roles of priest and physician has reached a point of dysfunction. Each profession in its own way has come to ignore vital aspects of total human existence. The priest must retain certain nonspecific medical functions, and the physician must retain certain nonspecific spiritual functions. We have fractionated these functions and lost the person in distress in the process. To adequately address the vexing issues of medical ethics, we must return to our concern with people.

III. HUMAN VALUES IN MEDICAL ETHICS

Before proceeding further, a distinction should be made between medical etiquette and medical ethics. Medical etiquette concerns the patterns of interpersonal relations within the profession that are the social code of the medical world. Medical etiquette is concerned with internal rules on the way doctors work with each other. But medical ethics is concerned with patient care and human values. Therefore, ethics is not an internal medical process, but an external process of the practice of medicine, which must always be a public process.

The practice of medicine has often been subsumed under its scientific base. As a consequence, medical ethics has often been set apart from "scientific medicine" and shunted aside as an area of personal religious values. But this view fails to recognize, as outlined in the first section, that medical practice is a social enterprise in which the whole society has a stake. And as a social enterprise it is thereby a humanistic and moral enterprise, not solely a technical scientific enterprise.

Basic medical ethics underlie all medical care decisions. Since we have long established ethical values, we tend to take such ethical decisions for granted and so proceed according to covertly accepted and reinforced values (Barton). It is only when times and circumstances change, when new technologies appear, that we then face a lack of social consensus in our community regarding medical decisions; and that lack of social consensus is then reflected in the internal questions that physicians have to address. Thus, conflicts in medical ethics reflect ambiguities and competing values in our society centered on that issue of ethics.

Therefore, when a question of medical ethics is faced it must be faced by the physician, and it cannot be passed on to the clergyman. A question of medical ethics is a question about the care of the patient. There is no such thing as a decision based on scientific alternative or religious alternatives, because a patient has only *a* problem, which has scientific, religious, and social facets. Any decision is a composite of these facets and may be said to be a *social decision,* that is, a decision which takes into account each facet. Of course, in different ethical decisions each facet may bear different weight, but no facet can be ignored (Lasagna).

It sometimes appears that the mere fact that we can technically accomplish medical goals gives us an ethical sanction to do so simply because we can. Examples of cancer cell injection in senile patients, organ transplants, artificial insemination, and radical surgeries, all present ethical decisions based not on what we *can* do, but what we *ought* to do.

Nor can decisions in medical ethics be decided solely in terms of the interests of the patient and his doctor. For each individual case reflects social ethical concerns and social ethical commitments of the society. Therefore, each ethical decision involves a responsiblility of the physician to himself, to the patient, to the family, and to the larger society.

This implies that decisions in medical ethics cannot be decided unilaterally, but must be open to the social process of discussion, evaluation, arbitration, and eventual social consensus, according to scientific, religious, and social criteria. Practically, this implies the need for public forums where representatives of the law, the church, medicine, government, etc., share competing and convergent values to the end of resolving ethical questions in a manner consonant with the requirements of physician, patient, family, and society.

The consensus of our society is not going to necesarily be the consensus reached in other societies in the world. Certainly one of the important observations of the worldwide practice of medicine is that the scientific knowledge of medical science must be applied and practiced according to the mores and customs of each country. To ignore this fact leads to frustration and failure as has been repeatedly experienced in the work of medical pioneers in primitive societies, as well as in Hindu, Moslem, and Buddhist cultures. To place folk medicine in opposition to scientific medicine is a fallacy, because all medical practice is in a sense folk medicine, that is, dependent upon the culture, its beliefs, structures, and views of man, God, and the world. This is not less true of Western medicine which is based on a Judaeo-Christian heritage and stands upon certain humanistic premises. These humanistic premises, or views of the nature of man, are worth reviewing as a general meeting ground for people of various specific religious persuasions and commitments.

We shall discuss five views of man that underlie medical practice. Taken in isolation any one view of man is a caricature and can lead to a distortion of human life. Each view of man gives a vantage for looking at medical practice. In ethical decision-making we cannot always satisfy all human values simultaneously—sometimes human values are opposing in emphasis, sometimes impossible to implement, and sometimes at too great a cost in terms of other values. Thus, we arrive at a position of balancing our values and commitments and arriving at compromises that we can accept at this time.

The Reality of the Human

Often we attempt to separate the body and soul in defining a human. But when is a human a human? When the child is but a gleam in the father's eye? When the sperm struggles through the vitelline membrane? When the fetus is viable? When the first breath is drawn? Is the helpless retardate child with an I.Q. of 25, or a feces-smearing psychotic, or an unresponsive "stroker" more or less human than we? When to define a biological organism as endowed with soul, psyche, personhood, what you will, is an arbitrary decision if it is even a legitimate question. Yet such arbitrary definitions are often used in medical decisions regarding abortion, rape, maternal and child welfare in delivery, euthanasia, etc.

Slavish devotion to an arbitrary intellectual definition, shrouded in metaphysical speculation, may only divert us from attention to the moral requirements of real human needs and actual life situations. Arbitrary devotion to rationalistic principle may confound rather than clarify. It may satisfy the letter of the law, but ignore the spirit of the law. The neglect of this principle was illustrated by Albert Schweitzer's high reverence for life per se which became a goading fetish instead of an illuminating virtue.

We face a paradox of two ethical principles: (1) the pursuit of idealistic norms, and (2) the fulfillment of actual reality needs. For example, we are committed both to potential life (a fetus, principle 1) and to actual life (a mother, principle 2). We cannot ignore either, but neither criterion can be followed to the exclusion of the other. The real needs of people are as morally imperative as the adherence to ideal ethical norms.

In summary, we deal with real humans in real life. For real decision-making we make arbitrary distinctions, but those arbitrary distinctions cannot be made into reality.

The Integrity of the Human

A basic right of each person is the inviolable privacy of the individual with his body, thoughts, and possessions. The physician is granted a privileged, but still limited, access to the privacy of a person's body and thoughts. The trust of this privileged access must be safeguarded and respected. At times, the personal values of the patient may be the determining factor in an ethical decision, and we must respect his values. A patient's attitudes may stem from membership in a particular cult, or it may be the unrealistic concern of the uninformed, or simply personal biases which may lead the patient to reject medical procedures or recommendations that we may deem medically appropriate. But the patient's right to decision must remain. On the other hand, patients may request operations or treatment that is not indicated or may be harmful. And here we must not succumb to the patient's demand, but maintain our medical integrity.

Nor can we allow our privileged access to be an occasion for abuse of the patient, or to use the patient for our own ends or benefits. In a little known, but superb address, Maurice Levine sums up these restraints: (1) to avoid hostile reactions that harm the patient, (2) to avoid self-aggrandizement that might lead to an operation or procedure for which one is not prepared, (3) to avoid sexually distorted attitudes that might lead to the abuse of the physician's role in the direction of heterosexual or homosexual seduction, (4) to avoid revealing the secrets of patients for the sake of gossip or to appear important in the eyes of one's wife or friends, (5) to avoid excessive therapeutic ambition that leads to unnecessary procedures, (6) to avoid unnecessary stimulation of anxiety in the patient.

The physician must retain and respect his own integrity and do the same for his patient (Szasz and Hollender).

The Unity of the Human

It seems almost unnecessary to reaffirm the fact that a human is an irreducible unity, who for convenience we divide into body, mind, and soul. Medical decisions cannot be made solely in terms of body, or mind, or soul. Neither the preservation of the soul despite what happens to the body nor the preservation of the body despite what happens to the soul is suitable. (I use soul here in the ancient Hebrew sense of "person"—the unique individual.) For example to treat sexual maladaptation as solely biological is just as unsatisfactory as treating it solely as a spiritual problem. Treatment deals with persons.

The Limitations of the Human

In assuming the role of physician one renounces the right to treat patients on the basis of personal preference or moralistic judgment, but must provide treatment on the basis of human rights and human dignity.

This principle is often neglected. For example, the poor, the minority person, the dirty, the uncouth, the arrogant or "uncooperative," and the "crock" are often dealt with as if they did not deserve care. Medical students used to ask me how I could stand to provide medical care in the prison to felons, thieves, murderers, rapists. Why express concern and care for the dregs of humanity? But this attitude ignores the limitations of each human in the expression of his humanity. Despite limitations and even gross distortions, each human being merits a basic respect for his human person.

Another limitation is the limitation of knowledge and judgment. Just as we may be tempted to assume divine prerogative of judgment, we may be tempted to assume divine prerogative of omniscience. To assume that we have always made the best or most correct ethical decision is foolish. In a sense, we must act in good faith on the basis of limited knowledge, with a full realization that in retrospect we might have made a different decision. And even in retrospect we may not be able to judge the adequacy of our decision.

The critical issue is to distinguish between blameability and responsibility. To assess our decisions is important, not to blame or praise ourselves, but rather to assess the consequences of our decisions. Ethical integrity does not devolve upon making 100 percent right decisions, but rather the willingness to commit ourselves personally to our decisions, and to accept and deal responsibly with the consequences of our decisions.

We must be able to say as Levine suggests: "I know that physicians are not perfect and need not be, but I profoundly respect the attempt of honest physicians to do a good job and to practice their profession in a self-respecting fashion. I know that I am far from perfect, but I am going to make a serious attempt to do a really decent job."

The Transcendence of the Human

Part of the motivation for the practice of medicine has always been the idealistic sense of overarching commitment to humanity and the common good. Medicine is not merely human veterinarianism, nor another applied science. In part, it is an ultimate commitment to help one's fellow man in the human dilemma. Erik Erikson reminds us that medical ethics is not only rational decision-making, but also a love of ideals toward which we strive: "ideals which hold up to us some highest good, some definition of perfection, and some promise of self-realization."

In this sense, the concrete immediate issues of medical ethics decision-making should not obscure the fact that our very concern for medical ethics is grounded in our continuing commitment to affirming the nature and substance of being human.

The Summation of Human Values

To bring together our discussion, we can outline some basic conclusions:

1. Specific religious moral values couched in traditional religious systems have led to obscurity rather than enlightenment.

2. The process of moral decision-making rests squarely with us.
3. We have absolute moral values/humanistic values to which we are committed in our culture. But those values provide us no substantive absolute answers.
4. We face competing and contradictory values.
5. Medical ethical decision-making is a process. We are involved in a process of reaching the best possible social consensus at this time in history.
6. We will seek to continue the process of evaluation, examination, and assessment. Rather than to determine praise or blame, our moral task is the personal commitment to decisions and the integrity to accept and deal responsibly with consequences of our decisions.

IV. MEDICAL ETHICS IN DEATH AND DYING

Appropriate medical care is by no means a clear-cut task. The current interest in the care of the dying patient reminds us that as physicians we often care for bodies but neglect people. And it is not just dying, but the problem of death in manifold medical decisions.

The issues of death and dying have long been taboo in American culture. It is not that they were ignored, but rather repressed, surfacing only in the pornography of death. While the Judeao-Christian heritage, which has formed the backbone of Western cultural attitudes, has failed to meet the challenge of a changing culture and technology, the tragedy of the demise of our Western religious heritage is not so much the loss of religiously moored meaning in life as it is the resultant scientism which has reduced man to anatomy and physiology, leading to a neglect of the human person in the practice of medicine. Our religious heritage has always emphasized the person, and in the discard of religion we often discard the person.

Before the advent of modern medicine, the ravages of disease, war, and punishment continuously faced people with death. And they reckoned with death in terms of religious beliefs. In the twentieth century the success of medical technology and the distant displacement of war left many in American culture with little direct contact with death until well into adult life. We have even sequestered our old people into retirement colonies so that the processes of aging and demise were removed from our eyes.

However, a number of factors have converged to challenge our cultural denial of the issues of death. Medical advances have prolonged life so that for the first time in our culture a major segment of aged remind us of the end of life. Medical technology prolongs the lives of many who live among us while they die. Thus, we face persons who are living on kidney machines, heart machines, anti-cancer agents, etc., that enable them to live a while longer, prolonging the inevitable, forestalling death for a

bit. And then we have decisions about life and death involving organ transplants, radical medical and surgical therapies, and the presence but not
ready availability of many life-saving medical measures. In total, we have
acquired a greater ability to decide when we die, although we have no
more capacity to influence the inevitability of death than before (Pattison,
1972).

   This poses a great perplexity in our society, for we not only face decisions of life and death in medical practice, but also a perplexity of meaning
and values in life in a culture bereft of a consensual value system. The
challenge to traditional values and their religious supports has left many
in American culture facing an existential problem of finding purpose in
living. This is reflected in the modern practice of medicine where medical
practice has been philosophically often reduced to the preseveration of life,
while death is viewed as an intrusion into a scientific quest for eternal existence. It is as if when we cannot find meaning in life, then the only value
left is to keep on living.

   The contemporary existential vacuum of meaning in life makes it
therefore difficult, if not impossible, to face the issue of death. For example,
a recent symposium on the ethics of death attitudes in medicine began with
a proposal that we must evaluate medical procedures in terms of cultural
cost effectiveness (Morison). The rebuttal was that a cardinal principle
of medicine is that doctors must not kill (Kass). Too simplistic. Doctors
do kill. We kill inadvertently; we kill by risk-taking procedures. We kill
by providing geographic and social class maldistribution of care. We kill
by disinterest, by racism, by sexism, by self-interest.

   How can we face the fact that we kill if life per se is the dominant
value? This should not occasion denunciation of the medical profession or
medical self-flagellation. But it should pique our self-scrutiny. And it
should remind the medical profession of the importance of self-correction
by continuing dialogic involvement with our constituency. As the current
jargon has it, the decisions of medical practice are too important to be
left solely to doctors.

   In this sense we must then examine how we may go about the practice
of medicine in response to the ethical issues of death and dying. In a traditional sense this has been thought to be the province of religion. But just
as medical decisions are too important to be left to medicine alone, they
are also too important to be left to religion alone. Recent studies on the
influence of religious beliefs on dying behavior indicate that formal religious beliefs give us minimal cues about a person's responses to death
and dying. Rather, religious beliefs, values, and life styles are imbedded
in much broader sociocultural aspects of medical experience (Martin and
Wrightman; Spilka et al.). Indeed, the most problematic issues in medical
ethics reflect on our values in living life and our attitudes toward facing
death.

V. SUMMARY

In this chapter we have focused on some of the religious dimensions of medical ethics. I have attempted to illustrate in the first section how traditional religious approaches to morality as a culturally bound absolute process has been replaced by a culturally relative view of morality as a central psychosocial process; in the second section how religion and medicine are ineluctably intertwined in the care of the patient; in the third section how general humanistic values, certain overarching religious values if you will, play a determinative role in medical ethics; and in the fourth section the central focus of attitudes toward death involved throughout the texture of decision-making in medical ethics.

My central thesis is that medical ethics is not a provincial concern of religion. Medical ethics is at core the concern for the care of patients and thus central to the practice of medicine.

REFERENCES

Adorno, T. W., E. Frenkel-Brunswick, D. J. Levinson, and R. N. Sanford. 1950. The Authoritarian Personality. New York, Harper.

Barton, R. T. 1965. Sources of medical morals. *J. Amer. Med. Ass.* **193**:133–138.

Blumgart, H. L. 1964. Caring for the patient. *New Engl. J. Med.* **270**:449–456.

Erikson, E. H. 1963. The Golden Rule and the Cycle of Life. Harvard Medical Alumni Bulletin (winter).

Kass, L. R. 1972. Death as an event. *Science.* **173**:698–702.

Kluckhohn, C. 1966. Introduction. *In* Reader in Comparative Religion: An Antropological Approach. W. A. Lessa and E. Z. Vogt, eds. 2d ed. New York, Harper and Row.

Kohlberg, L. 1964. Development of moral character and moral ideology. *In* Review of Child Development Research. M. D. Hoffman and L. W. Hoffman, eds. Vol. I. New York, Russell Sage Foundation.

Lasagna, L. 1965. The mind and morality of the doctor. II. The physician and the microcosm. *Yale J. Biol. Med.* **37**:361–378.

Levine, M. 1948. The Hippocratic Oath in modern dress. *Cincinnati J. Med.* **29**:257–262.

Martin, D., and L. Wrightsman. 1964. Religion and fears about death; a critical review of research. *Religious Education.* **59**:174–176.

Morison, R. S. 1972. Death: process or event? *Science.* **173**:694–698.

Pattison, E. M. 1968. Ego morality: an emerging psychotherapeutic concept. *Psychoanalytic Rev.* **55**:187–222.

Pattison, E. M. 1969. Clinical Psychiatry and Religion. Boston, Little, Brown.

Pattison, E. M. 1972. Help in the dying process. *In* American Handbook of Psychiatry. Rev. ed. S. Arieti, ed. New York, Basic Books. In press.

Peabody, F. W. 1927. The care of the patient. *J. Amer. Med. Ass.* **88**:877–882.

Rieff, P. 1966. The Triumph of the Therapeutic: Uses of Faith after Freud. New York, Harper and Row.

Rokeach, M. 1969. Religious values and social compassion. *Rev. Religious Research* **11**:3–40.

Shapiro, A. K. 1960. A contribution to a history of the placebo effect. *Behavioral Sci.* **5**:109–135.

Spilka, R., R. J. Pelligrini, and K. Dailey. 1968. Religion: American values and death perspective. *Sociological Symposium.* **1**:57–66.

Szasz, T. S., and M. H. Hollender. 1956. A contribution to the philosophy of medicine: three basic models of the doctor-patient relationship. *Arch. Int. Med.* **97**:585–592.

CHAPTER 24

MARRIAGE: WHENCE
AND WHITHER?

DAVID R. MACE

Man, having practiced marriage for at least a million years, has seriously studied it for less than a hundred. Edward Westermarck's massive three-volume *The History of Human Marriage,* first published in 1891, was not the first scientific study of the subject; but it is by far the best-known of the earlier writings, and the only one still given any serious attention. Westermarck was 28 years of age when his monumental work was completed—and he never married!

Westermarck defined marriage as "a relation of one or more men to one or more women which is recognized by custom or law and involves certain rights and duties both in the case of the parties entering the union and in the case of the children born of it." Given a definition as broad as that, it is not surprising that he reached the conclusion that marriage has been a universal human institution.

A SHORT HISTORY OF MARRIAGE

Second only to the miracle of life's emergence was the transition from asexual to sexual reproduction. Early in phylogenetic development, simple, one-celled organisms multiplied by division, a process of one becoming two. Then, one momentous day, somehow this process reversed itself, and two became one, leading to such cataclysmic consequences as sex, evolution, individual consciousness, relationship—and marriage.

In early phylogeny the sexual encounter was blindly performed as the closing act of individual life. The eggs from which the young would develop hatched of their own accord, and the new generation survived either because they were fighting fit from the start, or because they emerged in such massive numbers that they could endure fantastic casualties. But as the process of evolution produced increasing complexity, the young manifested increasing dependency, and the parental instinct became necessary for the protection and provision apart from which their survival was threatened. Generally, maternal care emerged first; but notably among the fishes, it was sometimes the father that assumed the duties of guardian and nursemaid. When the burden of caring for the young became excessive, a point was inevitably reached at which the combined efforts of both parents were needed. This is especially true of most of the birds. The resulting cooperative effort of male and female brought about the association, destined finally to develop its own intrinsic values, that was the genesis of marriage. It was to this that Westermarck referred in his often-quoted statement: "Marriage is rooted in the family, and not the family in marriage."

Man shares his ancestors with the primates, whose typical family system consists of a dominant male with several females and their young. Surplus males hover hopefully in the wings, furtively snatching sexual opportunities, until one of them deposes the jealous patriarch. This polygamous system, with male dominance and the females viewed as desirable property to be fought over, could have been the immediate precursor of the human family; and certainly such patterns are recognizable in *homo sapiens.*

However, archeological evidence now demonstrates an extended intermediate stage with an important change of pattern. Desmond Morris describes early man, the hominid, as the "naked ape." Forced by climatic changes in Africa to descend from the trees and live on the ground, he used his superior brain to emulate the predatory animals and formed hunting groups which, substituting efficient cooperation for the absence of natural weapons, managed to survive. The new way of life, however, demanded effective teamwork among the male hunters. This required a rough basis of equality among them, which could exist only if they were given equal access to the females. Monogamous family groupings formed, with occasional polygamy when a surplus of females occurred. This, we may suppose, became the marriage system of prehistoric hunting man; and it may well have continued for a million years or more.

As agriculture replaced hunting, man's social arrangements underwent appropriate adaptation. The farm family replaced the hunting band as the unit of survival. The polygamous marriage now had distinct advantages, because women and children became valuable workers instead of relatively idle dependents. But the sex ratio denied polygamy to all but the powerful potentate, and monogamy continued to be the majority pattern. The poor peasant and his wife, laboring together on their land, found comradeship in a common cause and developed marriage as something more nearly approaching a relationship of equals.

Urban development brought further social changes. In large communities custom could no longer regulate behavior, and laws, with prescribed penalties for wrongdoers, had to be enacted. Marriage arrangements could no longer be flexibly adapted to suit individual and family requirements, but were subject to impersonal rules, rigidly imposed from above, and based on broad majority interests. Even so, urban life provided ample opportunity to evade or defy the law, while it weakened the restraining power of both family and neighborhood groups.

Throughout these periods of transition, marriage continued to serve three major purposes: to secure procreation under conditions which assured the young of the protection and provision essential for their early development and socialization; to confine sexual activity within prescribed channels and prevent it from disrupting social life by generating jealousy and competitiveness; and to provide companionship and cooperation in the management of the basic social unit. Experience proved, over and over again, that failure to achieve these purposes led to disturbing and even disastrous results. Marriage was seen to be the foundation of the family, which in turn was the foundation of society. The preservation of marriage, and its proper regulation, were therefore seen to be of paramount importance to the community and to the state.

MARRIAGE IN TRANSITION

As we are reminded *ad nauseam,* the emergence of the new technology during the past 200 years has forced radical changes in man's total way of life. This has been as true of marriage as of our other institutions, although our traditional deep respect for the sanctity of the family has delayed until recently our full awareness of what is happening.

The major shift in emphasis has been from the concept of marriage as a duty undertaken for familial and social reasons, to that of a means of seeking personal and interpersonal fulfillment. The traditional practice has been for the choice of marriage partners to be made, or at least approved, to meet family criteria. Once married, the primary tasks of the couple were to produce children to continue the family name and line; preserve the family tradition by cultivating the land, or taking over the craft or business; and to continue the customary religious and social practices. Marriage was in fact the intergenerational link that preserved the continuity of the family identity. Today, these goals have receded into the background and have been replaced by the desire of the couple to satisfy each other's needs for individual happiness and emotional security. This radical change has come gradually but relentlessly and has been brought about by a complex combination of factors, some of which are mentioned below by way of illustration.

A progressive movement of populations has taken place, in Western society, from the land to the city. This has broken the continuity of tradition and custom and fostered pluralism in values and standards. It has also required geographical mobility and scaled the family unit down to the nuclear group of parents and children. Extended public education and the pervasive power of the mass media have created a "generation gap," which has further undermined the continuity of family tradition and the restraining power of parental authority. The movement for women's emancipation has opened gainful employment opportunities to the married woman, ending her economic dependence on her husband and the need for her to tolerate a state of subjection to him. The woman's new freedom has greatly increased sexual opportunity outside marriage, supported by contraception and abortion, which have enabled procreation to be subject to individual control. The threat of overpopulation has meanwhile wrought a dramatic reversal in the value placed on procreation, so that the renunciation of parenthood, hitherto viewed as the refusal of a primary human responsibility except for religious reasons, now ranks as a commendable virtue.

The cumulative consequence of these and other changes has been to devalue the first two of the traditional reasons for marriage—procreation and the regulation of sexual opportunity—which had always been given the greatest emphasis in the past. At the same time, the third reason for marriage—the development of the man-woman relationship—has received greatly increased emphasis and has now become the primary goal of marriage.

The pursuit of happiness is an occupation highly esteemed by Americans, for it is writen into the Declaration of Independence. It is not an easy task, however, to switch the primary goal of a basic social institution from duty to pleasure, without risking considerable dislocation in the process. Supposing, for example, we were to announce that going to school, or going to work, or service in the armed forces, was to be regarded henceforth primarily as a pleasant and rewarding individual experience and that no one was under any obligation to persevere in any of these activities if he did not find happiness in doing so! The long-term result might ultimately represent cultural gain, but the imagination boggles at the upheavals we might have to suffer before the goal was finally attained.

We are already experiencing this kind of upheaval in marriage. The increasing ease with which divorce can be secured has encouraged increasing numbers of people to take this course, either to give up marriage altogether or, in most instances, to pursue happiness afresh with a new partner. The resulting high incidence of marital failure has, indeed, seriously raised the question whether marriage should be regarded as an obsolete institution, and this argument has been used to justify widespread experiments in a quest for "alternative life-styles."

The new life-styles have received a great deal of publicity. They consist primarily of four patterns. The first is successive or seriatim monogamy: the possibility of a series of marriage relationships in the course of a lifetime, a new one being embarked upon when the existing one seems to have exhausted its potential for providing happiness to the individuals concerned. This, in fact, merely gives formal recognition and sanction to the current state of affairs; one suggested form, for example, would bypass divorce by requiring renewal or cancellation of all marriage contracts at three-year intervals.

The second pattern is that of the "open" marriage, which would eliminate the traditional exclusiveness of the husband-wife relationship, sexually and otherwise. "Wife-swapping" or "swinging" is the most provocative form of this plea for "civilized adultery." The argument is that the routine of married life often becomes boring and that periodic extramarital experiences would relieve the tedium without, as was formerly thought, damaging the relationship.

Third, attempts are being made to revive polygamy and group marriage as new forms of association for husbands, wives, and their children. The contention is that the availability of multiple partners for the adults and of multiple parental figures for the children will offer a wider variety of interactive experiences in meeting individual needs.

The fourth pattern, the homosexual marriage, need not concern us here, since it represents not a new form so much as the recognition of marital rights for a hitherto deprived and unrecognized minority.

MARRIAGE AS RELATIONSHIP—THE NEW FOCUS

In the past, the interpersonal aspects of the husband-wife relationship were largely ignored. Emphasis was so concentrated upon procreation and sexual regulation that the distinguished Protestant theologian Karl Barth accused the Catholic Church of having developed no theology of the marriage but only of the wedding. While sociologists studied marriage intensively as a social institution, little or no corresponding study was undertaken by psychologists of marriage as an interpersonal interaction. This field of investigation lay largely unexplored until very recently, with the result that we know surprisingly little about it.

Now, however, the interaction patterns of married couples are seen to be of major significance, if only because it is grimly realized that marriages can no longer be sustained by external coercion, but only by internal cohesion. The critical question, therefore, is what marriage has to offer, in relational terms, that is unique in itself and unavailable elsewhere.

The issue is confused by the fact that for at least half a century the promise of personal fulfillment in marriage was grossly overstated and oversold. A romantic aura was shed upon the husband-wife relationship which promised ecstatic bliss as the automatic result of the wedding ceremony. This myth has now been exploded, resulting in widespread skepticism and cynicism among modern youth. The public image of marriage has gone sour.

We should have anticipated this danger. Social psychology leaves us in no doubt about the fact that close relationships between persons, while they offer mutual support, can easily explode into mutual conflict. Such conflict can, however, be avoided or resolved when it arises in three ways. All are quite familiar in marital interaction.

The first solution is to structure the relationship in terms of a dominance-submission pattern. The clash of conflicting wills can be avoided if one of the wills is made subject to the other. This device is employed as a means of enabling human society to work smoothly in a multitude of hierarchical power structures: ruler and subject, master and servant, employer and employee, teacher and student, and parent and child. It was naturally employed also in marriage, the traditional doctrine being that the husband is the head of the home and his dutiful wife must meekly obey him. This concept has provided a firm foundation for stable marriage for countless generations. With the emergence of the new egalitarian concept of marriage, however, it has become increasingly unworkable. From a one-vote system, marriage has progressed to a two-vote system, and thereby it has become infinitely more difficult to manage. Dominance-submission patterns are still found in modern marriages, but they are increasingly ineffective as means of avoiding or resolving conflict.

The second way of dealing with interpersonal conflict in marriage is to put distance between the partners. The closer a relationship is, the more painful any conflict between the partners is likely to be. Our social relationships are therefore generally structured to provide adequate defenses against such hurts. Business partners go their several ways at the end of the day and over the weekend. For the married couple, the shared life involves relentlessly continuing intimacy, and achieving geographical distance is impracticable. The problem can, however, be resolved by achieving *psychological* distance by the raising of invisible barriers of coldness and mutual exclusion. While still living together, a couple can "drift apart" from one another, until nothing but an empty facade of pseudointimacy remains. This is by far the most common means of dealing with conflict in modern marriages. The conflict is only avoided, however, at the cost of attrition of the desired closeness and intimacy. For most couples, in time this becomes so frustrating that the pretense is finally abandoned, and the marriage breaks down.

The third way of dealing with conflict is highly effective, but it is difficult. It requires the patient resolution of conflicts by negotiation, compromise, and readjustment. The procedures are similar to those employed in attempts to resolve industrial and international disputes: bringing the issues out into the open; hearing out of both sides; prolonged, painful, and sometimes acrimonious disputes; and final movement, aided by arbitration if necessary, toward a mutually acceptable solution. This process of mutual adaptation, never easy, is particularly difficult in marriage, where only two persons try to negotiate in private. There is a powerful tendency to break off negotiations and seal off the area of disagreement. Repetition of this process leads inevitably to use of the distance-creating mechanism already described, rendering the relationship increasingly superficial and tenuous.

Yet if persevered in, the resolution of marital conflict by mutual adaptation can be highly effective, especially if both partners are actively seeking the goal of intimacy. Each successful experience of conflict resolution reinforces mutual confidence that further disagreements can be settled by the same procedures. Close and continuing mutual affection and support in marriage are not easy goals to achieve; but their achievement represents the reward which is eagerly sought by most people who marry. Those who give up have not ceased to desire what they originally sought; rather they have abandoned hope that it is attainable, at least at a price which they are able or willing to pay.

Our society has made little effort to teach its young people anything about resolution of interpersonal conflict, which arises inevitably in most marriages. By this omission we have doomed large numbers of persons to marital failure, which often leads to disillusionment and bitterness. At a time when the focus of marital expectation was shifting to interpersonal fulfillment, we committed a series of tragic errors. We fostered a glamorized concept of marital happiness effortlessly obtained. We failed to explain that success in egalitarian marriage, while theoretically highly rewarding, was much more difficult to achieve than in the traditional hierarchical pattern. When the romantic dream failed and the couple was confronted with the harsh realities of interpersonal conflict, we had provided them with little equipment for resolving this conflict. If we had deliberately and maliciously set out to entrap our youth in marital misery, we could hardly have done it more efficiently. There is a grim relevance for our own time in the old wisecrack that the troubles of Adam and Eve were caused not by a red apple but by a green pair.

MARRIAGE ATTACKED AND DEFENDED

There are those who affirm that marriage has no future in the new kind of human society that is evolving today. Some express regret but declare that it has served its purpose and must now wither away. Others are openly iconoclastic and insist that the marriage bond was always a form of slavery and a means of exploitation and that with its demise new and better relationships between men, women, and children will become possible (Cooper, 1970).

We have seen that marriage evolved, in human and even in subhuman society, as a means of achieving certain purposes essential for human survival. It cannot therefore be abolished unless achievement of these purposes is adequately met through other means. It is pertinent to ask what these other means would be.

Many replies are forthcoming. Procreation, it is conceded, will always be necessary for our human continuity, but this is seen as no problem. Indeed, it is argued that genetic improvement of the race could be achieved by confining reproduction to selected men and women of exceptional endowment, rather than permitting it indiscriminately to all. The scientific eradication of hereditary defects, it is claimed, is no more than a new front that must now be opened up in the conquest of disease. And quite apart from qualitative control, the threat of overpopulation will, in the view of many, necessitate quantitative control as well. The right to parenthood, the argument runs, can no longer be taken for granted.

The human child will obviously continue to need protection and provision during his long years of dependency. Hitherto this need has been met almost exclusively in the "cultural womb" which the family provides; and attempts to create alternative settings for the socialization of children have hitherto been conspicuously unsuccessful. However, it is contended that we could approach this problem today with much greater sophistication than in the past, because of our more adequate understanding of child development. Moreover, the personality patterns of those who live in our new "open" societies will have to differ considerably from those appropriate to the older cultures, in which familial prototypes were the models for all kinds of human groupings, large and small; so that new forms of early conditioning will have to be developed which may be best provided through agencies other than the family. If this all sounds highly precarious, the more conservative critics of marriage will reply that a carefully selected minority of men and women, possessing parental qualities in high degree, can be trained for, and supervised in, the specialized function of raising such children as are needed to maintain desirable population levels. The remainder will thus be freed from parental duties and consequently from marital obligations.

Turning next to the question of sexual regulation, it is affirmed that this will increasingly be unnecessary in the new society, except of course where gross exploitation is involved. Our traditional laws controlling sexual behavior, it is pointed out, are already being ignored and will progressively be repealed. Increasing support is being given to the principle that private sexual encounters of any kind between consenting adults should be considered as lying outside the sphere of the law. In support of this new approach, those who are experimenting with the new life-styles report that sexual jealousy is not the destructive force it is currently assumed to be and that it certainly was both in our human and subhuman past. Therefore, it is suggested, the traditional sexual exclusiveness of the marriage bond makes little sense today, and this raises the question of whether the bond is necessary at all.

So far as companionship between men and women is concerned, the contention is that this can develop better freely than within a legally structured relationship. Indeed, obligations imposed by society do not produce the best atmosphere for good relationships, because creativity is essentially spontaneous. Marriage as a solemn commitment made for life is therefore, say the critics, an undertaking that should not be required of young people because they are incapable of comprehending all that it implies and therefore of entering into it in any realistic sense.

These arguments against marriage are neither frivolous nor superficial. They must be taken seriously, and they demand answers. What *can* be said on the other side?

Those who defend the future of marriage point out that an institution that has been the foundation of man's social life for more than a million years cannot with impunity be jettisoned, even in a time of cataclysmic cultural change. They would support the conclusion of Edward Westermarck (1936), that while undoubtedly much has been suffered in and through marriage, yet more might be suffered in its absence. They would sound a solemn warning against the dismantling of a complex social structure to which mankind has so long been habituated, with the plea that the human personality, as suggested by Alvin Toffler in *Future Shock,* can tolerate only a limited amount of change in its living patterns without the danger of mental and emotional derangement. And they would deplore the making of experiments, the outcome of which must be regarded as far from certain, in such fundamental areas of human life that their failure could lead to irretrievable disaster.

The defenders of marriage would contend that the case against it is based on a preoccupation with marital failures, and the assumption that the increase in their number indicates that they were and are inevitable. But another viewpoint would see many of today's marriages as not having had a proper chance because they were caught in a crisis of transition in which the older criteria for effective functioning were no longer valid, while the new criteria were not yet comprehended. In other words, marriage today is in a fluid and apparently insecure state precisely because it is healthily adapting to social change by reformulating its criteria for success, a process which inevitably results in a period of confusion when casualty rates are bound to be abnormally high. What is needed, therefore, is not to abandon ship, but to repair the damage done by the storm and set a new course until the weather improves.

Even the most pessimistic marriage critics must concede, if they are ready to face the facts, that in our society today there are some very good marriages that can demonstrate their effectiveness in any reasonable test. Even if the number of these good marriages is small, should they not be investigated to discover why they have succeeded where others failed? Why is it that so many people deeply desire to love and to be loved? Is it not because the warmth and tenderness, the security and support, that each partner receives as a result of such love, given and received, is a fundamental requirement for mental health? Is there not much truth in what Havelock Ellis once said, that to live is to love and to love is to live? Scratch any average human being, and you soon find evidences of heart-hunger for closeness and intimacy and the shared life as the only dependable sources of a sustained sense of self-esteem and of personal worth.

In our modern world, with its great cities in which the individual is lost in the impersonal human throng, this need for real involvement, for relationship in depth, is greater than ever before in human history. The prevailing *malaise* of our era is the sense of rootlessness, of aloneness, of being merely a number on a list, a cog in a wheel, one unnoticed face amid a sea of faces. What can cure this sorry condition? Only the vital experience of being a real and significant part of the life of another, having a dependable comrade who will care for you and believe in you and stand by you whatever happens, and to whom you are devoted in the same way.

No doubt this fundamental need can be met, in part at least, in a variety of ways. There is an eager quest for intimacy in our time, eloquently manifested in the popularity of sensitivity training and encounter groups. Such experiences are appealing because they enable us to strip off the elaborate and cumbersome defenses we build up to protect ourselves from one another. To go away for a weekend with a group of total strangers and to plunge headlong into undefensive self-giving and unrestrained involvement offers alluring experiences of "instant intimacy" which vividly show us what we are missing and what we truly need. But is true intimacy, of a kind that will really meet our need, actually attainable without long and continued association, mutual acceptance despite difference and disagreement, tried and tested loyalty and "commitment," which the President of Boston University says has today become a dirty word?

In other words, is it possible that we are making the mistake of trying to cast away the very thing we most deeply need? Does not marriage at its best offer uniquely the very experience most of us crave—a deeply satisfying, dependable, and lasting relationship of complete openness, complete trust, complete sharing of life with one other loved person of the opposite sex, combining the companionship of congenial minds with the stimulus of fulfilled masculine-feminine reciprocity? Is not this the quintessence of what we vainly seek in the more casual and superficial relationships we experience as we thread our tortuous way through the human throng, constantly hoping and constantly suffering disappointment? Is our turning away from marriage just possibly a manifestation of our exasperation because it tauntingly beckons us to a desirable but seemingly unattainable goal?

CONCLUSION

The new "alternative life-styles" seem to be based upon a central premise: that the marriage bond holds people too close for comfort and that it must therefore be wedged open to provide opportunities for variety and change to relieve what would otherwise become an intolerable tedium. We must not, however, overlook the opposite premise: that marriages are failing today not because the bond between husband and wife is too close, but because it is not close enough—because they cannot achieve the enduring intimacy that would make their relationship dynamic, creative, and meaningful. And why not? Because they have never been taught that love and the expressions of love cannot be sustained except in a relationship in which conflict is recognized and resolved in the only workable way—by the painful but ultimately rewarding process of maintaining openness and coming to terms with difference in a persevering process of mutual adaptation that draws its strength from a commitment not outwardly imposed, but inwardly accepted.

Marriage in our time has reached a crisis point at which it is no longer a compelling social obligation, no longer even necessary to fulfill many of its traditional functions. In these circumstances it is easy to conclude that it therefore has little or nothing to offer us. In fact, it holds out, for those who will pay the price to attain it, the most desired and desirable of all human experiences. All will not see it in these terms. The experiments to find alternatives will go on, and we shall learn much from them. It may be that for many people, even for most people, the alternatives will be found to meet human needs more deeply than marriage ever did. But it will not be surprising if events turn out otherwise; if as in the search for the Holy Grail, we return in the end weary and travel-stained to find what we sought at the point where we began our quest; if the stone rejected by the builders of the brave new world is finally brought back to become again the foundation of human society.

REFERENCES

Barth, K. 1947. *Die kirkliche Dogmatik*. III/4. Zurich.
Cooper, D. 1970. The Death of the Family. New York, Random House.
Morris, D. 1967. The Naked Ape: A Study of the Human Animal. New York, Delta Books.
Silber, J. R. 1971. The pollution of time. *Center Magazine*, September-October.
Toffler, A. 1970. Future Shock. New York, Random House.
Westermarck, E. 1925. The History of Human Marriage. Vol. I. London, Macmillan.
Westermarck, E. 1936. The Future of Marriage in Western Civilization. London, Macmillan.

CHAPTER 25

CHANGING VIEWS ON HOMOSEXUALITY, TRANSVESTISM, AND TRANSSEXUALISM

JOHN L. HAMPSON

INTRODUCTION

It has become a cliché to say that we are in the midst of a sexual revolution. Revolution or not, enormous changes have taken place and are continuing to take place in our attitudes toward human sexuality. This movement toward an emancipation from traditional sexual mores began in the 1920's, but it took the Kinsey reports of 1948 and 1953 to bring a kind of scientific respectability to the topic of human sexuality and thus make it at least possible to discuss such matters as homosexuality and even heterosexuality in the newspapers and other communications media. Whereas earlier such phrases as "immoral practices" and "indecent behavior" were used to cover a multitude of things, gradually such words as "homosexuality," "transvestism," "lesbianism," and "gay" began to be seen with increasing frequency in articles, novels, plays, etc.

By 1966, homosexuals were protesting the discrimination imposed upon them by the armed services. Homosexual organizations have become more vocal in seeking equal rights for homosexuals. A great many films and plays dealing with homosexuality, such as "The Fox," "The Killing of Sister George," "Staircase," "The Boys in the Band," and "Midnight Cowboy," have served not only to mold public attitudes but also to exemplify the increasing understanding and tolerance—albeit still incomplete—that society has developed over the past several decades toward unusual forms of sexual expression. Paralleling these social phenomena, intensive research is being conducted in human sexuality which is contributing to our comprehension of the social and biological forces that enter into gender indentity, gender role behavior, and sexual behavior in general.

In the pages to follow we will briefly examine *homosexual behavior, transvestism,* and *transsexualism* as well as some of the related social dilemmas posed not only for the individual but also for society.

HOMOSEXUALITY

The Homosexual Spectrum

Over the past 10 to 15 years there has been increasing public and scientific interest in the matter of homosexual behavior. Some of this has been forced by the demands of the "gay" community, which has become more vocal in demanding greater equality of treatment of homosexuals in society. They object strenuously to being labeled "sick" or "abnormal."

At the outset it should be pointed out that homosexual behavior is simply behavior involving sexual activity between members of the same biological sex, whether male or female. Homosexuality and heterosexuality do not represent a clear-cut dichotomy, however, for all combinations of hetero- and homosexuality are known to occur. Kinsey, in fact, described five intermediate degrees of homoerotic behavior between exclusive heterosexuality and exclusive homosexuality.

With respect to the occurrence of homosexual activity in the United States, the best estimates indicate that 37 percent of postpubertal males and 13 percent of postpubertal females have had one or more homosexual experiences to the point of orgasm. Probably another 13 percent of postpubertal males and 8 percent of postpubertal females have had homosexual psychologic responses without actual sexual involvement. About 4 percent of males and nearly as many females are exclusively homosexual in their erotic interests and/or activity throughout their lives.

These statistics are explained by the fact that those who engage in homosexual activity do not all do so for the same reasons. Recent disclosures in the press regarding forced homosexual behavior in prisons at once illustrates the point. It is also fairly common knowledge that when men or women find themselves in situations of sexual deprivation for long periods of time, and where only members of the same sex are available, homosexual activity is not an infrequent outcome. Certain men find homosexual prostitution a lucrative way of earning a living although their personal sexual preference may even be heterosexual. Preadolescents and teen-agers frequently experiment with homosexuality out of sheer curiosity, boredom, and rebelliousness. Certain sociopathic individuals, retardates, and, occasionally, psychotic persons may also at times experiment with homosexual behavior.

It is not these groups of individuals, however, that society looks at so askance. Somehow we have been able to tolerate the adolescent experimenter and the emotionally disturbed individual who becomes involved in homosexual activity. Rather, it is the 3 or 4 percent of the population

308   *John L. Hampson*

both male and female, whose sexual interest *at all times* is for a sexual partner of the same sex. These exclusively homosexual individuals comprise the gay community which seeks to gain the acceptance of the point of view that homosexuality is a normal, healthy, and perhaps even desirable variation of sexual expression. They correctly point out that homosexuality has occurred in all societies throughout the ages. In support of their arguments they cite Ford and Beach's findings, which indicate that in nearly 65 percent of the 76 contemporary preliterate societies studied, homosexual activities were considered normal and socially acceptable for some members of the community. Spokesmen for the gay community also point to the fact that in our society there are homosexuals in virtually every walk of life, in all ethnic groups, among city dwellers and rural population alike, and at all socioeconomic levels. They argue that with 6 to 8 million Americans preferring a homosexual life style, there can be no justification for regarding this as an illness or for tolerating the condemnation and prejudice which now exist toward these individuals.

Homosexuality: Is It an Illness?

There can be no denying the fact that our society has traditionally taken a very dim view of homosexuality. The very words we have used to describe or explain homosexuality amply to attest to this: "unnatural," "perverted," "immature," "neurotic," "abnormal," "psychopathic," to list a few. Some professionals in the mental health field still continue to regard the homosexual as "a sick person." Viewed historically, the "sickness" concept may have served the useful purpose of evoking enlightened concern and tolerance for the homosexual. Now, however, "sick" has come to have a pejorative and belittling connotation to which the gay community quite rightly objects. Of equal importance, though, is the dubious scientific merit of the sickness concept of homosexuality. The issue, of course, is not whether a homosexual person can become emotionally sick—depressed, anxious, neurotic, etc.—but whether his homosexuality itself is a sickness.

Recent research does seem to shed some light on this matter. The bulk of the research evidence suggests that a "developmental" conceptualization of the problem is more useful than an "illness" conceptualization. Most behavioral scientists now agree that all psychosexual orientation, whether heterosexual or homosexual, is acquired gradually in the course of early life-learning experiences. To date, no unequivocally specific biologic causes for either a heterosexual or a homosexual orientation have been demonstrated. Biologic factors, such as physical appearance and the secondary sexual characteristics brought about by puberty, do have an indirect influence insofar as they cue the social environment to respond in certain appropriate or sometimes inappropriate ways. Even so, social learning appears to be the most powerful influence affecting an individual's sexual preferences. There is, of course, disagreement on the details of the learning process, but the essential findings of contemporary research suggest that a homosexual orientation is a logical and, indeed, almost predictable outcome of certain nonstandard life experiences occurring at particularly critical or sensitive periods in the lifetime of that person. Most commonly these experiences occur in the context of family life and involve child-rearing practices. Further, evidence from clinical research suggests that a person's gender identity and psychosexual orientation become manifest so early in life that it is now possible to identify the prehomosexual and pretranssexual individual in childhood. A redirection of social influences could conceivably lead to a heterosexual outcome. (More will be said about this later.) The militant homosexual, however, regards such research as irrelevant, and perhaps for him personally it is, for by adulthood the critical learning periods have passed and the possibilities for his acquiring an exclusively heterosexual orientation are increasingly remote.

Our national emphasis on rehabilitation and educational approaches to personal change is predicated on the psychologic and psychosocial plasticity of humans. In some areas of behavior though—gender identity and sex role being examples—human beings are not infinitely plastic and adaptive. The period of maximum plasticity for lower animals and humans alike is during very early life. Thereafter change can occur only with great difficulty, if at all. The implications of this for preventive intervention are obvious.

In view of these things, should we regard homosexuality as an illness requiring some kind of treatment, or is it, as the gay militancy asserts, simply an "alternative life style"? Since the words "sickness," "illness," and "disease" have come to have such depreciatory connotations, the point may be well taken that we do need a different term, or a reconceptualization to describe the person whose sexual preferences differ so sharply from those of the majority. Inasmuch as an exclusive homosexual orientation results from atypical psychosexual development, homosexuality would seem to be more than simply an alternative life style, for the individual has no more choice in the matter than does the heterosexual person.

The Legal Aspects

In countries where homosexuality is viewed with more understanding than in ours, homosexuals do not suffer from the self-condemnation and guilt so prevalent in the American gay community. The exclusively homosexual person seems fully entitled to the greater tolerance and acceptance by the rest of society that he now demands. On the other hand, it seems unlikely that our society will ever come to agree with the gay liberationists that homosexual love is a valid alternative to heterosexual love for everyone. To link acceptance of homosexual behavior with improved social relationships within a society, and to insist that homosexual love is identical with and as equally desirable as heterosexual love, seems biologically and socially unsound and scientifically inaccurate. Even so, there is no justice in viewing homosexuality as a crime, as is the case in most of the United States today. In addition, there is no evidence that relaxation of our punitive legal attitude toward homosexuality will result in increased numbers of homosexuals. In those countries where homosexuality is no longer a crime and where homosexual activity between two consenting adults is legally sanctioned, there has been no change in the *incidence* of homosexuality. Our laws do not condone public solicitation, the seduction of minors, and other activities by homosexuals or heterosexuals, nor should they. But private sexual activity with mutual consent should not be the concern of our legal system.

Erotic Reorientation of the Homosexual

Assertions of gay liberationists notwithstanding, some homosexuals do come to psychiatrists and other professionals, seeking help with problems related to their homosexuality. Some want help with depression, some want to resolve interpersonal difficulties that they are experiencing, some are threatened by a breakup of an important homosexual relationship, and so on. There is not the slightest justification for insisting that homosexuals "seek help" to become heterosexual, and most psychiatrists would never think of so doing. A few homosexuals, however, do genuinely want to become heterosexual, and there is no longer any question that certain homosexuals—depending on their motivation and the underlying causes for their homoerotic orientation—can become heterosexual. For although homosexuality is frequently unmodifiable, this is not always the case.

Although the literature on the subject is confused by methodological problems relating to research design, critieria for success, and follow-up, it does appear that perhaps as many as one-third of all male patients who attempt the shift from homoerotic to heterosexual erotic orientation can, with professional help, succeed. To achieve even this modest rate of success, the patient should ideally be under middle age, have been heterosexually responsive at some time in his life, have an assertive personality devoid of effeminacy and passivity, and his homoeroticism should be fairly recent in origin. Clearly, only a relatively few homosexuals qualify if these critieria for success continue to prove valid indices. The cry of gay liberationists to "stop looking for cures . . . we're not sick" must not be allowed to deter continuing research into improving our techniques for helping the reorientation of those homosexuals who do want help.

TRANSVESTISM

There are in our society three major groups of individuals who, with some regularity, dress in clothing considered more appropriate to members of the opposite biologic sex. This kind of behavior is called "cross-dressing" and is characteristic of a few (though by no means all) *homosexuals, transsexuals,* and *transvestites*. The tendency to lump all cross-dressing individuals together and call them transvestites only obscures our efforts to understand the problem. The homosexual who cross-dresses does so to attract attention to himself as a desirable homosexual partner. The transsexual, as will be discussed later, cross-dresses in order to feel "appropriately" dressed, for the transsexual is a person whose gender identity (sense of masculinity or feminity) is at variance with the biologic sex of his body.

Varieties of Transvestism

Transvestism is a more complex problem than the literature on the subject would lead one to suppose. It is frequently stated that in the transvestite cross-dressing is *fetishistic;* that is, the transvestite dresses in women's clothing to achieve an erection or to facilitate genital erotic activity. There is no denying that fetishism is an important dynamism in many transvestites, but it by no means represents a total explanation of transvestism. There is a second group of transvestic cross-dressers whose behavior is more nearly like that of a *compulsion*. For these individuals, cross-dressing behavior occurs in the context of certain specific types of psychologic stress and seemingly serves to relieve a dysphoric effect, such as anxiety or depression, or serves as an elaborate temporary erotic disguise for a wounded masculine self-image.

A third and perhaps the largest group of transvestites may share some of the fetishistic and compulsive elements, but in the main their cross-dressing is *expressive* in nature; that is to say, such transvestites view their dressing as women more simply as a matter of "expressing the feminine part of the personality." The men in this group—and they are all men—do not consider that they are women trapped in a man's body, as does the transsexual. They do not despise their male bodies. For the most part they function in traditionally masculine professions, are usually heterosexual, and frequently are married. The important distinction between this expressive form of transvestism and the fetishistic and compulsive forms is that these individuals assert their love of feminine things and of feminine gender role behavior, except for its erotic component. Indeed, one spokesman for such transvestites prefers the term "femmiphile."

Virginia "Charles" Prince, a well-educated transvestite who has written on the subject, has listed four factors that contribute to expressive transvestism: (1) the need to acquire virtue and to experience beauty ("This goodness and virtue is not expressful in masculine attire. It is out of place, but in feminine attire it is in order."); (2) the need for adornment and personality expression ("Some men find they can fulfill their natural desires by entering into the feminine world of color, fabric, decoration, and design."); (3) relief from the requirements of masculinity ("He cannot express all of his true self in masculine attire due to the social requirements and limitations placed on men and the feminine attire provides an outlet for the other part."), and (4) relief from social expectancy ("Most people cannot get away from themselves—the femmiphile, as his feminine self, can.")

Individuals in this group do not ordinarily come for psychiatric help unless pressured by others (perhaps a discontented wife) to do so. Their major satisfaction from cross-dressing appears to stem from successfully passing as a woman, and from a rather narcissistic display of themselves in convincingly feminine wigs, make-up, clothing, and manner. They thoroughly enjoy their successes in emulating the behavior and appearance of the opposite sex. Although this might suggest that this kind of transvestism is largely a matter of personal choice, there is good evidence to suggest that this is not the case. Research indicates that early life social experience is again largely responsible in having markedly affected gender identity and gender role behavior. For such individuals, the desire to cross-dress is compelling and sometimes troublesome. He must explain it to himself, to his spouse, and occasionally to other members of society. It is not an easy or comfortable thing for a transvestite to explain such unusual desires on the basis of the research literature alone. Instead, he tends to rationalize that such self-expression is normal and healthy, however atypical it is felt to be by the rest of society.

Perhaps more than any other group in our society, transvestites lead a double life. One survey of nearly 400 transvestites showed that 70 percent were married and 70 percent of these were fathers. Virtually all groups in society are represented in the transvestite world. Transvestism cuts through every socioeconomic bracket with some earning their livings at low-paying jobs and others being well-paid semiprofessionals and professionals. Many of the wives of transvestites know of their husbands' need to cross-dress; some have grown tolerant of it and may even actively aid and participate in the activity. Just as homosexuals and heterosexuals have their social groups, so, too, many transvestites have organized into social groups that meet regularly and frequently include their wives in the social activities. There are a number of publications, both books and magazines, intended for a transvestite audience. These publications are composed primarily of short stories, articles, case histories, pictures of attractively cross-dressed men, and advertisements for wigs, bras, and feminine underclothing. Some of the articles are aimed at the transvestite's wife, in an attempt to help her to understand and be more tolerant of her husband's compulsion to cross-dress. Other articles take issue with the scientific literature regarding the etiology of cross-dressing, because the transvestite, like the homosexual, is troubled by the slightest implication that his cross-dressing represents an illness or an abnormality.

The counterpart of this form of cross-dressing behavior in women has not been reported in the literature, though, of course, cross-dressing by females does occur in the instance of female transsexualism. Fetishistic transvestism or the more compulsive variety of transvestism seen in heterosexual men also does not seem to occur in women or, if it does, it is well disguised by the more liberal and permissive clothing styles allowed women in our society.

Helping the Transvestite

The compulsive cross-dresser, like the compulsive hand-washer, can be helped through sensitive, careful psychotherapy so that he is no longer pressured by a need to cross-dress. On the other hand, those individuals who cross-dress for fetishistic or expressive reasons have not been so successfully treated. Indeed, even the professional literature on the subject of treatment is scanty, for the low rate of success has dampened enthusiasm in this area of psychotherapy. If one can generalize, it does seem fair to say that single-garment fetishism (partialism) and cross-dressing in younger patients seem most responsive to current treatment methods, whereas those individuals with significant problems involving inappropriate "core" gender identity are not successfully treated. The common belief that a lengthy, in-depth psychoanalytic approach will succeed where other methods fail is not supported by the research literature.

TRANSSEXUALISM

The Development of Gender Identity

In the usual course of events sex chromosomes are responsible for "programming" the differentiation and functioning of gonadal tissue in the embryo. These embryonic gonads in turn determine whether fetal androgen will be secreted, and it is the presence or absence of fetal androgen that determines the maleness or femaleness of the external genitalia. Parents, in turn, respond to the appearance of the genitalia of the neonate by calling the child a boy or a girl and thereafter raising that child in ways that are culturally appropriate to its biologic sex. In most instances, a child who is developing normally begins to develop a concept of himself as a boy or of herself as a girl by the age of approximately two years. This self-concept is supported and reinforced by the ways in which the parents and other significant people in the child's life behave toward the child. In this way parents encourage a boy to behave in ways that are characteristic and appropriate for males in our society, and in like manner girls are encouraged to behave in ways that are feminine. The process itself involves "identification"—a process that resembles its near-counterpart of "imprinting" in lower animals. The little boy is encouraged by the father to act and think as males in our society act and think; the mother discourages emulation of her while encouraging identification with the father or other male figures. The result of all these interpersonal transactions during the first few years of a child's life is a sense of being a boy or a girl: gender identity.

If an individual's sense of identity is to serve him well throughout his life, the models from whom he or she has learned male or female gender role must have been clear, distinct, and appropriate to the culture in which that individual is to live. His or her gender models must have been unambiguous and the reinforcement consistent and progressive. Somewhere between the ages of three and five, gender identity becomes fully differentiated, insofar as its basic directions are concerned. The hormonal events of puberty serve only to activate eroticism. Even if there has been a hormonal failure or if there is an intrusion of inappropriate hormones (as in some forms of hermaphroditism), the person's gender identity remains consistent with the way in which he or she was reared. Sex chromosomes and sex hormones, per se, do not determine psychosexual orientation or the direction of an individual's erotic interest.

In rare instances, the process of gender identification, for one reason or another, goes astray. In the case of the person who becomes a transsexual, several elements seem to be required. Stoller's work illustrates clearly that to create a transsexual, a particular kind of mother, a particular kind of father, and particular kinds of child-rearing experiences are required. It is probable that one even needs a particular kind of appearance or responsiveness on the part of the child as well, to trigger the necessary social interactions. An intense closeness between mother and male child, perhaps triggered by the child's physical beauty, and uninterrupted by a passive, ineffectual, or absent father is the critical setting in which the process of gender identification can falter and go astray in a male's infancy and childhood. In the case of female infants who are to become transsexuals, a frequent finding has been a mother-infant relationship disrupted by maternal depression or emotional coldness, further complicated by a father who permits his daughter to be his substitute in providing loving care and attention for his depressed or disturbed wife. In significant degree, too, he substitutes his daughter as his closest companion and confidant, thereby providing her with a ready-made opportunity to identify with him; sometimes this is precisely what happens. The result of such incongruous identification can be transsexualism.

A disordered gender identity begins to be manifest very early in a child's life. By the age of three or four, the boy who is to become a transsexual begins to display feminine gracefulness and interest. For example, he plays with dolls and fantasies that he is their mother. He chooses girls for his playmates, and so convincing is he in his feminine demeanor that the girls accept him as a girl in their play activities. Later on, whenever he has a chance, he dresses up in girl's clothing, and frequently this behavior is not only tolerated but even approved of by the important adults in his life. During the early school years such a child feels marked confusion about his identity, and the confusion is further heightened at puberty by the advent of eroticism that, to the child's puzzlement, is triggered by the physical presence of other boys. The young teenage transsexual begins to think of himself now as perhaps being a homosexual. Some act upon these erotic impulses; many others carry it as a guilty secret, perplexed and puzzled because they feel themselves to be feminine and more like girls than boys except for their bodily status. Indeed, it is his own genitalia that are a daily reminder that he is a male despite his feminine sense of personal identity. From this comes the gradual conviction that he is really a woman trapped in a male body. (Transsexuals have even castrated themselves to rid themselves of the despised organs.) He despises his virilized male body as being out of keeping with how he feels as a person.

It is in this setting, then, that the wish to have his genitalia removed and altered to simulate female genitalia begins to grow.[1] In view of these things, is the transsexual's sense of incongruous gender identity an illness? A disease? A delusion? Is the transsexual's desire to dress according to his sense of identity and the wish for surgical transformation of the genitalia only further evidence of a disturbed individual? The author's admittedly biased view is that transsexualism is not an illness in the usual sense but once again an anomalous outcome of the process of psychosexual development.

Although most transsexuals have cross-dressed surreptitiously and many cross-dress more or less regularly, the author has seen many transsexuals who rejected the idea of cross-dressing and living as a member of the opposite sex as being somehow immoral unless they were first surgically converted. When the transsexual does cross-dress, however, it is never for fetishistic reasons; that is to say, he does not become sexually excited by women's clothes any more than does the average woman. When dressed as a man, the transsexual male feels as strange and inappropriately dressed as the average man would feel if he were to put on women's clothes and make-up. If the transsexual male has feminine features, he is aided in passing in society as a woman. His sexual interest is in normal heterosexual males, and an attractive, convincing transsexual usually has no difficulty establishing a love relationship as a woman with a heterosexual male. Surprisingly, even after the transsexual has disclosed his or her biological identity, it is not infrequent that the heterosexual lover will want to continue the relationship nonetheless, and may actively support efforts to obtain conversion surgery.

To those who have never seen or talked with a transsexual person the phenomenon of transsexualism may sound like the manifestation of

---

[1] Surgical conversion of transsexuals will be discussed further in the next subsection of this chapter.

a psychotic state. But the transsexual is not psychotic. He is quite aware of his true biologic status and shows no other signs to suggest a psychotic disorder. His tragedy is that he learned to feel, think, and act like the opposite biologic sex instead of like his own sex.

Helping the Transsexual Through Surgical and Hormonal Therapy

At the present time there is no known technique, either psychotherapeutic, pharmacologic, or re-educative, that will reverse an adult's core gender identity once established. This is true for transsexuals and nontranssexuals alike. The therapy of transsexualism has been revolutionized in recent years, however, by an increasing acceptance of the idea of approaching the problem by bringing the individual's body into greater conformity with gender identity by surgery. Sex conversion surgery, though not a new idea, has been systematically employed and researched for less than 10 years. Currently there are several university-based medical centers in this country and abroad developing the necessary surgical techniques and doing follow-up studies. Both biologic males and females have been converted by plastic surgery so that their bodies more closely simulate the sex corresponding to their gender identity. For the male, the process involves castration, construction of labia and an artificial vagina, breast augmentation by hormones and/or implants, and electrolytic removal of facial hair. For the biologic female transsexual, the process involves breast removal, virilization of the body with male sex hormones, and usually castration, hysterectomy, and vaginal closure. Although it is possible to construct a simulant artificial penis by plastic surgery, such a penis is not tumescent and erectile nor is it capable of evoking orgasm. For cosmetic purposes, a scrotal sac with plastic "gonads" is also surgically feasible.

So far the evidence suggests that nearly all of the transsexuals so converted have been benefited to the extent that they are happier and better satisfied with themselves as human beings. Despite the imperfections inevitable in such surgery, these patients seem to lead more comfortable lives, free from the previously present fear of discovery and of "living a deceitful life." Some have married and a few are functioning as parents to their spouses' children with apparent success. The time may come when such surgery will no longer be considered elective but a wholly reasonable and desirable approach to the resolution of the transsexual's life dilemma. This is not to say that everyone who requests conversion surgery will, or should, in the future, obtain it. Increasing numbers of pseudotranssexuals—troubled homosexuals and transvestites, not to mention a significant number of overtly psychotic persons—are seeking surgical conversion. The pseudotranssexual should never be considered a candidate for conversion surgery for he (she) does not qualify as a person with an inversion of gender identity. Only the much rarer true transsexual should ever undergo surgical and hormonal sex conversion therapy.

Ultimately, though, our goal should be prevention of transsexualism and the development of therapeutic methods which can help children whose gender identity is still in the process of formation.

SUMMARY AND CONCLUSIONS

We have reviewed, in an admittedly sketchy and superficial way, three varieties of atypical sexuality. Homosexuality either directly or indirectly touches the lives of millions of Americans. Transvestism and transsexualism, though far rarer behavior patterns, are nonetheless of deep concern to the individuals involved and to their families. In a society that attempts to base its behavior and attitudes on the findings of science, it is important that we utilize such findings to enhance our understanding and tolerance of those individuals whose sexuality deviates from the usual. There is still much to be learned and many problems to be solved before behavioral scientists and the public alike can be entirely comfortable with even the three varieties of sexual deviants discussed here. For example, how should we handle the homosexual's demand that persons of the same biologic sex be permitted to marry and enjoy the same legal advantages that heterosexual marriage provides? Legal adoptions by transsexuals who wish to raise children will pose a problem for adoption agencies. In neither instance— homosexual marriages or transsexual adoptions—has behavioral or social science provided much of a data base from which one can extrapolate answers. Instead, we now have controversy among lawyers and others concerned with individual civil rights regarding the pros and cons of a homosexual marriage, while social scientists can only speculate concerning the advantages or disadvantages of transsexuals attempting to provide healthy parental models for their adopted children. In time, no doubt, it will be more common for homosexual marriages to occur and for transsexuals to raise adopted children; the world can then make a judgment regarding the outcome. Meanwhile it seems prudent to maintain an open mind on these and other issues related to unusual forms of human sexuality. Sexuality has always been a matter that has tended to polarize emotions and attitudes for many Americans. In a country that prides itself on its scientific accomplishments we should insist that further research be pursued in this important area.

REFERENCES

Psychosexual Development and Gender Identity

Biller, H. B. 1971. Father, Child and Sex Role. Lexington, Boston, D. C. Heath Co.
Gadpaille, W. J. 1972. Research into the physiology of maleness and femaleness. *Arch. Gen. Psychiat.* **26:**193–206.

Hampson, J. L., and J. G. Hampson. 1961. The ontogenesis of sexual behavior in humans. *In* Sex and Internal Secretions, 3rd ed. W. C. Young, ed. Baltimore, Williams & Wilkins.

Marshall, D. S., and R. C. Suggs. 1971. Human Sexual Behavior. New York, Basic Books.

Stoller, R. J. 1968. Sex and Gender. New York, Science House.

Stoller, R. J. 1972. The "bedrock" of masculinity and feminity: bisexuality. *Arch. Gen. Psychiat.* **26:**207–212.

Homosexuality

Freund, K. 1960. Some problems in the treatment of homosexuality. *In* Behavior Therapy and the Neuroses. H. J. Eysenck, ed. New York, Pergammon Press.

Marmor, J. 1971. "Normal" and "deviant" sexual behavior. *J.A.M.A.* **217:**165–170.

Marmor, J., ed. 1965. Sexual Inversion. New York, Basic Books.

Weltge, R. W., ed. 1969. The Same Sex. Philadelphia, Pilgrim Press.

Wyden, P., and B. Wyden. 1968. Growing Up Straight. New York, Stein and Day.

Transvestism

Gelder, M. G., and I. M. Marks. 1969. Aversion treatment in transvestism and transsexualism. *In* Transsexualism and Sex Reassignment. R. Green and J. Money, eds. Baltimore, The Johns Hopkins Press.

Prince, C. V. 1965. Survey of 390 cases of transvestism. Delivered at the Western Divisional Meeting of the American Psychiatric Association, Honolulu.

Stoller, R. J. 1971. The term "transvestism." *Arch. Gen. Psychiat.* **24:**230–237.

Transsexualism

Green, R., and J. Money. 1969. Transsexualism and Sex Reassignment. Baltimore, The Johns Hopkins Press.

Green, R., L. E. Newman, and R. J. Stoller. 1972. Treatment of boyhood "transsexualism." *Arch. Gen. Psychiat.* **28:**213–217.

Stoller, R. J. 1972. Etiological factors in female transsexualism: a first approximation. *Arch. Sex. Behav.* **1.**

Stoller, R. J. 1968. Sex and Gender. New York, Science House.

CHAPTER 26

EQUALITY AND INEQUALITY: FACTS AND VALUES

MELVIN M. TUMIN

The disparity between the ideals of equality and the facts of inequality is a dominant fact in our lives today—in the United States and throughout the world. This is not to say that everywhere there is uniform endorsement of the ideal of equality, or that the actual inequalities are everywhere the same. Rather, legal and moral claims of entitlement to unequal portions of the good things of life can no longer be publicly advanced without showing that one has "earned" that right through some unequal contribution to the community.

At the same time, unequal shares of the good things of life—property, power, prestige, and all forms of psychic gratification—are visible everywhere. They divide the poor from the rich (individuals, groups, and nations), the black from the white, the young from the old, the female from the male, and the "low born" from the "well born." These disparities in actual shares often do not seem justified by anything except the power to preserve privileges which have been acquired over the centuries.

Accordingly, new demands by the "dispossessed"—the poor, the blacks, the young, the women, and the "underdeveloped" nations—for more equal shares of the good things of life are everywhere being made with increasing vigor and militance. Both the legitimacy and the morality of present-day inequalities are being challenged, and every major government of the world is under pressure to devise newer and more egalitarian forms of redistribution of opportunity, wealth, and power. Adults, males, whites, and wealthy individuals and nations are being pressed to share more equitably with their traditional underdog counterparts.

By contrast with inequality, equality seems such a natural, reasonable, and moral ideal that it is difficult to recall that inequality was considered the legitimate, moral, and natural condition until relatively recently in human history. Our lack of historical perspective also makes it difficult to understand why so much inequality should actually be present in the world today.

Two major questions emerge when one confronts the apparent para-

dox of widespread actual inequality in societies with the ideal of equality:
(1) What are the actual *natural* inequalities among humans? and (2) To
what extent must organized societies take account of these inequalities in
their patterned arrangements 'for distributing property, power, and
prestige?

The "natural differences" among humans, in which many believe, fall
into two classes: those that set apart various categories and groups, and
those that distinguish among individuals.

The group differences fall into three subdividisions: those between
high and low born, as exemplified in the Indian caste system among others;
those between males and females; and those between racial groups, including certain ethnic, religious, and national groups that are treated as
though they were separate races.

The low-born vs. high-born difference is one that no society need take
account of since there is no conceivable evidence to support any such
claims. These are matters sheerly of belief. Of course, when people act
in terms of such beliefs, as they do in various caste systems in the world,
then the consequences are serious and severe. But it is evident that the
differences in which people believe are mythical.

The differences between sexes and races, however, *seem* to have certain evidential supports. Men and women are constituted differently, look
different, and everywhere behave differently. And everywhere there are
differences among groups of people in average skin color, height, shape
of head, amount of body hair and beard, facial features, and other such
phenotypical features. When these differences in appearance are accompanied by differences in cultural patterns, as they often are, it seems quite
reasonable to most people to link the two sets of differences, such that
the differences in behavior are assumed to flow either from the differences
in appearance, or from some factor common to both appearance and behavior. This "logic" underlies most existing beliefs in natural and important differences between sexes and races.

Systematic and decisive evidence in these matters is only now beginning to be secured. All trends in that evidence suggest that with certain
minor exceptions, men and women are interchangeable members of the
human species for all relevant *cultural* functions.

Yet existing norms of sex differentiation do not embody this awareness. To the contrary. Thus, the fact that the female of the species has
ovaries, a womb, and the mammary equipment for nursing children is
used to justify the notion that women *should* be the rearers of children
and specialists in domestic service. To reason this way, however, is to use
neutral biological facts—the presence of ovaries, womb, and breasts—to
justify highly consequential *value decisions* regarding the proper division
of labor between men and women, on the grounds that these decisions
are in line with nature's intentions.

In fact, however, *biological* maternity and *social* maternity are eminently separable—as are biological and social paternity. Many societies throughout the world practice some such separation, as for instance, when the mothers' brothers and *not* the women's husbands are assigned the role of social fathers to their sisters' children.

Of course, since only women can breast-feed children, if no other supply of milk is available and milk is considered essential nourishment for the babies, then it makes sense to assign that limited function to women. Aside from such limited "natural" accommodations in culture to the facts of biology, the differences between men and women do not otherwise seem naturally to suggest the rightness of any one version of a division of labor over any other. The naturally greater average strength and speed of men over women may be culturally relevant in hunting bands, but become increasingly irrelevant with every technological innovation. Indeed, in many technologically primitive societies, women do heavier work than men.

The appeals to "nature" which many make in support of existing cultural arrangements between men and women are themselves a very special and limited form of cultural rationale. Nature presents the human species with certain geographic, climatic, and biological facts to which the human being then responds in a variety of ways. This variety of responses—often quite different from one culture to another—derives from learned values and knowledge and their adaptation to resources and technology. All of these are themselves natural products of a natural creature, called the human being, and they exemplify a central fact about that being, namely, that he (she) is a *uniquely cultural animal*. Culture, as manifested in "acts and artifacts," is as natural as trees, streams, mountains, minerals, skin color, ovaries, and gold. Hence, to appeal to "nature" to justify certain time-and-space-bound cultural decisions is to assign to physical and biological nature a "directionality" that it does not have and a priority over human nature that cannot be justified. Moreover, any examination of the variable ways in which humans respond to facts of biological and physical nature throughout the world will reveal that there is always great selectivity in the choice of which facts are observed, which are responded to, and what the character of the responses is.

Now, can the dominance of one society over others—whether this dominance is technological, military, economic, scientific, or whatever—be brought forth as evidence of the correctness of superiority of one set of responses to nature as against others? Such cultural dominances are temporary facts of human historical life, and, in any event, to adduce them in justifying the "way of life" of the temporarily dominant people is to engage in the self-confirming hypothesis.

It is ironic how little noticed is the fact that those groups in the world which, because of the absence of the requisite values, knowledge, and technology, live "closest" to physical nature in their economic pursuits are those which are least technologically advanced. If anything, then, this would suggest that human "progress" depends on the deliberate subversion of nature by culture. But that argument is as specious as its opposite. The only reasonable conclusion one can draw here is that the facts of biological and physical nature are "value neutral" and nondirectional and do not naturally call for or justify any one form of cultural response over any other. All societies are very selective, we repeat, regarding which "natural" facts they notice and how they respond to these facts.

What has been said about the cultural interchangeability of women and men must be said with equal force about the so-called races of mankind. There is no evidence that will support any conclusion about race differences more reasonably than the conclusion that the races are randomly varying, trivially differentiated specimens of the same human species. The relevant scientists are now generally agreed that a race consists of a breeding group (a *cultural* fact) that exhibits one or more distinctive gene frequencies. By this definition, there are hundreds or thousands of races of mankind—the number finally depending on how many different genetic characteristics one wishes to take into account and how "distinctive" must the "distinctiveness" of these characteristics be.

Moreover, because there are groups of the breeding population that constitute cultural facts (based as they are, on beliefs, values, preferences, and choices), races as they exist at any one time must be seen as *temporary* aggregations, whose constituency and characteristics will surely change under the impact of subsequent contacts with other breeding groups, for these contacts always result in interchange of genes. Given this fact, the only possible condition under which a pure race could exist, as Ralph Linton once pointed out, is a condition in which the men of the group were too cowardly to seize the women of other groups, and/or the women of the group were too repulsive to be desired by the men of the other group.

Current efforts by a limited group of scientists in the United States to revive the formerly dominant belief in significant differences between blacks and whites, especially in regard to culturally relevant intelligence, have been met with contrary superior evidence and logic mustered by the dominant majority of the concerned scientific community. That evidence and logic command the conclusion that any contention about significant racial differences between black and white, here or elsewhere, shall be judged unproven. Until black and white color can be made neutral cultural facts in this and other societies, and until some reliable instrument for testing natural intelligence (assuming that concept has some significant meaning) has been developed, the best conclusion one can draw from existing data is that black and white are interchangeable members of the human species.

If certain groups appear at this historical moment to have dispropor-
tionate percentages of members who are specially talented—intellectually,
athletically, musically, or whatever—the appearance must be subjected to
rigorous tests of reality. If those tests should verify the apparent differences,
then explanations must first be sought in the special cultural histories
and situations of the groups, including their political exclusion from other
lines of effort, that lead them to specialize in one or another cultural function, such as intellectual profundity, athletic and musical entertainment,
grace in social affairs, or preference for blooded sports.

On the basis of what we now know, it is most probable that all such
apparent "natural" differences between groups will be found to be explain-
able mostly if not totally in terms of each group's special cultural histories
and situations. Any residue of unexplained variance is likely to be due to
subtle cultural inhibitors and facilitators that we have not yet conceptual-
ized because we have not felt pressed to do so.

If the major *group* differences among humans seem relatively inconse-
quential, as they do, what then of individual differences? Here we confront
quite another realm of facts. For it is undeniable that there are wide ranging differences among humans, without regard to color or sex, in factors
highly relevant to cultural functions, such as intelligence, creativity, and
temperament. The human species is highly variable in these and other matters, just as is apparently every other animal species.

What, then, is to be done about the demands for equality now being
heard so widely today? If humans are in fact unequal in their culturally
relevant abilities, what forms and amounts of inequality in property,
power, and prestige do these differences justify, if any? Posing the question
this way indicates, as we mean to do, that even if, and when, all existing
inequalities between sexes and races were to be obliterated, we would still
have to face the problems presented by inter-individual variability.

Any answers to the question of "what should be done" necessarily
presuppose certain restrictive cultural values and goals that one desires
to achieve, along with certain beliefs—true or otherwise—about the
greater efficiency of certain social arrangements over others in the pursuit
of these values and goals. For example, it is widely argued that humans
of superior natural endowments, which are relevant to desired cultural
goals, will not be motivated to train and utilize their talents in the desired
ways unless they are "motivated" to do so by the promise of unequal rewards. This is the traditional argument advanced by some sociologists regarding the "unavoidability of social stratification." But serious doubt has
been cast upon this claim. When examined, it proves to rest upon a theory
of human nature derived from the model of the marketplace of goods
and services and the fluctuation of supply and demand in that marketplace. This example illustrates how special sets of beliefs and values can
and do distort scientific theories.

In any event, individual differences in human talents, like group differences, are *neutral* biological facts to which cultures may or may not wish to attend and respond. Thus, the practice of rewarding the more naturally talented people with unequal shares of the good things of life is only one special practice among many possible others. To give unequal shares of life's valued things to people who by accident are born with greater genetic potentials must be seen for what it is: namely, the substitution of an aristocracy of the genes for the former aristocracy of family and noble descent.

It cannot be denied that the response to differences in talent in human societies almost always results in social inequalities. But what has been true in human history so far can hardly be cited in support of the claim of the rightness or efficiency of such arrangements. One must also avoid the mistake of equating the *practical political* difficulties of altering existing social arrangements with the *theoretical* impossibility or difficulty of making those alterations.

Yet, since most people take existing ways of thinking and believing as "human nature," the argument that existing forms are always theoretically subject to modification is not normally very persuasive. Nevertheless, when we are considering the range of possibilities in human affairs, the *theoretically* possible must always be taken as the primary guide. Here, then, again one must be aware of the separability of biological superiority and social advantage. The fact that societies throughout the world practice very different kinds and degrees of social inequality is strong persuasive evidence that biological and social inequalities are eminently separable.

In light of these considerations, the present demands for greater equality in property, power, and prestige must be seen as one special version of changeable and changing social morality. If the current of affairs today makes the demands for equality seem so much more eminently legitimate and moral than the claims for inequality, that current ideological trend must not be mistaken for an eternal verity. The facts of biological nature do not justify social inequality, but do they justify social equality? Equality and inequality in social situations are values that have to be justified, if at all, in terms of other values and goals desired.

Should we reward humans according to their abilities, or according to their needs, or some combination of both, or by some other as yet unannounced criteria? These are questions we are in the midst of debating and contesting often with great vehemence, and, more frequently these days, with some degree of violence. More often than is salutary for rational consideration, this debate is put in terms of the mediocrity of egalitarianism vs. the oppressiveness of elitism. These are obviously simpleminded and hence dangerous formulations of very complex questions.

Crucial concerns are at stake in this debate. These include the utilization of human talents; efficiency in the production of goods and services;

the struggles between sovereign national powers, and hence questions of war and peace; marital and family stability and functioning, depending on sex-role assignment; the rearing of children; the conduct of the schools; the modes of recruitment for specialized tasks; the division of the world's natural resources; the presence of poverty and hunger midst affluence and satiation; and the ecological balance between physical nature and human productivity. Also at stake are fundamental moral and ethical concerns, involving theories of entitlement, obligation, fairness, political rule, and the qualities of human interchange.

We approach these issues knowing that numerous and diverse possibilities are open to us and that we are not bound by the facts of physical or biological nature to one solution more than to any other. We know, too, that cultures go *against* physical nature on behalf of cultural values as often as they "conform" to that physical nature. Any set of solutions to any of these problems necessarily entails losses and costs along with such gains and profits—material, psychological, spiritual, moral, and social—as may emerge. Since any solution is sure to be diverse in its balance of positive and negative outcomes, we should at least be armed with a knowledge of the limits and possibilities, including such information about the consequences of existing patterns as may enable us to make more enlightened choices in the future.

CHAPTER 27

EPILOGUE

ROBERT H. WILLIAMS

In this chapter I will recapitulate some of the points made in this book and add some of my own thoughts on the subjects covered by other contributors. At the end I will summarize some major conclusions regarding life and death.

BODY, MIND, AND SOUL IN LIFE, DEATH, AND THE HEREAFTER

The prime function of the body is mentation; all parts are subservient to this function (Chapter 2). Without mentation the body does not serve a useful function and need not continue to live; in the future some of its organs will be used more often for transplantations. Mentation and behavior are affected by the chemical and physical status of the brain. All abnormalities in mentation are presumably associated with altered cerebral metabolism. This abnormal metabolism may result from primary disease in the brain, from disorders in other parts of the body, or from environmental influences. Specific biochemical changes in the brain are associated with sleep, rage, learning, memory, and other mental states. A single primary biochemical abnormality can produce marked mental retardation and bizarre behavior.

The soul has been described in many ways. The characterization I find most comprehensible is that the soul is a special aspect of mentation (Chapter 3). Presumably, with no mentation there can be no soul, no active communication with God, no moral actions, and no personality. People who have abnormal actions of the soul apparently have abnormal mentation. Qualitative as well as quantitative abnormalities in the functions of mind and soul exist.

Many of us have been told since earliest childhood that we must live righteously and productively, doing our best in every way to gain glory in Heaven. The Hereafter has been pictured in many ways, and some of these characterizations embody extensive and colorful conjectures. As in the case of the soul, some people regard the Hereafter as consisting of many mystical aspects. My own concept is that the Hereafter consists of memories and other reminders of the characteristics and activities a person has displayed during his lifetime—things he has said, experiences (good and bad) that he has had, actions he has or has not taken, his physical appearance, recordings of some of his statements, photographs, drawings, sculptures, etc.

We tend to honor our great men and women after they have died. The buildings that we dedicate and the monuments and portraits we commission all bring great pride to the family, but the person being honored knows nothing of them. The large amounts we spend for embalming, caskets, graves, tombstones, and flowers have a value only for those left behind, since the deceased apparently never knows anything about them. Even for the survivors, it seems pleasanter to think more on the full spectrum of the person's life and less on the cold dirt and stone in the cemetery.

When the body is not preserved as with embalming fluid, it decomposes rapidly and minute amounts of certain constituents are acquired by plants and animals, some of which are devoured by man and incorporated into his body. With cremation these constituents are also reutilized in infinitesimal amounts, but we do not see evidence of a significant amount of reincarnation.

Some thoughts regarding the Hereafter can be crystallized if we consider certain consequences of brain transplantation (see the next section for details). If John Doe, age 30, with a long criminal history, receives the brain of Thomas Brown, who has normal mentation, John Doe's subsequent behavior will be normal, assuming that the nonbrain portion of his body is normal. When John Doe dies 20 years later, what will the Hereafter be like for him? What will it be like for Thomas Brown? When would the Hereafter begin for each? Would the many sins of John Doe be forgiven in view of his subsequent 20 years of righteous living? Would he experience the tortures of Hell or the grandeurs of Heaven? As I see it, John Doe's aberrant behavior was conditioned by chemical abnormalities in his first brain, so that after receiving the normal brain he would behave normally. For John Doe the Hereafter would actually begin at the time of the brain transplant, because his mentation and soul would cease then. For Thomas Brown, the Hereafter would begin 20 years after the brain transplant because during these 20 years the mentation and soul, although lodged in the body of John Doe, were really those of Thomas Brown. Thomas Brown's prime function, mentation, prevailed in two people and certain associations would be made with each. Throughout the 20 years after the transplant, relatives, friends, and the public could be less critical and more forgiving of John Doe than if he had had no transplant.

SOME MAJOR EFFECTS OF ORGAN TRANSPLANTATION

Future progress probably will permit transplantation of several organs into one body; with enormous advances possibly even the brain (or head) can be transplanted. Although we cannot be sure that such transplants will be successful, this approach serves as an interesting format for discussion. It was stated in Chapter 3 that if the heart of Moses Jones, the kidneys of Ho Chinn, the liver of Joe Murphy, and the brain of Rebecca Goldstein were transplanted into John Doe, the mentation and soul would be essentially those of Rebecca Goldstein (Fig. 1, Chapter 3). Now I will discuss some of the results that might be anticipated from transplantation of brain, heart, liver, or gonads. In each category the donors and recipients were 30 years old. Except for the donor in Fig. 1, all of the body functions of the donors had been normal and all of the body functions of the recipient, except for the organ replaced, had been normal or became normal after transplantation.

Since the organ transplantations discussed below have not yet been done successfully, my discussion of the probable results of such transplants is conjecture based upon observations of somewhat related phenomena. Much of the rationale in conjecturing brain function is presented in Chapter 2. However, I emphasize that *we cannot be sure of the results,* especially over long intervals, until we actually observe them. Certain psychologic reactions to receiving an organ of another person would influence the results, but these effects are assumed to be less significant than those discussed below. The name applied to each recipient is the same as was always applied to his body, despite marked personality changes; the only exception is the person subjected to transsexual operation.

(a) *Effect of Transplanting a Normal Brain from a Woman (Rebecca Goldstein) into a Man (John Doe) on his sex interests and actions.* Since sex assignment is generally based upon the genitalia, after replacement of John Doe's brain by that of Rebecca Goldstein, he will continue to be designated as male because of his male genitalia (Fig. 1a). Each body cell continues to be male, except for the brain cells, which are female. Since these cells are responsible for the thinking and emotional reactions of the body and have been conditioned for many years for a female role, this pattern will prevail despite the male physiognomy (Chapter 25). Indeed, experiences with patients have demonstrated that even when sex assignment has been erroneous, it usually cannot be changed satisfactorily after it has prevailed for several years. Therefore, John Doe's sex desires are now more like those of Rebecca Goldstein, because they are greatly influenced by the many years of conditioning along feminine lines. However, the larger quantity of androgen in John Doe's body stimulates more sexual desire than Rebecca Goldstein had. Some of John Doe's sexual activity may be decreased by psychological conflicts (produced by having a woman's brain in a man's body), and possibly by the fact that the levels of androgen in Rebecca Goldstein's original body, at the time when her sexual desires were being conditioned, were lower. Since Rebecca Goldstein long had a female sex role and a male

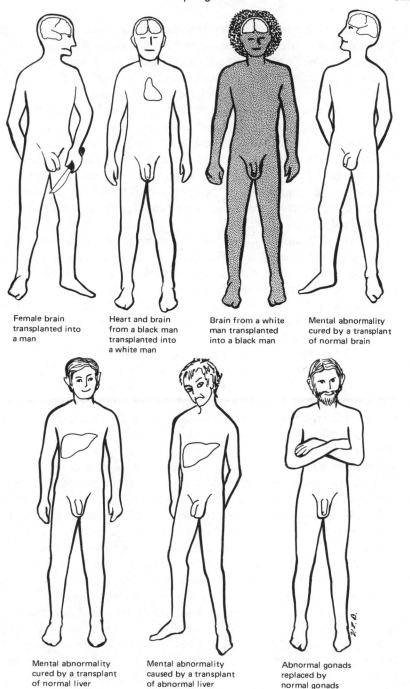

Female brain transplanted into a man

Heart and brain from a black man transplanted into a white man

Brain from a white man transplanted into a black man

Mental abnormality cured by a transplant of normal brain

Mental abnormality cured by a transplant of normal liver

Mental abnormality caused by a transplant of abnormal liver

Abnormal gonads replaced by normal gonads

Fig. 1. Transplantation of brain, heart, liver, and gonads. In the text, conjectures of the effect of each of these operations upon behavior are presented. We cannot predict the extent of future success with these transplantations.

mate, John Doe now presumably has reactions of homosexuality (male) and transvestism (desire for female clothes) and wants transsexual conversion (to female). Although the recipient is still designated as John Doe, the thinking patterns and personality tend to be those of Rebecca Goldstein. Therefore, John Doe will think and act femininely. He will want to wear feminine clothes and get rid of his gonads, genitalia, beard, and other masculine features. He probably will seek breast enlargement (through hormone treatment and plastic bag insertions), surgical creation of a vagina, and other female characteristics. Then the person will be designated Rebecca Goldstein despite the fact that all body cells, except those of the brain, are male. No longer will her feminine dress be considered transvestism or her sexual indulgence with males be called homosexuality.

(*b*) *Effect of Transplanting a Heart or Brain from a Black Man (Moses Jones) into a White Man (John Doe) on his Reactions of Racial Prejudice and Discrimination.* Transplanting Moses Jones's heart into John Doe would have no significant effect on John Doe's feelings of racial prejudice if it were not revealed to him and others that he had a heart from a black person. Even if it were known, the reactions probably would not differ very much.

If Moses Jones's brain were transplanted into John Doe (Fig. 1b), but it was not revealed to others that the brain from a black person was used, John Doe would encounter much less prejudice than Moses Jones had because John Doe's skin would not be black. However, some unfavorable reactions would result from John Doe's new problack bias—for example, his tendency to associate more closely with black people than with whites. John Doe would now hyperreact to racial discrimination and prejudice because Moses Jones had been conditioned by so many previous experiences. As the years passed he probably would become less race sensitive because his white skin would have caused fewer psychologic reactions in him and others. If it were generally known that Moses Jones's brain had been transplanted, some members of the white public would probably exhibit more prejudice and discrimination, but less than Moses Jones would have experienced before transplantation. Much of the response of the black public would depend upon the extent to which John Doe was prowhite or problack.

(*c*) *Effect of Transplanting a Normal Brain from a White Man (John Doe) into a Black Man (Moses Jones) on his Reactions of Racial Prejudice and Discrimination.* Had John Doe's brain, when normal, been transplanted into Moses Jones (Fig.1c), the result would be difficult to predict. John Doe's brain would not have been conditioned by years of racial oppression and discrimination. Such conditioning is accompanied by anxiety regarding the existence of racial prejudice but also by some refractoriness in responding to it. With John Doe's brain,

Moses Jones would be expected to have less of each of these reactions. He would prefer associating with white people because he would have memories of having done this for many years (while the brain was in John Doe). However, he would increase his associations with blacks, because of his black skin, because he would be received better by black people, and because he would be rejected by some white people. On the other hand, the fact that he would tend to think and act like a white man might decrease his associations with some black people. Hopefully, he would be stimulated to work with whites and blacks to overcome discrimination and prejudice.

(*d*) *Effect upon Abnormal Mentation of Transplanting a Normal Brain.* Transplanting a normal brain into a person with abnormal mentation but with normal function of nonbrain organs should produce normal mentation (Fig. 1d). Thus, an insane person could be converted to one who is sane, a criminal to a noncriminal, a sinner to a nonsinner, and a sexual deviant to one with normal sex interest.

This example is given to emphasize once again that normal mentation and behavior depend upon normal brain function. When the primary functions of nonbrain structures are normal but those of the brain are abnormal, the abnormal mentation that results can be corrected by implanting a normal brain.

(*e*) *Effect upon Abnormal Mentation of Transplanting a Normal Liver.* Many diseases are accompanied by abnormal mentation even though there is no primary disorder in brain function. This occurs with certain abnormalities in function of the liver, pancreas, or other body organs which cause abnormal biochemical constituents to accumulate in the brain. If this situation can be corrected before the brain has changed irreversibly, the mental abnormality can be corrected too. Perhaps in the future some mental abnormalities can be abolished by replacement of an abnormal liver, or other affected organ, with a normal one (Fig. 1e).

(*f*) *Effect upon Normal Mentation of Transplanting an Abnormal Liver.* A person who has normal mentation and a normal brain may develop permanently abnormal mentation if he receives an organ transplant, such as a liver, that produces an appreciable amount of abnormal metabolites of certain types (Fig. 1f). The organ donor would have had a similar type of mental abormality, but the association might not have been recognized.

(*g*) *Effect of Gonad Transplantation upon the Progeny.* Some people are sterile, and others can reproduce but have a genetic disorder that carries a high risk for the offspring. In the distant future, such situations might be corrected by transplanting normal gonads (Fig. 1g). Sex desire and capacity to reproduce can be expected to be normal. The genetic characteristics transmitted to the progeny would be those of the gonad donor and the gonad recipient's mate. If a couple's infertility is due to male gonadal deficiency, artificial insemination could supply offspring with some genetic characteristics of the female. In time, however, gonad transplantation in the male could have the same result but could permit the male to feel that he has played a role in the reproduction.

CREATION AND PROPAGATION OF LIFE; POPULATION INCREASE

The earth was created about 4.5 billion years ago, apparently through the condensation of cold cosmic dust. It required more than a billion years to cool sufficiently to be compatible with life. Life presumably appeared according to natural laws of chemistry and physics (Chapter 4). It has been shown recently that when some of the gases that accumulated on the outer surface of the earth (hydrogen, methane, ammonia, and water vapor) are subjected to electrical discharge, within a week more than 20 of the common elements of the living systems are produced in large quantity. In the course of the evolutionary process numerous enzymes were formed, and they greatly accelerated the formation of more complex forms of life. In time, matter was formed in such a way that it could lead to a duplication of its structure, this being a fundamental attribute of a living system. When one polynucleotide of a given type was produced, it preferentially interacted with another chain of complementary structure. In this manner genetic information began to be stored, chiefly in DNA, and a self-replicating system was produced. Mutations occurred that made the organisms better adapted to their environment and simultaneously aided their survival and perpetuation. On the earth it took about 1.5 billion years for life to appear and twice that long for man to develop. It is estimated that life exists on 0.1 percent (150 million) of the planets. The sun has fuel for about 7 billion more years, but life on earth may well become extinct before then.

The DNA of the nuclear chromatin of germ cells contains a large number of messages which are transmitted through messenger RNA to the protein manufacturing center, the ribosomal system (Chapter 5). The amount and type of protein synthesized greatly influence body functions. The nature of the messages directs the formation and function of various body organs. If as little as one ten-millionth of the DNA is abnormally structured it can cause a pronounced alteration in mental or physical behavior. It is estimated that from 5 to 25 percent of patients have genetic diseases, many of which are relatively insignificant. Ideally, it is desirable to detect the nature and location of the abnormal gene in the DNA molecule and to replace it with a normal gene. However, even if one can ascertain this information, it is difficult to get the correct parts of DNA to penetrate the cell wall and to be incorporated appropriately in the DNA of the cell nucleus. Since bacterial viruses have a unique property of binding specifically to certain cells and of becoming incorporated intact in the nuclear DNA, it is hoped that by attaching the needed normal gene to a certain type of virus the gene can become incorporated into the appropriate location of DNA and promote normal action. Much remains to be done before this approach can be used satisfactorily. Meanwhile, various other measures are being used to decrease the frequency of genetic abnormalities and to decrease their ill effects.

Increased efforts are being made to prevent gene mutation by X ray, atomic radiation, and various chemicals. More attention is being given to avoiding mating of two people who are carriers of certain genetic abnormalities that are likely to cause major diseases such as diabetes and sickle cell anemia. Artificial insemination is used in some instances when the father is the carrier of the undesirable traits; adoption is encouraged when the mother is a carrier. During early pregnancy, some fluid bathing the fetus can be removed by needle and syringe (amniocentesis), examined, and cultured. In this manner many genetic abnormalities can be detected, and when indicated the pregnancy is terminated. The fetus of a subsequent pregnacy may be normal. Efforts are made to avoid pregnancy when the woman is more than 35 years of age because of the frequency of mongolism; by the age of 45 it is 2.5 percent.

Many endocrine diseases caused by genetic abnormality are managed satisfactorily by removing the gland that produces excessive hormone or by administering sufficient hormone to correct the hormone deficiency. In certain genetic disturbances associated with the accumulation of products that alter brain or other organ functions, dietary measures are sometimes helpful. For example, brain alterations in people with phenylketonuria are decreased by dietary restriction of phenylalanine, and those of galactosemia are decreased by omitting milk from the diet.

In the past century numerous changes have occurred that affect the quality and quantity of people propagated, their pattern of living, and the time and cause of death (Chapters 6, 7, and 16). Especially prominent in producing these changes are technologic developments. They have offered both advantages and disadvantages, providing improved farm implements, transportation, communication, clothing, food, shelter, preventive and therapeutic health aids, and many other items. They have greatly decreased the death rate at all ages, but especially in the young. They have provided means for contraception and abortion, but also for increasing fertilization. They have caused ill-health and death as a result of pollution of air, water, food, and other components; automobile accidents; drug toxicity; and in other ways.

A marked population increase has resulted chiefly from increased survival. With the increase in young survivors there is a significant increase in the number of people having children. To avoid excessive increase in population and to improve its quality, we should systematically institute many measures to produce widespread participation in various well-organized programs. Some detailed considerations are presented in Chapters 5, 6, and 7.

TOO MANY AND TOO FEW LIMITATIONS
FOR CHILDREN

In dealing with our children we have been distinctly superconventional, overwhelming them with our own ambitions and failing to recognize that children can have different patterns. Consequently, we have not appropriately respected the fact that different courses in life are desirable. At the same time, we have extended so much freedom in certain ways that some of the children have been overwhelmed and frustrated by the many decisions they have had to make (Chapter 14). The resulting anxiety, fears, and frustrations have caused some of them to withdraw from reality, resorting to drugs, sometimes dropping out of school, leaving home, and in other ways avoiding pressure. Many have received too little love, patient attention, understanding from their parents with regard to their concepts, and assurance.

EXCESSIVE FEARS, ANXIETIES, AND FRUSTRATIONS

Man differs from other animals in his greater capacities in many ways, including perception, interpretation, memory, integration, association, communication, and emotional responses to experiences (Chapter 17). The nervous system has billions of cells and extensive intercommunications for accomplishing these functions. This system alerts man to his surroundings, permitting him to interpret various events and to respond appropriately. A multitude of memories, associations, and interpretations are often involved in man's ability to initiate various activities, creative thoughts, and actions.

Some of the greatest accomplishments and pleasures in life occur during periods of great emotional stress, but some of the strongest suffering can occur at such times, too. The nature of emotional responses depends very much on the individual's past experiences and on the patterns of response that he has established. When he has been subjected to many stresses, especially major ones, that have been very threatening, he may have become conditioned to respond excessively with fear, anxiety, and frustration. Such reactions are associated with hyperactivity of the autonomic nerve system and many endocrine glands, which may produce marked changes in the vascular, respiratory, gastrointestinal, muscular, and other systems. In this manner, numerous psychosomatic disorders can result (e.g., abdominal cramps, nausea, vomiting, hay-fever-like symptoms, headache, sensation of suffocation). In the United States psychosomatic problems have apparently increased significantly in ghettoes of big cities;

some of this presumably has been associated with increased density of population and the increased competition in social, economic, emotional, and other activities. Man often feels uncertain about how well he registers in the minds of others and feels threatened by competition from them. He is challenged frequently to make adjustments to actions of others, and often these challenges promote feelings of insecurity, anxiety, and frustration. The accumulation of these reactions has been the basis for increased campus unrest, demonstrations, and protests; career problems; and crime. These problems are now briefly discussed.

(a) *Campus Anxieties, Frustrations, and Protests*

Farnsworth has carefully reviewed many factors that have caused the campus uprisings, protests, anxieties, and frustrations, and also some of the reasons for their being less frequent in the last 1–2 years (Chapter 18).

During the past decade, a significant number of young people have lost confidence in their elders, themselves, our government, and the ideals in which they were brought up to believe. Many have been disturbed by apparent incongruities of ideals and actions of their elders. Affluence has increased for many even while the problem of poverty has remained unsolved. As the population has increased, more education has been needed to get good jobs. Education and communication media have increased knowledge of social injustices and have spread disillusionment among the young. Some of the young have become so disturbed that they want to withdraw from these problems and seek unconventional comforts. Discouraged in dealing with their elders, young people have sought ways to achieve warm relationships with their contemporaries, leaning more heavily on one another, concentrating on the present and discounting lessons of the past. Discouragement and anxiety have led many to use psychedelic drugs.

Some groups of young people devoted themselves to stimulating discontent. Protests and violence on campuses increased. But problems were not solved in this destructive manner. More constructive and less violent forms of protest are returning, prompted especially by wise, well-balanced, and dedicated activities of other young people. Therefore, these problems of life are going through the same pendulum pattern as many others (Fig. 2, Chapter 1)—underactivity, overactivity, antiactivity, and then a fairly optimal level of activity.

(b) *Careers*

Career failure often causes great unhappiness. Such failure frequently is caused by improper selection of a career (Chapter 15). For optimal performance, it is important for a person to choose a career in which he has both interest and ability. These areas tend to be the same. When the goals seem to be in excess of capacity, anxiety, distress, and frustration develop.

(c) *Crime*

A crime consists of breaking the law. Since this can range from parking a car illegally to murder, there are marked differences in crimes and criminals. Many criminals are never charged with more than one crime, while some are involved with repeated crimes throughout their lives. My comments in this section refer predominantly to criminals who commit one or more major crime or to those who commit many crimes, small or large. Menninger (Chapter 20) emphasizes that the increasing maladaption and maladjustment in society have increased the frequency and consequences of crime. Many criminals have a distorted view of society, and vice versa. Criminals and society often display hostility and revenge toward each other. Poverty, oppression, crowded living conditions, frustrated ambitions, genetic abnormalities and various other types of illness, and improper rearing are prominent factors contributing to crime. Juvenile delinquency is promoted when parents vacillate between excessive permissiveness and strictness (Chapters 14 and 20).

Management of criminals has consisted chiefly of punishment and confinement. Imprisonment increases reactions of dependency, violence, and dehumanization; these reactions increase with the duration of imprisonment. Not much opportunity for decision is offered to prisoners. Play, work, and other activities are routinely programmed. Resentment and sometimes violence are stimulated by constant regimentation, repression, demeanment, impersonal relationships (prison numbers, uniforms), restricted communication and correspondence, disinterest, and neglect.

Recently, there has been increasing emphasis upon rehabilitation, but the amount has been meager (Chapters 20 and 21). The transition from imprisonment to a normal life outside of prison is too big a jump for many, especially those with many unsolved emotional problems. Various economic, sociologic, neurotic, or psychotic problems may require some degree of professional assistance. As I have discussed in the Prologue, each prisoner must be carefully evaluated and managed in accordance with his problems. Proper management of these problems necessitates a large personnel with varied specific training, which is costly. However, we are already paying high costs with relatively little return.

TECHNOLOGY IN THE WELFARE OF MAN

The enormous technological advances that have occurred in the last half century (Chapter 16) have brought both happiness and unhappiness. Improved farm machinery has made it possible for less than 10 percent of the population to supply a great abundance of food for the entire United States, plus significant surpluses that are exported. We have brisk transportation and instant communication both nationally and internationally. Our homes, yards, offices, and industrial plants are filled with machines that have reduced the long hard physical labor of the past to 40 hours per week, with indications that further reductions to 30–35 hours may occur. We have a great array of mechanical devices for dealing with health problems, including artificial kidneys, respirators, facilities for total intravenous alimentation, and artificial devices for locomotion, seeing, and hearing. Technological progress has presumably increased our happiness and has certainly increased our physical comforts, but also seems to have increased the incidence of mental problems, suicide, homicide, thievery and other crimes, drug addiction, alcoholism, and other problems. The pride of craftsmanship and satisfaction for a job well done are often not enjoyed by individuals on an assembly line.

Mankind has become highly competitive, yet in the establishment of big businesses many small competitors have been crowded out of business. The big business leaders then find themselves heading drives to offer benefits for all, including those whom they have oppressed in business. Numerous farmers have left the farm to work in city factories, but many were not properly prepared for such work and have found themselves living in substandard housing and in poverty in central areas of cities. On the other hand, the rural areas contain about half of the nation's poor.

Better nutrition, housing, clothing, and various health measures have significantly prolonged the average length of life. Yet at the same time many old people are very unhappy.

Our great progress in utilizing machinery has caused widespread pollution of air and water. We hope that the technology that has caused so many of these problems can now be used to correct them (Chapter 16).

MARRIAGE

Mace has reviewed the history of marriage and a number of current plans that involve multiple choices for sexual intimacy (Chapter 24). Some plans designed to offer the spice of life prove to be the vice of life, leading to jealousy and broken marriages, along with anxiety and suffering for parents and children alike.

Throughout history, marriage has evolved as a prominent foundation of society. It has developed as the accepted channel through which to have and protect children, conduct sexual activity, and obtain close companionship. Past emphasis in marriage was on procreation and sexual gratification, and the interpersonal aspects of the husband-wife relationship were largely ignored. Now, however, marriage can no longer be sustained by external coercion but only by internal cohesion. Individuals today want to know what marriage has to offer in *relational* terms that is unavailable elsewhere.

In our modern world where the individual feels lost in the human throng, the desire for real personal involvement—relationship in depth—is greater now than ever before. The prevailing malaise of our era lies in our rootlessness, isolation, and loss of identity. Only the experience of being a significant part of the life of another can cure this condition. Regardless of the many alternatives proposed by the critics of marriage, marriage uniquely offers a deep and lasting relationship of openness, trust, and sharing with a loved person. Marriage fulfills much of what we seek as we drift through life, hoping and being disappointed by superficial relationships. On the other hand, many marriages have caused great unhappiness, causing failure in social and business relationships, failure of mental and physical health, suicide, and homicide. The dividends of marriage depend considerably on the extent to which we invest in its success.

SEX DEVIANTS

People with aberrant sexual behavior have suffered from discrimination and persecution. As discussed in Chapter 25, three of the major categories consist of homosexuality, transvestism, and transsexualism. Homosexuality is far commoner than the other two conditions. Since conditioning for the development of these deviations occurs chiefly in the first few years of life, they are best viewed as developmental deviations (unusual patterns of psychological conditioning regarding sex roles) rather than illnesses. There is no *specific* biologic cause of heterosexual or homosexual orientation. Homosexuality depends upon certain nonstandard life experiences occurring in a critical period of early life—often related to certain child-rearing practices. The amounts and types of sexual communication between homosexuals vary markedly. The persons involved are usually so strongly conditioned in this direction that in only a small proportion of instances can they be changed significantly (Fig. 1a). Most of them are not interested in a change, and even in those requesting a change the problem is difficult. Their pattern of sex indulgence is as normal for the manner in which they have been conditioned as are heterosexual activities for others. This form of sexual communion should be legalized and matrimony permitted.

Transvestism is rare, occurring chiefly in males, many of whom are married, have children, and continue to engage in heterosexual activities. Many transvestites have interests that are not homosexual, but they derive erotic sensations from wearing female clothes and gain pleasure from displaying a feminine type of personality.

The transsexual is one who, in the first few years of life, begins to feel, think, and act like one of the opposite biologic sex. The gender identity is at variance with the biologic sex. This type of development usually results from the way in which the parents have dealt with the child, a daughter acquiring a self-image of her father, a son assuming a self-image of his mother. The latter occurs more often than the former. After puberty a boy may detest his male organs and other characteristics, seeking surgery and other treatments to eliminate male characteristics and to create a vagina, breasts, and other feminine characteristics. Requests for these changes are being granted with increased frequency, since efforts to change the desires of transsexuals are futile after they have become deeply embedded.

In conclusion, since it is clear that deviant sexual patterns, once established, are almost impossible to alter, the only hope for prevention would lie in avoiding the development of these distorted self-images by avoiding abnormal living patterns and child-rearing practices on the part of parents—a feat that would be difficult to accomplish.

MANAGEMENT OF THE SICK AND DYING

The state of health is all-important in decisions about who should live and die, as well as when, why, and how death should occur. The physician, the person confronted with imminent death, and his close relatives all play important roles in these decisions. To be sick in any way a person has to have one or more abnormalities, varying from a minor chemical change to gross anatomical alterations. Some emotional reaction is often stimulated by sickness.

Careers in medicine have changed markedly in the past 40 years (Chapter 15). Medical education, diagnostic and treatment facilities, and preventive medicine have improved greatly. However, there has been a tendency to concentrate on the *science* of medicine to the neglect of the *art* of medicine. Physicians and allied personnel are involved so extensively with gadgets, pills, and infusions that they fail to permit humanistic, realistic, and free communication with the patient. Mutual respect between physicians and patients has diminished. Physicians, allied medical professionals, ministers, and others should be far more helpful in preparing patients and their families for death and in managing the various stages of death.

Ross properly stresses that physicians, nurses, family, and others do not talk freely and honestly enough with dying patients and do not provide the most appropriate settings for these patients to talk freely about life and death (Chapter 12). Now that so many patients are in hospitals they suffer from isolation from family and close friends. There is too little consideration of the patient's innermost thoughts, wishes, and feelings. Far too many fears have been associated with dying. Dying marks the end of suffering for the patient.

EUTHANASIA

In polls that I have conducted (Chapter 7), approximately 80 percent of physicians and laity favored negative euthanasia. Positive euthanasia was favored by 18 percent of physicians and 35 percent of laity. However, my estimate is that negative euthanasia is applied either (a) too late, (b) too little, or (c) not at all in more than 99 percent of the instances where it should be. Positive euthanasia appears to be applied very rarely, and probably should not be applied until public attitudes have been conditioned and the laws been changed. The public must be oriented with regard to many of the major problems of euthanasia. I am pleased with the current extensive discussions of the situation in schools, colleges, churches, public forums, newspapers, magazines, and journals. Some programs on television and radio have also been helpful. It is good that coverage has dealt predominantly with major principles and guidelines. Reasonably good agreement in these areas will make it easier to formulate detailed plans. Although strong conflicting opinions prevail in some regards, each person should respect the opinions and rights of others and not try to force others to conform to his own concept of dealing with euthanasia.

Two important factors involved in decisions regarding euthanasia are (a) man's authority from God to make such decisions and (b) man's mental and emotional capacity to make appropriate decisions and to apply them effectively. Many of us believe that man has been granted this authority by God and that man has the ability, responsibility, and duty to apply euthanasia in certain situations in the manner that will be best for individuals and society. As stated in Genesis, God created man in His own image and gave him dominion over all of the earth and over everything that moveth upon it. In Psalms it is stated that man has been made "a little lower than the angels," and "to have dominion over the works of Thy hands." It is good to recall that in creating the world God created man as the greatest benefactor, and as the partner of God man has been endowed with knowledge and power to influence life's phenomena, including propagation, the manner in which we live, and when and how we die.

Even in the past, we have been making difficult decisions regarding life and death. For example, certain operations are associated with more than 50 percent mortality. We also make decisions concerned with killing when we deal with wars, capital punishment, release of prisoners, and management of patients who have attempted suicide. It is better for us to judge and act as best we can than to turn our backs in sinful neglect.

General guidelines for euthanasia decisions can be offered after extensive consideration by a wide variety of leaders in society, including physicians, paramedical personnel, psychologists, ministers, attorneys, sociologists, and others. Barring wars and civil defense, most decisions regarding termination of life involve sick people. In making a decision involving euthanasia it is important to learn the desires of the patient, certain relatives, the patient's physician, and others as indicated. Careful evaluation of the diagnosis, treatment, and prognosis are highly important, but these aspects must be considered in conjunction with many others, including the patient's age, general psychology and emotional status, amount of mental and physical suffering (past, present, future), abilities, and responsibilities, viewpoints about life and death, desires, and other points that evolve in frank discussions with the patient. Similar evaluations must be made of key members of the family. Reactions of the public and effects upon society (immediate and long range) must also be appraised. The main decision is based upon the balance between net advantages and net disadvantages in applying euthanasia. A reasonably good appraisal can be made in many patients concerning past and present suffering, as well as of other problems of the patient and his family. A fairly good estimate of the probable future course can often be made, although the possibility of unexpected events always exists. Because of some uncertainty, hope is sometimes maintained for miraculous recovery, but a remote possibility must be balanced against the very strong probability that the miracle will not occur and that the disease process will advance. Moreover, in the elderly there often is a good possibility that additional complications will appear. Thus, the amount of unhappiness will probably exceed the amount of happiness.

Today, with all the drugs, mechanical devices, and other measures that are available, a situation is created that is more appropriately designated as procrastination with regard to death rather than prolongation of life! Moreover, this procrastination is not infrequently against the wishes of the patient and his family, especially when a clear picture of the true status and probable outcome are presented. This has prompted the rapidly increasing custom of signing the "Living Will" (Chapter 9), which attempts to avoid unreasonable prolongation of life. The time and money that we devote to delaying death pointlessly would be better spent helping the elderly to enjoy life while they still can. It is estimated that more than 12 million people over age 65 in the United States have incomes averaging less than $2,000 per year. Many live in substandard housing and suffer from various ailments, especially inattention, loneliness, and insecurity.

Dyck favors negative euthanasia under certain conditions but not positive euthanasia (Chapter 10), but Fletcher points out the justification and benefits of positive euthanasia in certain situations (Chapter 9). Fletcher states that the purpose of negative and positive euthanasia is the same—to bring about the patient's death; the former is an act of omission while the latter is an act of commission. Each results from a positive decision concerning action. Fletcher emphasizes that we are morally justified in our acts of euthanasia and states that its consequences are good or evil according to whether and how much they serve human values. He says: "It is harder morally to justify letting somebody die a slow, ugly death, dehumanized, than it is to justify helping him to escape from such misery." Humanness and personal integrity are of higher value than biological life and function in determining when a person is dead or should die. Religious leaders are agreeing that we are no longer morally obliged to preserve life in all terminal cases.

Fletcher presents fundamental inconsistencies in some present policies, such as: You are permitted to end your neighbor's life for your own sake (self-defense), but not for his sake. You may end your own life for your neighbor's sake (sacrificial heroism), but your may not end your life for your own sake.

NEED FOR ADJUSTING GUIDELINES IN LAW AND RELIGION

Rieke states (Chapter 22): "Law is a catalyst in a social organization; a mechanism for the identification, implementation, conservation, and transmission of ethical values; a means of distributing the benefits and burdens of society among persons." Certain rules supposedly are for the good of society and its individuals, but many deviations develop that necessitate judicial opinions. The marked increases in the use of drugs, equipment, operations, and other measures affecting health increase both advantages and disadvantages for individuals and society. Unduly long lag periods have existed in changing laws and interpretations to meet the current problems in health. Some examples of legal delinquency: negative euthanasia is illegal in some areas; abortions have been excessively restrictive in most areas until recently. Closer collaboration between the legal and medical professions should permit much improvement.

A recent survey in the United States revealed that 128,505,084 people were affiliated with some church, and there were more than 400 different religious groups. A few of the many deviations in religious policies, recently summarized for me by Reverend Thomas McCormick, include (a) Christian Science—avoidance of various phases of medical care, (b) Catholic—resistance to antifertility drugs and abortion, (c) Jehovah's Witnesses—resistance to blood transfusion, (d) Seventh Day Adventist—prohibition of meat-eating, (e) Jewish—avoidance of eating pork.

The existence of a large number of religious denominations and their numerous differences in interpreting what is morally best for society and individuals emphasizes the difficulties in dogmatically maintaining that certain religious policies hold the right answer. As discussed in several chapters, there is a great need for revising policies and codes in religion to deal most effectively with current problems. Pattison (Chapter 23) has emphasized the need for changing many of the traditional religious approaches to morality to embody more psychosocial considerations. He also stresses the net benefits to patients and society of more integration of religious, medical, and other activities, centered on helping the patient as a whole.

EQUALIZATION OF UNEQUAL PEOPLE

When I consulted Dr. S. F. Miyamoto, a professor of sociology, on the subject of equalizing unequal people, he emphasized that social equality must be considered in two phases: (a) equality of attributes and (b) equality of treatment. The former means that certain characteristics of persons are the same: age, sex, race, intelligence, skills, income, property holdings, interests, etc. Humans differ markedly in the quality and quantity of individual attributes. In several chapters of this book the disadvantages to individuals and to society of considering all people equal are presented. One person has certain attributes far superior to those of another, but may have some that are inferior. We cannot equalize attributes, but we can help to compensate for some of the differences. Equality of treatment refers to the sameness of opportunities, conditions, and benefits, as well as of duties, restrictions, and liabilities. We must aim for equality of treatment in many ways. Some people seek equal status in areas such as family, housing, economics, politics, education, security (regarding law, police, fire, insurance), health, welfare, religion, recreation, transportation, communication, and social affiliations. Sociologists consider that basic needs should be assured for everyone. Included in these needs are food, shelter, health, protection, training, self-expression, development, and affection. In the past, many individual needs were met within the family members of a family working together, taking recreation together, having each member participate in accordance with his desires and abilities, and pooling various resources and rewards. In this manner the more capable members compensated for the less capable ones and aided them in somewhat subtle ways, yet each member of the family felt that he was an integral and important component.

Today, when greater training, specialization, and ability are required for maximal performance, there are many who surpass others in capacity. With a great array of powerful machines for much larger and more efficient production, fewer people are required for certain tasks. In some spheres of work it is economically more efficient to have certain capable and skilled individuals do the work and to divide the rewards equally between workers and a certain number of nonworkers than it is to try to train and use equally some other people. However, such a scheme makes some nonworkers very unhappy because it degrades their pride, dignity, feelings of worthiness, and other personal satisfactions. Therefore, we are faced with problems far greater and more complex than simply equalizing basic needs.

FINAL SUMMARY AND CONCLUSIONS

The supreme function of the body is mentation. As far as I can comprehend, even the soul is a special aspect of mentation. Without menta-

tion the body is not of significant use. With no mentation there is no pleasure or pain. Abnormal mentation can produce enormous suffering. The
type and amount of mentation depend upon the chemical and physical
status of the brain. In turn, this depends upon many internal (cerebral
and extracerebral) and environmental factors. Since behavior depends upon
mentation, there are numerous factors that influence behavior, some of
which can be controlled by the individual and some of which cannot.

The extent to which one wishes to live or to die depends somewhat
on the amount of happiness or unhappiness one has experienced. Many
of us believe that man has the moral and logical right and responsibility
to play a much greater role regarding (a) patterns of propagation, (b)
patterns of living, and (c) timing and manner of death. Decisions should
be based upon what is considered best for individuals and society. Since
the desires of certain individuals and groups concerning actions affecting
life and death often differ from those of other individuals and groups, we
should attempt to grant the wishes of each mentally competent person
unless such actions are too damaging to others. This permissiveness should
apply to both active and passive roles of man. Adoption of these policies
necessitates changes in laws, religious formulations, and public traditions.

We have made too few plans for attaining better quality and quantity
of propagation. The increase in population in some regions is marked. An
increase of 10-fold, 1,000-fold, or 1,000,000-fold will not proportionately
increase happiness; indeed, such increases would probably cause much
unhappiness. Simple and effective antifertility measures should be made
readily available to everyone. Moreover, in many instances appropriate
inducements (including money) should be offered for their use. Abortion
should be provided readily when it affords sufficient benefit to the health
and welfare of the progeny, parent(s), and society. Amniocentesis is of
rapidly increasing benefit in selecting subjects for abortion.

Innumerable mistakes in child-rearing, particularly with young children, have caused enormous problems in subsequent years for the individuals involved, for their families, and for society. These mistakes have had
deleterious effects upon careers (Fig. 3, Chapter 15), marriage, and other
phases of life. Parents, physicians, educators, and many other groups have
erred in child-rearing policies. There has been hyperconventionality in
some spheres and excessive freedom in others. Frequently, too little interest, love, and personal attention are displayed by parents and others. Discouragement, anxiety, and frustration have often resulted, sometimes
leading to drug addiction, depression, panic, violence, and crime (Fig. 3,
Chapter 1).

Progress in various avenues of science and technology has increased
significantly the average duration of life, but this has both advantages and
disadvantages. We have been provided with a great array of machinery
in homes, yards, offices, and industrial plants. We have much elaborate

equipment for progress in health measures and many other areas. However, this progress has also brought pollution in various ways, along with sickness and death.

Man's genetic pattern is such that usually for many years before death there are progressive anatomical and functional degenerative changes in body tissues. Despite a variety of therapies that improve certain aspects of body function, incapacities accumulate, producing mental and physical suffering. Nevertheless, death often can be postponed for weeks, months, or years by many types of treatment, such as use of an artificial respirator, hemodialyzer, pacemaker (Fig. 1, Chapter 7), or organ transplantation. Physicians often apply these measures without adequately learning the wishes of the patient and his family. Moreover, it has been common policy for physicians, allied professional personnel, and others not to present the prognosis to the patient in what is considered the most accurate perspective. Unfounded optimism is combined with highly improbable hope. The agonies, horrors, and disadvantages of dying have been overemphasized. There are many times when death should not be put off any longer. At such times, after appropriate discussion and approval by the patient and/or his nearest relative, certain therapies should be withheld and major attention devoted to the patient's comfort and happiness. This constitutes negative euthanasia.

At present we are not prepared to institute positive euthanasia; first there must be changes in laws, religious policies, and orientation of the public, as well as support by the public. For positive euthanasia, there must be appropriate guidelines, safeguards, and careful planning in many directions.

Much progress can be made in preventing suicide. Information is accumulating rapidly concerning chemical changes in the brain associated with depression, and about methods for correcting them. Moreover, significant progress can be made regarding contributory effects of patterns of living and environmental factors. Since most people who commit suicide are sick, we should be less castigating and far more active and straightforward in dealing with the specific problems. We must also admit that some people who commit suicide are not mentally sick and not cowards—indeed, they are wise, courageous, unselfish, and kind. However, euthanasia may be preferable to suicide.

In my judgment, the answer to the question "When should one live or die?" depends upon the balance of the advantages and disadvantages of living or dying to the individual, his friends and relatives, and society. Representative opinions from each of these groups are important. For net good, sacrifices by one or more components are often needed. Some decisions need to be made on estimates of the probable course of events, because some prognostic uncertainties in individual instances may exist.

Finally, in this book we have dealt with many major problems of life and death—problems that will be even more prominent in the future unless we become active in preventing and managing them. Most major changes, whatever their type, trigger strong emotional reactions—indeed, reactions that temporarily interfere with wise analysis. With continued enlightenment, however, broad support should be obtained eventually. Patience, good temper, consideration, and wisdom are very much in order.

My Life Prayer

Oh, for more quality and less quantity in propagation;
Oh, for less suffering and more wisdom in termination.